PHYSIOLOGICAL AND FUNCTIONAL ASSESSMENT OF PROFESSIONAL FOOTBALL PLAYERS

W0235000

Physiological and Functional Assessment of Professional Football Players presents a science-based approach to enhance athletes' performance and prevent muscle injuries. Professional football players undergo a rigorous competitive season with frequent and numerous competitions, exposing them to significant stress that can detrimentally affect their performance and lead to serious injuries in extreme cases. In order to avert such negative outcomes, coaches and team staff must formulate preventive training programs tailored to the unique characteristics and needs of each player.

The execution of these individualized training programs necessitates a comprehensive assessment of players' health status, evaluation of their functional and fitness performance, analysis of their muscular structure, identification of muscle imbalances or movement dysfunctions, and detection of potential injury risk factors. Furthermore, it is imperative to monitor the weekly training and competition load using appropriate indicators of external and internal load, adjusting workloads accordingly.

In addition, recovery training programs must be meticulously designed for each injured player. This process involves isolating the factors causing the injury and assessing the injury's severity in the initial stage. Subsequently, recovery training programs must be thoughtfully planned, incorporating various assessment tools and procedures to verify the restoration of players' functional ability and inform decisions about the return to play.

Physiological and Functional Assessment of Professional Football Players delves into the utilization of appropriate testing protocols and emphasizes that understanding the reported data is crucial for the success of professional football training. This groundbreaking book is essential reading for researchers and practitioners in the fields of soccer, sports science, recovery, data and performance analysis, and soccer coaching.

Moisés de Hoyo Lora is a Professor in Physical Education and Sports at the University of Seville (Spain). He is a former strength and conditioning coach for professional soccer teams (Sevilla FC, Levante UD, Deportivo de la Coruña, CD Leganés, and Watford FC). He is working as fitness coach in Villarreal CF. His major research interests are centered on resistance training programs and training load control in team sports.

Borja Sañudo Corrales is a Full Professor in the Department of Physical Education and Sport at the University of Seville and teaching in numerous master's degree programs in Health and Sport Sciences in Spain. He is a member of the BIOFANEX (Biological and Functional Analysis of Exercise) research group. His major research interests are centered on the role of exercise and other lifestyle factors for promoting improvements in physiological function and return to play in sports.

Redha Taiar is a Professor at the University of Reims Champaign, France. He is a specialist on biomechanics of health disease and rehabilitation. His studies focus on the industry engineering for medicine and high-level sport.

Luis Carrasco Páez is a Senior Researcher of the BIOFANEX Research Group (CTS-972; Andalusian Research Program). He is also an Associated (Tenured) Professor in the Department of Physical Education and Sport, University of Seville, and at International Andalusian University.

PHYSIOLOGICAL AND FUNCTIONAL ASSESSMENT OF PROFESSIONAL FOOTBALL PLAYERS

Edited by
Moisés de Hoyo Lora, Borja Sañudo Corrales,
Redha Taiar, and Luis Carrasco Páez

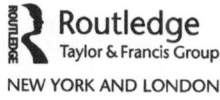
Routledge
Taylor & Francis Group

NEW YORK AND LONDON

Designed cover image: Tuadesk / Getty Images

First published 2025
by Routledge
605 Third Avenue, New York, NY 10158

and by Routledge
4 Park Square, Milton Park, Abingdon, Oxon, OX14 4RN

Routledge is an imprint of the Taylor & Francis Group, an informa business

Library of Congress Cataloging-in-Publication Data
Names: de Hoyo Lora, Moisés, editor. | Corrales, Borja Sañudo, editor. |
Taiar, Redha, editor. | Páez, Luis Carrasco, editor.
Title: Physiological and functional assessment of professional football
players / edited by Moisés de Hoyo Lora, Borja Sañudo Corrales,
Redha Taiar, and Luis Carrasco Páez.
Description: New York: Routledge, 2024. |
Includes bibliographical references and index. |
Identifiers: LCCN 2024028623 (print) | LCCN 2024028624 (ebook) |
ISBN 9781032636993 (hbk) | ISBN 9781032623450 (pbk) | ISBN 9781032637006 (ebk)
Subjects: LCSH: Soccer players—Selection and appointment. | Physical
fitness—Testing. | Soccer—Statistical methods. | Soccer—Physiological aspects. |
Soccer—Psychological aspects. | Sports sciences.
Classification: LCC GV943 .P49 2024 (print) | LCC GV943 (ebook) |
DDC 796.33206/93—dc23/eng/20241014
LC record available at https://lccn.loc.gov/2024028623
LC ebook record available at https://lccn.loc.gov/2024028624

ISBN: 978-1-032-63699-3
ISBN: 978-1-032-62345-0
ISBN: 978-1-032-63700-6

DOI: 10.4324/9781032637006

Typeset in Times New Roman
by codeMantra

CONTENTS

List of figures   *vii*
List of tables   *xi*
List of contributors   *xii*

1 Body composition and nutrition in professional football   1
Antonio Jesús Sánchez-Oliver, Francisco Javier
Martín-Almena and Raúl Domínguez

2 Evaluation of muscle structure and function   19
Alejandro Muñoz-López and Manuel García-Sillero

3 Cardiorespiratory fitness testing   43
José Naranjo Orellana

4 Assessment of range of motion in football players   54
Sergio Hernández-Sánchez, José Luis Hernández-Davó
and Víctor Moreno-Pérez

5 Strength and muscle power testing   77
Eduardo Sáez de Villarreal Sáez and Rodrigo
Ramírez-Campillo

6 Assessment of football-specific endurance   109
Alejandro Rodríguez-Fernández and Javier
Sánchez-Sánchez

7 Static and dynamic neuromuscular balance field-based
assessments 119
*Marc Madruga Parera, Rodrigo Ramírez-Campillo
and Víctor Moreno-Pérez*

8 Kinematic and kinetic assessment in professional
football players 133
Javier Courel-Ibáñez and Raúl Domínguez Herrera

9 Assessment and quantification of external load 157
*Moisés de Hoyo Lora and
Miguel Ángel Campos Vázquez*

10 Assessment and quantification of internal load 175
Moisés de Hoyo Lora and Borja Sañudo Corrales

11 Typology and severity of football injuries: data from
incidence studies 195
Sergio Tejero García and Beatriz Martínez Sañudo

12 Identification of injury risk factors for lower extremity
muscle injury and preventive training guidelines 207
Luis Suárez-Arrones

13 Fitness testing and functional assessment of football
players during injury periods 219
*Francisco Javier Núñez Sánchez and
Alberto Torres Campos*

14 Genotypic analysis of football players 239
Luis Carrasco Páez and Inmaculada C. Martínez-Díaz

15 The use of Big Data in football players' evaluation 252
Borja Sañudo Corrales and Moisés de Hoyo Lora

16 Comprehensive evaluation of football players: the
biopsychosocial model 268
*Tomás García-Calvo, Jesús Díaz-García, Ana
Rubio-Morales and Miguel Ángel López-Gajardo*

Index 283

FIGURES

1.1   Skinfold map of two soccer players. Measurements are in mm   5
1.2   Nutrition in elite football: competition day   11
1.3   Nutrition in elite football: training day   12
2.1   Technologies that can be used to monitor the muscle structure
       and function   20
2.2   Displacement–time curve of a muscle measure with TMG.
       Muscle contractile properties are calculated using this relationship   21
2.3   TMG muscle chain custom report. Column "Int" shows the
       intervention for the muscle based on a combination of low,
       normal, or high Tc or Dm values for each muscle   24
2.4   Load range concept   26
2.5   Conventional electrode montages (extracted from Cavalcanti
       Garcia and Vieira [43])   30
2.6   Biceps femoris EMG signal evolution during a soccer match
       (extracted from Marshall et al. [51])   31
2.7   Quadriceps EMG during soccer instep kicking to each target
       area (adapted from Scurr et al. [54])   32
2.8   Biceps femoris (BF) to medial hamstring (MH) nEMG
       relationship for the (A) concentric and (B) eccentric phases of
       each exercise (adapted from Bourne, et al. [65])   35
2.9   Practical recommendations for the implementation of
       ultrasound-based imaging in the elite sports context (adapted
       from Sarto et al. [71])   36
3.1   Mechanical efficiency of an elite soccer player in an incremental
       test. The slope of the line indicates that 0.27 L/min of O2 are
       consumed for every km/h that speed increases. By equating the

units of time (in hours) and eliminating them, we obtain that the
efficiency is 16.2 L (author's data).   48

3.2 HR–VO$_2$ relationship of an elite soccer player in an incremental
test (author's data)   49

4.1 Weight-bearing lunge test [27]   56

4.2 The use of inclinometer during the weight-bearing lunge test   57

4.3 The simplified version of the weight-bearing lunge test proposed
by Cejudo et al. [30]   58

4.4 Ankle dorsiflexion range of motion measurement using
smartphone technology during the weight-bearing lunge test   59

4.5 Goniometric assessment of ankle dorsiflexion ROM   59

4.6 Leg motion device   60

4.7 Active Knee Extension test [43]   62

4.8 Maximal Hip Flexion Active Knee Extension proposed by
Whiteley et al. [47]   63

4.9 Passive straight leg raise test   64

4.10 Bent knee fallout test   65

4.11 Hip internal and external rotation test   66

4.12 Hip abduction ROM test   67

4.13 New device for assessment of the sagittal plane tilt   68

4.14 Assessment of the shoulder rotation range of motion: testing for
glenohumeral internal rotation position and for glenohumeral
external rotation position   69

5.1 Vertec vertical jump tester   85

5.2 Squat Jump test   86

5.3 Countermovement jump test   87

5.4 Abalakov jump test   88

5.5 Drop jump test   89

5.6 Standing long jump test   89

5.7 Throwing-in test   92

5.8 10 × 5 m Shuttle Test   93

5.9 Diagram of the course used in the zigzag test. Each straight
sprint is 5 m and each turn at a flag is 100°   94

5.10 Diagram of the course used in the Illinois test   95

5.11 Diagram of T-test. Adapted from Semeick [52]   95

5.12 Diagram of 5-0-5 agility test. Adapted from Gabbett et al. [54]   96

5.13 Diagram of L-run test. Adapted from Gabbett et al. [54]   96

5.14 Hexagonal agility test   97

7.1 Y-Balance Test (modified from Plisky et al. [9]. A: anterior;
B: posterolateral; C: posteromedial)   120

7.2 Four single-leg hop tests. A: single hop for distance; B: triple
hop for distance; C: cross-over hop for distance; D: 6-m timed
hop [16]   122

7.3   Landing Error Scoring System   124
7.4   Tuck jump test   125
7.5   Muscular-based core stability tests   127
7.6   Double leg lowering test   128
7.7   Three-plane core test, A: sagittal plane; B: transverse plane;
       C: frontal plane   129
8.1   Three common agility and Change of Direction (COD) tests in soccer   136
8.2   The soccer-specific, Y-shaped COD speed and reactive agility test   136
8.3   An example of jumping phases and force–time–velocity curves
       from a Countermovement Jump (CMJ). TOV: Take-off velocity   137
8.4   Countermovement Jump (CMJ)   141
8.5   Squat Jump (SJ)   141
8.6   Abalakov jumping test   142
8.7   Drop Jump (DJ)   142
8.8   Loaded Squat Jump   143
8.9   Example of an FVP profile in jumping using the 2-load method and
       the available online Excel sheet   144
8.10   A graphical representation of the FVP profile in sprinting. Taken
       from a free Excel sheet   145
8.11   Rate of Force Development (RFD) measures from the force–
       time curve during an isometric ballistic test   146
8.12   Isometric midthigh clean pull test (left) and isometric knee
       flexion test (right)   148
9.1   Evolution of metabolic power (black line) and oxygen
       consumption (gray line) during a 5 versus 5 small-sided game
       (3 × 4 min, 2 min rest period)   160
9.2   Evolution of maximum intensity periods (MIP) using total
       distance as criterion variable (m·min-1) along competitive
       season, for a professional center forward. Grey zone (mean ±
       95% confidence interval). 1, 2, 3,... 1st, 2nd, 3rd round   161
9.3   Illustration of the importance of individual thresholds for two
       athletes possessing similar Maximal Aerobic Speed (MAS), but
       different Maximal Sprinting Speed (MSS). During a training
       session, if we use an absolute sprint threshold (> 25.1 km/h),
       Player B with a greater Anaerobic Speed Reserve (ASR) will
       work at a lower percentage of his ASR, and will therefore
       achieve a lower exercise load compared with Player B (adapted
       from Buchheit and Laursen [62])   164
10.1   Conceptual Banister's model of the dose–response relationship
       (adapted from Calvert et al. [3])   176
10.2   Player load monitoring outlining the cyclical nature in which
       physiological and biomechanical load leads to adaptation of the
       biological system as a whole, as proposed by Vanrenterghem et al. [2]   177

10.3   Perceived wellness questionnaire   178
10.4   CK evolution after an official football match in started (line with
       diamonds) and non-started players (line with squares)   179
10.5   Poincaré Plot: (a) after 10 min of high-intensity training; (b) after
       8 hours of sleep. The SD1 axis is reduced after a fatiguing
       training and recovery a normal length after 8 hours of sleep   184
10.6   Thermal responses in posterior chain (with the permission of
       ®ThermoHuman)   186
12.1   The intervention exercise with the elastic band (17)   209
12.2   The Copenhagen adduction exercise with different levels (22)   210
13.1   Tensiomyography. S: sensor; E: electrostimulator; L: laptop;
       e: adhesive electrodes   221
13.2   Numerical variables obtained through the TMG   222
13.3   Player positioning for TMG measurement   223
13.4   MTT of the hip external rotator muscle chain [5]   226
13.5   MTT of the hip internal rotator muscle chain [5]   227
13.6   MTT of the supine hip abductor muscle chain [5]   227
13.7   MTT of the hip abductor muscle chain in a lateral position [5]   228
13.8   MTT of the hip abductor muscle chain in a lateral position with
       hips and knees flexed [5]   229
13.9   MTT of the supine adductor muscle chain [5]   230
13.10 MTT of the supine ulnar hip flexor muscle chain [5]   231
13.11 MTT of the supine hip extensor muscle chain [5]   232
13.12 MTT of the hip extensor muscle chain in the prone position [5]   232
13.13 MTT of the supine knee extensor muscle chain [5]   233
13.14 MTT of the flexor muscle chain of the prone knee [5]   234
13.15 MTT of the supine knee flexor muscle chain [5]   235
13.16 Using a dynamometer in MTT   236
14.1   Human gene structure   240
15.1   Data analytics framework in sports (adapted from
       Claudino et al. [5])   254
15.2   Example of inputs used to predict injuries using data mining   256
15.3   Quantification of variables and presentation of data during a
       typical week in La Liga   257
15.4   Example of data representation using Microsoft Power BI   258
15.5   Main machine learning approaches to assess injury risk or
       performance in football (adapted from Claudino et al. [5])   260
15.6   Graphical representation of the first classifier of the predictive
       model for muscle injuries   261
16.1   Biopsychosocial model applied to football   269

TABLES

3.1 Results of a stress test performed on a treadmill by a
professional football player 50

8.1 Examples for sprinting outcomes in soccer players 134

8.2 Performance, kinetic, and temporal jumping metrics. Modified
from Cohen et al. [32] 139

8.3 Examples for jumping outcomes in soccer players 140

8.4 Common metrics for RFD assessment 145

13.1 Muscle reference values for TMG analysis in professional
soccer players 224

13.2 Subjective assessment equivalence criterion 235

CONTRIBUTORS

List of authors in alphabetical order (by surname).

Miguel Ángel Campos Vázquez, Fitness Coach Youth National Teams, Royal Spanish Football Federation.

Luis Carrasco Páez, Department of Physical Education and Sport, University of Seville, Seville, Spain.

Javier Courel-Ibáñez, Department of Physical Education and Sport, Faculty of Education and Sport Sciences, University of Granada, Melilla, Spain.

Moisés de Hoyo Lora, Department of Physical Education and Sport, University of Seville, Seville, Spain. Performance and Fitness Coach Aston Villa FC, Birmingham, UK.

Jesús Díaz-García, Faculty of Sport Sciences. University of Extremadura, Cáceres, Spain.

Raúl Domínguez Herrera, Department of Human Motricity and Sports Performance, Faculty of Educational Sciences, University of Seville, Seville, Spain.

Tomás García-Calvo, Faculty of Sport Sciences, University of Extremadura, Cáceres, Spain.

Manuel García-Sillero, Department of Human Physiology, Physical Education and Sport, Faculty of Medicine, University of Málaga, Spain.

José Luis Hernández-Davó, Faculty of Health Sciences, Isabel I University, Burgos, Spain.

Sergio Hernández-Sánchez, Translational Research Centre of Physiotherapy, Department of Pathology and Surgery, Faculty of Medicine, Miguel Hernandez University, Alicante, Spain.

Miguel Ángel López-Gajardo, Faculty of Sport Sciences, University of Extremadura, Cáceres, Spain.

Marc Madruga Parera, Department of Physical Therapy, International University of Catalonia, Barcelona, Spain. reQ, Return to Play and Sports Training Center, Barcelona, Spain.

Francisco Javier Martín-Almena, Food, Nutrition and Public Health Strategies Research Group, University of Alcalá, Alcalá de Henares, Madrid, Spain; Department of Biomedical Sciences, Faculty of Pharmacy, University of Alcalá, Alcalá de Henares, Madrid, Spain.

Inmaculada C. Martínez-Díaz, Department of Human Motricity and Sports Performance, University of Seville, Seville, Spain.

Beatriz Martínez Sañudo, Virgen del Rocio University Hospital, Seville, Spain.

Víctor Moreno-Pérez, Department of Behavioral Sciences and Health, Faculty of Medicine, Miguel Hernandez University, Alicante, Spain.

Alejandro Muñoz-López, Department of Human Motricity and Sports Performance, Faculty of Educational Sciences, University of Seville, Seville, Spain.

José Naranjo Orellana, Department of Sport and Computing Science, Faculty of Sports Sciences, Pablo de Olavide University, Seville, Spain.

Francisco Javier Núñez Sánchez, Department of Sport and Computing Science, Faculty of Sports Sciences, Pablo de Olavide University, Seville, Spain.

Rodrigo Ramírez-Campillo, Exercise and Rehabilitation Sciences Institute, Faculty of Rehabilitation Sciences, Universidad Andres Bello, Santiago, Chile.

Alejandro Rodríguez-Fernández, University of Leon, León, Spain.

Ana Rubio-Morales, Faculty of Sport Sciences, University of Extremadura, Cáceres, Spain.

Eduardo Sáez de Villarreal Sáez, Department of Sport and Computing Science, Faculty of Sports Sciences, Pablo de Olavide University, Seville, Spain.

Antonio Jesús Sánchez-Oliver, Department of Human Motricity and Sports Performance, Faculty of Educational Sciences, University of Seville, Seville, Spain.

Javier Sánchez-Sánchez, Pontifical University of Salamanca, Salamanca, Spain.

Borja Sañudo Corrales, Department of Physical Education and Sport, University of Seville, Seville, Spain.

Luis Suárez-Arrones, Department of Sport and Computing Science, Faculty of Sports Sciences, Pablo de Olavide University, Seville, Spain.

Sergio Tejero García, Virgen del Rocio University Hospital. Department of Surgery, University of Seville, Seville, Spain.

Alberto Torres Campos, Villarreal CF Fitness Coach, Villarreal, Spain.

1

BODY COMPOSITION AND NUTRITION IN PROFESSIONAL FOOTBALL

Antonio Jesús Sánchez-Oliver, Francisco Javier Martín-Almena and Raúl Domínguez

1.1 Body composition of the professional football player

1.1.1 Anthropometric traits and sport performance

Appropriate anthropometric traits, such as body mass, body composition, or the ratio between different body segments, are essential for good sports performance because they are related to the execution of most of the gestures of each sport discipline [1]. Football players, due to the speed requirements and the distances that are covered during a match, tend to benefit from a light and lean complexion that increases the muscle mass/fat mass ratio, even though their fat mass values are not as low as seen in endurance athletes. Body fat levels present an inverse relationship with performance for sprints, although there is no specific value that is considered optimal because professional football players have values in the range of 6–20% of fat mass [2].

At specific times of the season, when a change in the body is expected or during injury recovery, anthropometric assessment is a basic tool that will allow us to control and quantify the changes that are happening. Mostly, body composition changes will aim to increase musculoskeletal mass and reduce fat mass, probably based on previously established reference values. However, we must take these reference values with caution and not become obsessed with achieving them because each player has an optimal body composition value in which their sporting performance is maximized, and that does not always coincide with the values documented in other football players [3]. For this reason, it may be of interest to ask the player if he knows the values of any of his anthropometric traits, for example, percentage of fat mass, when he presented best sports performance, and use it as his reference. Even so, we must not forget that the normal aging process implies changes in body

DOI: 10.4324/9781032637006-1

composition and trying to emulate the values recorded 5 or 10 years earlier may imply a substantial decrease in sports performance as well as a significant risk to the football player's health.

Once the athlete's body composition has been assessed, we cannot ignore that it will vary depending on the playing position, the category in which the player competes, as well as the individual characteristics of each player. Likewise, a reduction in fat mass and an increase in musculoskeletal mass are usually observed as the season progresses. Therefore, as previously commented, we must objectively assess which will be the most favorable body composition for the player which is realistic for himself or herself, because exceeding certain values that are not healthy can decrease his performance [1–3].

1.1.2   General considerations for anthropometric data collection

There are a wide variety of validated tools and methodologies that are useful for evaluating football players as long as they allow detecting changes in body composition. Given the characteristics of this sport and of the athletes who practice it, it is advisable to use methodologies that allow us to quantify the fat, muscle, and bone content of the football player, so it is necessary to use a body composition model (with four or five compartments fat mass, muscle mass, bone mass, and residual mass [4] or adipose mass, muscle mass, bone mass, skin mass, and residual mass [5].

Laboratory techniques, such as dual X-ray absorptiometry (DXA) or hydrostatic weighing, have great precision and accuracy, but their price is usually high, and it is not easy to perform these techniques. Likewise, some of these techniques, even in low amounts, apply radiation to the subject being evaluated, which also implies greater requirements from the healthcare professionals who perform and interpret the test [3]. The UEFA Consensus document advises the use of DXA for the assessment of body composition due to a reduction in its costs in recent years [3]. However, authors of this chapter consider that many football teams, even in the First Division from National Leagues, will suffer difficulties to access this methodology because its price may still be excessive for many players and teams and there are not so many healthcare centers that have the required equipment, so they have to travel long distance to be able to carry out the test.

Conversely, we can also use other techniques, such as anthropometric measurements or bioelectric impedance analysis, that, despite a lower accuracy than DXA or hydrostatic weighing, if it is applied following rigorous and standardized protocols, allow to assess the player's nutritional status properly at an affordable cost. For this, the anthropometric measurements must be carried out by a professional who has learned the measurement techniques in depth and follows standardized protocols such as those established by the International Society for the Advancement of Kinanthropometry (ISAK) [6]. If body composition is studied using bioelectric impedance analysis, it is essential to obey Lukaski et al. [7] protocol to ensure the precision and accuracy of the measurement [7]. However, the follow-up of this protocol among the sports population can be difficult because it requires no physical exercise in the hours before the measurement [8]. If these issues are taken into account, tools of acceptable quality will be available for the assessment of body composition at a lower cost [3].

As previously mentioned, it is important to follow a standardized protocol for taking measurements. In this case, we are going to briefly comment most important issues to consider according to the ISAK protocol [6], although these apply to any other measurement technique followed, such as the indications of the International Biological Program or those of NHANES. Even so, in sport studies, the ISAK standardized methodology is predominant, and its use will allow comparison of the results of our football players with the values published in the scientific literature.

Taking anthropometric measurements implies being very close to the football player and direct contact with him or her. Therefore, at least the first times that measurements are made for a player, it is important to explain the procedures to be carried out, so that the athlete understands them and does not feel uncomfortable during the measurement. On the other hand, either through the documentation of the team or the player himself, you must have the informed consent signed by him to perform the measurements. This aspect is even more important if possible in the case of those football players who are not over the legal age for whom it will be necessary to get the signed approval of their parents or legal guardians [6].

Measurements, whether in the laboratory or the field, must be carried out in a private, orderly place of sufficient size to be able to move around the player comfortably [6]. The tools to carry out these measurements must be specific for the measurements to be taken, and they must have precision and exactitude enough. Likewise, they must be periodically calibrated to ensure the reliability of the tools which are being used [6].

The football player must be barefoot and wearing as little clothing as possible to be measured. It is recommended that men must be measured wearing only sports shorts or swimming trunks. For women, it is recommended to wear sports shorts and a sports top or bikini. Therefore, it must also be ensured that the temperature of the room is comfortable for the subject who is going to be measured [6].

Regarding the measurement process, before starting it, the anatomical landmarks for taking measurements should be marked. These anatomical points must be established in the exact place that corresponds to them, and the measurement technique must be carried out as it is specified in the protocols. The variation of these parameters, for example, measuring a skinfold at a distance of 1 cm from the measurement site, produces significant differences in the registered measure. Hence, it is very important to follow standardized and protocolized procedures to be able to compare our results with those from other studies that can serve as a reference [6, 8].

On the other hand, to minimize possible measurement errors, once all the measurements have been made on the subject, a second complete measurement will be carried out following the same order of execution of the measurements. Once the second complete measurement has been finished, those anthropometric traits that differ by more than 5% for skinfolds and more than 1% for the rest of the measurements between the first and second time should be measured a third time. For this reason, it is useful to have a proforma in which all the measurements made are noted. In this proforma, measures must appear in the order that they are going to be carried out to facilitate taking measurements and to avoid possible oversights. The value of each anthropometric trait will be the mean of the two measurements or the median when the third measurement has to be made [6].

Last but not least, we must take into account the cultural and social factors of each person being measured to avoid them feeling uncomfortable or offended because the measurement process implies being very close to the subject [6].

1.1.3 Data treatment

Once the measurements have been made, it is necessary to interpret data to obtain all the information they provide us.

To estimate body compartments from anthropometric measurements, estimating equations are often used. Currently, there are multiple equations developed and validated to estimate different compartments, especially fat mass. These equations are specific to the populations in which they were researched and developed and, therefore, in this case, it should be used by those few that have been validated for the sports population [8].

1.1.3.1 Skinfolds: individuals or sum

Estimating fat mass in the same subject with different equations can generate very different results depending on the equation used [9]. For this reason, in recent years, Marfell–Jones's proposal [10] of using the values of the individual skinfolds as an estimate of adiposity and their distribution or the summation of skinfolds is getting more acceptance. Graphically, these measurements of skinfolds can be represented in a radial plot (Figure 1.1) that can be used to evaluate the progression of the football player or to compare him or her against the group or the reference value [8].

The collected anthropometric variables, if we want to evaluate the progression of our football player by comparing him with himself over one or more seasons, could be used through a table or a graph format, giving us very useful information. We could observe the variations of their skinfolds or even their body girths, and with these traits, we could infer if the fat mass and/or the muscle mass is being modified by the training and diet.

Another option would be the use of skinfold sums. There are different types of sums, but the most common are the sum of six skinfolds (triceps, subscapular, supraspinale, abdominal, thigh, and calf) or the sum of eight skinfolds (triceps, subscapular, biceps, iliac crest, supraspinale, abdominal, thigh, and calf) [11].

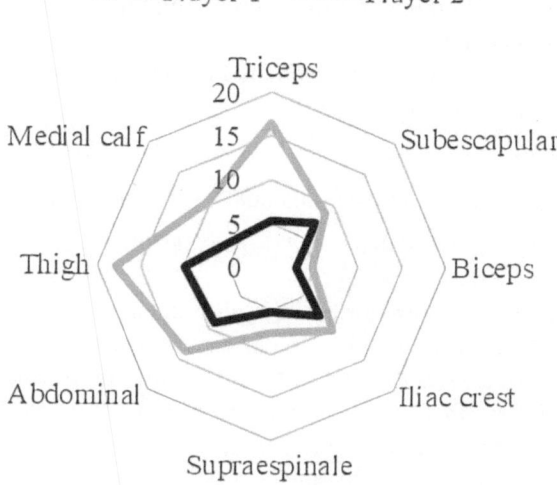

FIGURE 1.1 Skinfold map of two soccer players. Measurements are in mm.

1.1.3.2 Body composition equations

Body composition can be assessed by different compartment models. In the case of football players, the tetracompartment model is suitable to evaluate the required body tissues. Therefore, we will study the whole body mass through the following compartments: fat mass, muscle mass, bone mass, and residual mass.

As the Spanish Kinanthropometry Group recommends [12], these compartments can be estimated with the equations shown below.

Fat mass (FM): there are many equations to estimate this compartment, although the most common in the sports population is the Faulkner equation [13]. This equation only requires measurements made on the trunk or the arm, so it is easier to carry out.

Faulkner [13]:

Men: $\% FM = 0.153 * (Tri + Sub + Sesp + Abd) + 5.783$

Women: $\% FM = 0.213 * (Tri + Sub + Sesp + Abd) + 7.9$

where triceps skinfold in mm; Sub: subescapular skinfold in mm; Sesp: supraspinale skinfold in mm; Abd: abdominal skinfold in mm.

Another possible very useful equation is the Carter & Heath equation [14], which was developed from the anthropometric data of the athletes of the Montreal Olympic Games. This equation takes into account measurements of the whole body.

Carter & Heath [14]:

Men: $\% FM = 0.1051 * (Tri + Sub + Sesp + Abd + Thi + Mca) + 2.58$

Women: $\% FM = 0.1548 * (Tri + Sub + Sesp + Abd + Thi + Mca) + 3.58$

Tri: triceps skinfold in mm; Sub: subescapular skinfold in mm; Sesp: supraspinale skinfold in mm; Abd: abdominal skinfold in mm; Thi: thigh skinfold in mm; Mca: medial calf skinfold in mm.

Skeletal Muscle Mass (SMM): to estimate muscle mass content in the sports population, Lee's equation is used [15].

Lee et al. [15]:

$$SMM(\text{kg}) = Ht * \left(0.00744 * CAG^2 + 0.00088 * CTG^2 + 0.00441 * CCG^2\right)$$
$$+ 2.4 * sex - 0.048 * age + race + 7,8$$

Ht: height; CAG: corrected arm girth = arm girth in cm − (π*[triceps skinfold in mm/10]); CTG: corrected thigh girth= thigh girth in cm − (π*[thigh skinfold in mm/10]); CCG: corrected calf girth= calf girth in cm − (π*[medial calf skinfold in mm/10]); sex: 0 for female and 1 for male; race: −2.0 for Asian, 1.1 for African American, and 0 for white and Hispanic.

Bone Mass (BM): the bone compartment is estimated through the Rocha equation [16]. This equation is the same for men and women.

Rocha [16]:

$$BM(\text{kg}) = 3.02 * (H^2 * WB * FB * 400)^{0.712}$$

H: height in m; WD: wrist breadth in m; FD: femur breadth in m.

Residual Mass (RM): it is estimated by the difference between the total body mass and each of the calculated components.

Residual Mass:

$$RM(\text{kg}) = BoM - (\%FM * BoM(\text{kg}) + SMM(\text{kg}) + BM(\text{kg}))$$

BoM: total body mass; FM: fat mass; SMM: skeletal muscle mass; BM: bone mass.

In all these estimation equations, it is essential to take into account the units in which the anthropometric trait is measured and those required by each of the equations because it is a common mistake in body composition assessment.

1.1.3.3 Somatotype

Somatotype is the "numerical description of the morphological configuration of an individual at the time of being studied" [11], so it provides us information about the football player's body shape as well as an estimate of his body composition referred to the specific time in which he or she is being evaluated. Currently, the methodology used is the Heath–Carter somatotype whose main contribution to previous models was that the somatotype of a person changes over time and, therefore, is modifiable [14].

The somatotype is made up of three numbers that are always expressed in the same order and correspond to the endomorphy, mesomorphy, and ectomorphy values. The Heath–Carter methodology equations to estimate each component are specified below [14]:

Endomorphy: this component of the somatotype refers to the relative adiposity of the football player. Therefore, its estimation requires the measurement of some skinfolds.

$$Endomorphy = -0.7182 + 0.1451 * X - 0.00068 * X^2 + 0.0000014 * X^3$$

$$X = (Tri + Sub + Sesp) * \frac{170.18}{H}$$

Tri: triceps skinfold in mm; Sub: subescapular skinfold in mm; Sesp: supraspinale skinfold in mm; H: height in cm.

Mesomorphy: this component of the somatotype refers to the development of muscle and bone mass. It is calculated using the measurement of bone breadths and body perimeters.

$$Mesomorphy = 0.858 * HB + 0.601 * FB + 0.188^* A + 0.161 * C - 0.131 * H + 4.5$$

HB: humerus breadth in cm; FB: femur breadth in cm; A: corrected arm girth in cm = flexed arm girth in cm – (triceps skinfold in mm/10); C: corrected calf girth in cm = calf girth in cm – (medial calf skinfold in mm/10); H: height in cm.

Ectomorphy: this component of the somatotype refers to the relative linearity or thinness of the football player. For its estimation, it requires previously the calculation of the height–weight ratio (HWR).

$$HWR = \frac{Height\ in\ cm}{\sqrt[3]{Weight\ in\ kg}}$$

If HWR $\geq$ 40.75

$$Ectomorphy = (HWR * 0.732) - 28.58$$

If 38.25 < HWR < 40.75

$$Ectomorphy = (HWR * 0.463) - 17.63$$

If HWR $\leq$ 38.25

$$Ectomorphy = 0.1$$

When assessing each of the components, we can say that these are low values when the results of that component are between 0.5 and 2 somatotype units, mean values between 3 and 5 somatotype units, high values between 5.5 and 7 somatotype units, and as extremely high when they are greater than 7 somatotype units [14].

The somatotype can also be represented graphically on a somatochart. The somatotype has three dimensions so as to plot it is necessary to modify it to a two-dimensional system to obtain the X and Y coordinates [14]. For this, the following calculation is carried out:

$$X = ectomorphy - endomorphy$$
$$Y = 2 * mesomorphy - (endomorphy + ectomorphy)$$

1.2 Nutrition in professional football

Among the many factors that contribute to athletic success, nutrition plays a small but vital role concerning influence and performance in elite football [17]. A carefully planned nutritional strategy should increase performance during training and competition, improve and accelerate recovery, achieve and maintain optimal body composition and fitness, and minimize the risk of injury and illness. These aspects, are key themes in contemporary elite football [3, 18]. This can offer additional related benefits and provide a competitive advantage [3, 17].

The characteristics of football as an acyclical and intermittent sport (e.g. distances, intensities, and/or speeds that occur during a match) have implications for energy expenditure and nutritional strategies to take into account [19–22]. In addition, elite football has changed in recent years [23–25], directly or indirectly influencing the nutritional aspects to consider in this sport. Greater physical demand; changes in technical aspects; more demanding workouts; a greater number of games in the season, even with more than once per week; very different schedules due to the prominence of television broadcasts; continuous changes of geographic location; great cultural diversity of the players that make up the squads, etc., are some of the factors that may have an influence. Everything can get even more complicated due to European/World competitions and/or national team matches [18].

1.2.1 Energy requirements

Providing adequate energy to meet the demands of high-intensity intermittent exercise is essential in professional football since the main characteristic of football, like most team sports, is its intermittent dynamics, in which periods of high intensity are interspersed with other periods of rest or low intensity [26, 27].

Although daily energy expenditure varies greatly depending on individual (e.g. age, sex, height, weight, body composition, demarcation, or position on the field) or contextual (e.g. weather or team tactics) characteristics [21, 28–31], in several studies, the average daily energy expenditure of a professional male football player is between approximately 3400 and 4000 kcal, being able to spend around 1100 kcal during a competition [30, 32–35]. Research on elite female players is scant. This energy expenditure, in turn, can vary depending on the number of games, the phase of the season, or the training planning cycle in which the player is, hence emphasizing the importance of proper maintenance of energy balance and the importance of adequate nutritional intervention based on individual goals for performance optimization and health maintenance [30, 36, 37]. Furthermore, energy demands can also be influenced by temporary variations in basal metabolic rate, the thermic effect of food, or the thermic effect of activity [36].

However, expressing daily requirements as a percentage of total daily energy intake can be misleading, making it difficult to achieve these goals in real time. The provision of generic guidelines also becomes complex. Thus, it is recommended to use a periodized approach to facilitate feeding and recovery from specific training sessions and matches. This approach highlights the large daily variations in energy intake previously observed in professional football players in matches and training days, with a difference of up to 850 kcal [30, 32]. In addition, it must be taken into account that several nutritional challenges arise as a result of possible adaptations to footballers and their context since they may lose their appetite after training, eat poorly or skip meals regularly, or become hungry and resort to fast food or takeaway [38].

Finally, football training and competition must be accompanied by a higher energy intake to maintain performance capacity and prevent the development of excessive fatigue [39]. The use of technological devices (e.g. GPS, video analysis, or cardiac monitoring) in professional football can provide a more realistic estimate of the individual's energy expenditure, but the precision can vary greatly between systems, and the values should be interpreted with caution [40, 41].

1.2.2 Competition day

1.2.2.1 Pre-competition

Carbohydrates (CHO) are the key macronutrient when preparing a game as they are the main fuel for the muscles during high-intensity activities. CHO intake is similar both the day before the match and the day of the match prior to the competition (Figure 1.2). This intake is essential to increase glycogen stores in the muscles and liver. In addition, when there is more than one game planned in the week, normal in elite football, that same range must be maintained during the 2–3 days prior to the matches. It is important to influence this high CHO consumption, which is normally done at the cost of a lower fat intake [3]. To the aforementioned pattern, a meal richer in CHO should be included in the 3–4 hours prior to the match (Figure 1.2). This is essential to replenish liver glycogen stores, which are usually reduced by up to 50% after an overnight fast [3]. In addition, this food should be easily digestible to avoid gastrointestinal problems, and it should respect the taste and habits of the players so that they feel more comfortable with them [39, 42].

Finally, and just before starting the match, it is recommended to consume between 30 and 60 g of CHO after the warm-up due to its benefits during the warm-up [43].

This previous intake of CHO is important since there are many studies that support this high previous intake of CHO since it improves performance and delays fatigue in intermittent-intensity team sports [44]. Sequentially, it has been seen that players who start a match with a low muscle glycogen reserves perform less, especially in the second half of the match, than those with a high reserve, who are capable of running longer and faster [45, 46].

Hydration is the other aspect to consider before a football match due to its importance in the performance and health of the player [2, 39]. The advice to drink only when thirsty may be inappropriate since the need for fluids and the sensation of thirst may not coincide in various contexts, affecting the health and performance of the player. It is therefore recommended to develop individualized hydration plans, which should be accompanied by the education of the players for its better understanding and importance [3]. Finally, to guarantee that players who start the game are hydrated, they should drink liquids 2–4 hours before the game, following the guidelines that can be seen in Figure 1.2 [47, 48].

1.2.2.2   During competition

In the same way as before the match, sufficient CHO and fluid intake are the two most important aspects to consider during the competition. Numerous studies show benefits (shooting and passing performance or dribbling speed) when players consume CHO during the game [43, 49–52]. Therefore, it is recommended to consume CHO at rest, in the same way as after warming up (Figure 1.2) [3]. The use of gels or drinks with CHO can help, in both cases, the consumption of this without the appearance of gastrointestinal problems [3]. Another strategy in this regard is the use of mouthwashes with CHO since it could improve performance without these problems appearing [53, 54]. However, more studies are needed to support this theory in football [55].

Sweat rates vary greatly depending on the individual (e.g. distance traveled or speed) and context (i.e. environmental conditions or state of acclimatization) [56–58]. Sweat contains electrolytes, especially sodium, which vary greatly between players [57], and attention should be paid to their consumption during the game. The complexity is found by having to avoid hypohydration, on the one hand, and hyperhydration, on the other. Thus, players should try to drink enough fluids to prevent a deficit greater than 2–3% of body mass during exercise [59], while avoiding hyperhydration, ensuring maintenance of fuel needs through the consumption of sodium and CHO [48, 51].

It must be considered that both aspects, hydration and CHO intake, will need special attention when it comes to extra time. In addition, it is essential that both nutrition and hydration strategies, as well as the use of supplements (gels or drinks with CHO), should be tested in advance and on several occasions to know their details before use in a match [3].

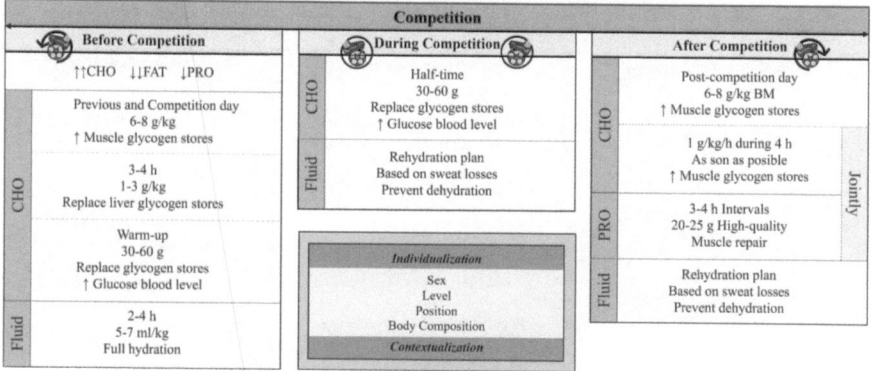

FIGURE 1.2 Nutrition in elite football: competition day.

1.2.2.3 After competition

Player recovery is one of the main post-match goals [60]. Rapidly replenishing CHO reserves is an essential part of this recovery [36]. The recommendation in this regard places CHO at 1 g/kg/h during the 4 hours after the competition [61]. In the event of not being able to reach these recommendations at these times (e.g. matches late in the day), it is recommended to follow the same CHO consumption guidelines that were given for the previous day and the day of the competition (Figure 1.2), and this should be the case for the following 2–3 days in the case of more than one match a week [3].

In addition to post-match CHO consumption, high-quality protein intake at 3–4 hour intervals is important for recovery to optimize protein synthesis (Figure 2.1) [62, 63]. This should be done together with the CHO intake for a better result [36].

Hydration (fluids and electrolytes), again, is another relevant aspect in recovery [36]; however, in most situations, normal post-match drinking and eating practices are sufficient [60, 64]. Post-competition liquids with alcohol are likely in team sports [60]. It is important to bear in mind that less alcohol consumption could interfere with glycogen resynthesis, protein synthesis, and rehydration [65, 66].

1.2.3 Training day

1.2.3.1 Carbohydrate requirements

Considering the importance of glycogen (muscle and liver) in the energy contribution during the match, it is important to take into account the CHO intake according to the training objectives [67]. Although everything will depend on the duration and intensity of the training session, the time of training in relation to the last meal or the search for physiological adaptations through nutritional strategies based on changes in CHO intake during training [30, 68], the CHO requirements in training

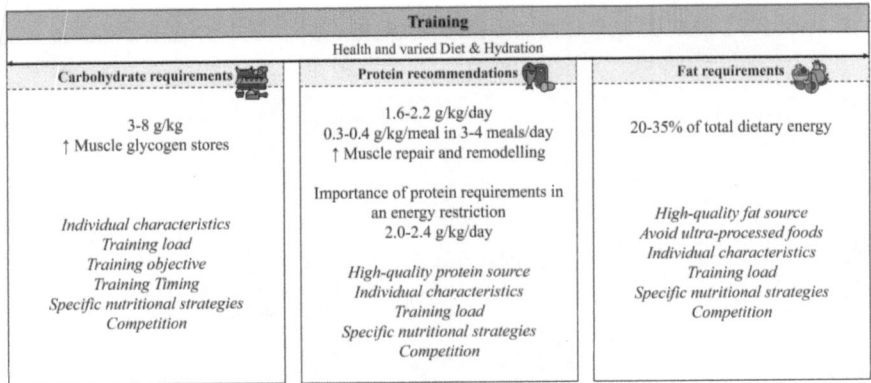

FIGURE 1.3 Nutrition in elite football: training day.

will be in a range of 3–8 g/kg/day, depending on the specific training scenario, the match schedule, and the general or specific training objectives for each player (Figure 1.3), [3].

1.2.3.2 Protein recommendations

Protein intake is important since the physical demand of daily training sessions in elite football influences the musculoskeletal and tendon tissue, creating the need to repair and remodel these [36]. Due to this requirement, the recommendations exceed that of the general population, ranging between 1.6 and 2.2 g/kg/day (Figure 1.3) [69]. This can be easily accomplished as long as a quality protein is consumed and the energy demands of training are met [3]. It appears that the ideal practice would be to include protein-rich foods (0.3–0.4 g/kg/meal) in 3–4 meals per day to provide a sufficient dose to stimulate protein remodeling/repair (Figure 1.3) [69]. Protein quality is important in this process, so the consumption of eggs, dairy, meat, or isolated vegetables such as soy is recommended [70].

The importance of protein requirements in the case of an energy restriction should be highlighted [71]. Although more studies are necessary, a protein intake in a range of 2.0–2.4 g/kg/day is recommended that will depend on the training load, the individual's weight loss, or an injury situation (Figure 1.3) [3, 72]. Although they are probably not necessary with a well-planned diet, protein supplements can be a comfortable and easy-to-digest alternative, especially after training. Among the existing ones, it seems that whey protein may be the most appropriate [3, 70].

1.2.3.3 Fat requirements

Despite beliefs, dietary fat is essential in the general diet of football players due to its use as an energy source, its important content and absorption of fat-soluble vitamins, as well as its contribution of essential fatty acids [36]. The recommendations are in a range of 20–35% of the total daily energy, although this is determined by the previous adjustment of the protein and CHO requirements according to the objectives (Figure 1.3) [36].

As with CHOs and proteins, foods high in fat should be of quality, avoiding ultra-processed foods due to their low nutritional content. To excessively restrict the consumption of these (< 15–20%) can cause some nutritional deficit or unnecessarily avoid foods with high nutritional value [3]. At the other extreme are currently ketogenic, high-fat, low-CHO diets [68]. Although there is still much to study in this regard, the current lack of evidence does not recommend the use of this type of diet in professional football [3, 73].

References

1. Cárdenas-Fernández V, Chinchilla-Minguet JL, Castillo-Rodríguez A. Somatotype and body composition in young football players according to the playing position and sport success. *J Strength Cond Res* [Internet]. 2019 July 1 [cited 2021 May 30];33(7):1904–1911. Available from: https://pubmed.ncbi.nlm.nih.gov/28723818/

2. Oliveira C, Ferreira D, Caetano C, Granja D, Pinto R, Mendes B, et al. Nutrition and supplementation in football. *Sports* [Internet]. 2017 May 12 [cited 2021 May 30];5(2):28. Available from: https://pubmed.ncbi.nlm.nih.gov/29910389/

3. Collins J, Maughan RJ, Gleeson M, Bilsborough J, Jeukendrup A, Morton JP, et al. UEFA expert group statement on nutrition in elite football. Current evidence to inform practical recommendations and guide future research. *Br J Sports Med* [Internet]. 2021 Apr 1 [cited 2021 May 19];55(8):416. Available from: https://pubmed.ncbi.nlm.nih.gov/33097528/

4. Matiegka J. The testing of physical anthropometry. *Am Phys Anth*. 1921;4:223–230.

5. Kerr DA. *An anthropometric method for fractionation of skin, adipose, bone, muscle and residual tissue masses in males and females age 6 to 77 years*. Theses (School of Kinesiology)/Simon Fraser University; 1988.

6. Esparza-Ros F, Vaquero-Cristobal R, Marfell-Jones M. *Protocolo Internacional para la Valoración Antropometrica*. Murcia, Spain: Universidad Católica de Murcia (UCAM); 2019.

7. Lukaski HC, Bolonchuk WW, Hall CB, Siders WA. Validation of tetrapolar bioelectrical impedance method to assess human body composition. *J Appl Physiol*. 1986;60(4):1327–1332.

8. Ackland TR, Lohman TG, Sundgot-Borgen J, Maughan RJ, Meyer NL, Stewart AD, et al. Current status of body composition assessment in sport: Review and position statement on behalf of the Ad Hoc research working group on body composition health and performance, under the auspices of the I.O.C. Medical Commission. *Sports Med* [Internet]. 2012 [cited 2021 May 30];42:227–249. Available from: https://pubmed.ncbi.nlm.nih.gov/22303996/

9. Vaquero-Cristóbal R, Albaladejo-Saura M, Luna-Badachi AE, Esparza-Ros F. Differences in fat mass estimation formulas in physically active adult population and relationship with sums of skinfolds. *Int J Environ Res Public Health* [Internet]. 2020 Nov 1 [cited 2021 May 30];17(21):1–13. Available from: https://pubmed.ncbi.nlm.nih.gov/33114260/

10. Marfell-Jones M. The *value of the skinfold background, assumptions, cautions and recommendations on taking and interpreting skinfold measurements*. In: 88a Conferencia Internacional de Ciencias del Deporte de los Juegos Olímpicos de Seúl. Seul, Korea; 2001, pp. 313–323.

11. Esparza F, Alvero JR, Aragonés MT, Cabañas MD, Canda A, Casajús JA, et al. *Manual de cineantropometría*. Pamplona, Spain: GREC-FEMEDE; 1993.

12. Alvero JR, Cabañas MD, Herrero A, Martinez L, Moreno C, Porta J. *Body composition assessment in sports medicine*. Statement Spanish Gr Kinanthropometry Spanish. *Fed Sport Med*. 2010;330–344.

13. Faulkner J. Physiology of swimming and diving. In: Falls H, editor. *Exercise physiology*. Baltimore: Academic Press Inc.; 1968.

14. Carter J, Heath B. *Somatotyping: Development and applications*. Vol. 5. Cambridge: Cambridge University Press; 1990.

15. Lee RC, Wang Z, Heo M, Ross R, Janssen I, Heymsfield SB. Total-body skeletal muscle mass: development and cross-validation of anthropometric prediction models. *Am J Clin Nutr*. 2000;72(3):796–803.

16. Rocha MSL. Peso ósseo do brasileiro de ambos os sexos de 17 a 25 años. *Arq anatomía e Antropol*. 1975;1:445–451.

17. Maughan RJ, Shirreffs SM. Nutrition for football players. *Curr Sports Med Rep* [Internet]. 2007 [cited 2021 May 19];6:279–280. Available from: https://pubmed.ncbi.nlm.nih.gov/17883961/

18. Oliveira C, Ferreira D, Caetano C, Granja D, Pinto R, Mendes B, et al. Nutrition and supplementation in football. *Sports* [Internet]. 2017 May 12 [cited 2021 May 19];5(2):28. Available from: https://pubmed.ncbi.nlm.nih.gov/29910389/

19. Arjol-Serrano JL, Lampre M, Díez A, Castillo D, Sanz-López F, Lozano D. The influence of playing formation on physical demands and technical-tactical actions according to playing positions in an elite football team. *Int J Environ Res Public Health* [Internet]. 2021 Apr 14 [cited 2021 May 19];18(8):4148. Available from: https://www.ncbi.nlm.nih.gov/pubmed/33919928

20. Bradley PS, Di Mascio M, Peart D, Olsen P, Sheldon B. High-intensity activity profiles of elite football players at different performance levels. *J Strength Cond Res* [Internet]. 2010 Sep [cited 2021 May 19];24(9):2343–2351. Available from: https://pubmed.ncbi.nlm.nih.gov/19918194/

21. Bangsbo J, Mohr M, Krustrup P. Physical and metabolic demands of training and match-play in the elite football player. *J Sports Sci* [Internet]. 2006 July [cited 2021 May 19];24(7):665–674. Available from: https://pubmed.ncbi.nlm.nih.gov/16766496/

22. Paul DJ, Bradley PS, Nassis GP. Factors affecting match running performance of elite football players: Shedding some light on the complexity. *Int J Sports Physiol Perform* [Internet]. 2015 May 1 [cited 2021 May 19];10(4):516–519. Available from: https://pubmed.ncbi.nlm.nih.gov/25928752/

23. Bush MD, Archer DT, Hogg R, Bradley PS. Factors influencing physical and technical variability in the english premier league. *Int J Sports Physiol Perform*. 2015 Oct 1;10(7):865–872.

24. Barnes C, Archer DT, Hogg B, Bush M, Bradley PS. The evolution of physical and technical performance parameters in the english premier league. *Int J Sports Med* [Internet]. 2014 July 10 [cited 2021 May 19];35(13):1095–1100. Available from: https://pubmed.ncbi.nlm.nih.gov/25009969/

25. Bush M, Barnes C, Archer DT, Hogg B, Bradley PS. Evolution of match performance parameters for various playing positions in the English Premier League. *Hum Mov Sci*

[Internet]. 2015 Feb 1 [cited 2021 May 19];39:1–11. Available from: https://pubmed. ncbi.nlm.nih.gov/25461429/

26. Gabbett TJ, Mulvey MJ. Time-motion analysis of small-sided training games and competition in elite women football players. *J Strength Cond Res* [Internet]. 2008 [cited 2021 May 19];22(2):543–552. Available from: https://pubmed.ncbi.nlm.nih. gov/18550972/

27. Carling C, Le Gall F, Dupont G. Analysis of repeated high-intensity running performance in professional football. *J Sports Sci.* 2012 Feb;30(4):325–336.

28. Anderson L, Orme P, Di Michele R, Close GL, Morgans R, Drust B, et al. Quantification of training load during one-, two- and three-game week schedules in professional football players from the English Premier League: implications for carbohydrate periodisation. *J Sports Sci* [Internet]. 2016 July 2 [cited 2021 May 19];34(13):1250–1259. Available from: https://pubmed.ncbi.nlm.nih.gov/26536538/

29. Oliveira R, Brito J, Martins A, Mendes B, Calvete F, Carriço S, et al. In-season training load quantification of one-, two- and three-game week schedules in a top European professional football team. *Physiol Behav.* 2019 Mar 15;201:146–156.

30. Anderson L, Orme P, Naughton RJ, Close GL, Milsom J, Rydings D, et al. Energy intake and expenditure of professional football players of the English Premier league: Evidence of carbohydrate periodization. *Int J Sport Nutr Exerc Metab.* 2017 June 1;27(3):228–238.

31. Briggs MA, Cockburn E, Rumbold PLS, Rae G, Stevenson EJ, Russell M. Assessment of energy intake and energy expenditure of male adolescent academy-level football players during a competitive week. *Nutrients* [Internet]. 2015 Oct 2 [cited 2021 May 19];7(10):8392–8401. Available from: https://pubmed.ncbi.nlm.nih.gov/26445059/

32. Brinkmans NYJ, Iedema N, Plasqui G, Wouters L, Saris WHM, van Loon LJC, et al. Energy expenditure and dietary intake in professional football players in the Dutch Premier League: Implications for nutritional counselling. *J Sports Sci* [Internet]. 2019 Dec 17 [cited 2021 May 19];37(24):2759–2767. Available from: https://pubmed.ncbi.nlm. nih.gov/30773995/

33. Osgnach C, Poser S, Bernardini R, Rinaldo R, Di Prampero PE. Energy cost and metabolic power in elite football: A new match analysis approach. *Med Sci Sports Exerc* [Internet]. 2010 Jan [cited 2021 May 19];42(1):170–178. Available from: https://pub-med.ncbi.nlm.nih.gov/20010116/

34. Rico-Sanz J, Frontera WR, Molé PA, Rivera MA, Rivera-Brown A, Meredith CN. Dietary and performance assessment of elite football players during a period of intense training. *Int J Sport Nutr Exerc Metab* [Internet]. 1998 [cited 2021 May 19];8(3):230–240. Available from: https://pubmed.ncbi.nlm.nih.gov/9738133/

35. Ebine N, Rafamantanantsoa HH, Nayuki Y, Yamanaka K, Tashima K, Ono T, et al. Measurement of total energy expenditure by the doubly labelled water method in professional football players. *J Sports Sci* [Internet]. 2002 [cited 2021 May 19];20(5):391–397. Available from: https://pubmed.ncbi.nlm.nih.gov/12043828/

36. Domínguez R, Mata-Ordoñez F, Sánchez-Oliver AJ. *Nutrición Deportiva Aplicada: Guía para Optimizar el Rendimiento* [Internet]. ICB Editores, editor. Malaga, España; 2017 [cited 2018 Aug 22]. 397 p. Available from: https://books. google.es/books?hl=en&lr=&id=ChkwDwAAQBAJ&oi=fnd&pg=PT12&dq= info:Sgp87ELWE5IJ:scholar.google.com&ots=O9vM0f0i1D&sig=1XtWeif5L n9S_O4lBquqZHJvTcQ&redir_esc=y#v=onepage&q&f=false

37. Bettonviel AEO, Brinkmans NYJ, Russcher K, Wardenaar FC, Witard OC. Nutritional status and daytime pattern of protein intake on match, post-match, rest and training days

in senior professional and youth elite football players. *Int J Sport Nutr Exerc Metab* [Internet]. 2016 Jun 1 [cited 2021 May 19];26(3):285–293. Available from: https://pubmed.ncbi.nlm.nih.gov/26630203/

38. Caruana Bonnici D, Akubat I, Greig M, Sparks A, Mc Naughton LR. Dietary habits and energy balance in an under 21 male international football team. *Res Sport Med* [Internet]. 2018 Apr 3 [cited 2021 May 20];26(2):168–177. Available from: https://pubmed.ncbi.nlm.nih.gov/29366354/

39. Caruana Bonnici D, Greig M, Akubat I, Sparks SA, Bentley D, Mc Naughton LR. Nutrition in football: A brief review of the issues and solutions. *J Sci Sport Exerc* [Internet]. 2019 May 12 [cited 2021 May 20];1(1):3–12. Available from: https://doi.org/10.1007/s42978-019-0014-7

40. Ranchordas MK, Dawson JT, Russell M. Practical nutritional recovery strategies for elite football players when limited time separates repeated matches. *J Int Soc Sports Nutrit*. 2017;14:41–42.

41. Ranchordas M. Nutritional needs. In: Strudwick A, editor. *Football science*. Champaign, IL: Human Kinetics Publishers Inc.; 2016.

42. Williams C, Serratosa L. Nutrition on match day. *J Sports Sci* [Internet]. 2006 Jul [cited 2021 May 30];24(7):687–697. Available from: https://pubmed.ncbi.nlm.nih.gov/16766498/

43. Rodriguez-Giustiniani P, Rollo I, Witard OC, Galloway SDR. Ingesting a 12% carbohydrate-electrolyte beverage before each half of a football match simulation facilitates retention of passing performance and improves high-intensity running capacity in academy players. *Int J Sport Nutr Exerc Metab* [Internet]. 2019 [cited 2021 May 31];29(4):397–405. Available from: https://pubmed.ncbi.nlm.nih.gov/30507267/

44. Holway FE, Spriet LL. Sport-specific nutrition: Practical strategies for team sports. *J Sports Sci* [Internet]. 2011 Jan [cited 2020 Oct 1];29(Suppl. 1):S115–S125. Available from: https://pubmed.ncbi.nlm.nih.gov/21831001/

45. Saltin B. Metabolic fundamentals in exercise. *Med Sci Sports Exerc* [Internet]. 1973 [cited 2021 May 30];5(3):137–146. Available from: https://pubmed.ncbi.nlm.nih.gov/4270581/

46. Briggs MA, Harper LD, McNamee G, Cockburn E, Rumbold PLS, Stevenson EJ, et al. The effects of an increased calorie breakfast consumed prior to simulated match-play in Academy football players. *Eur J Sport Sci* [Internet]. 2017 Aug 9 [cited 2021 May 30];17(7):858–866. Available from: https://pubmed.ncbi.nlm.nih.gov/28323574/

47. Nuccio RP, Barnes KA, Carter JM, Baker LB. Fluid balance in team sport athletes and the effect of hypohydration on cognitive, technical, and physical performance. *Sports Med* [Internet]. 2017 [cited 2020 Oct 1];47:1951–1982. Available from: https://pubmed.ncbi.nlm.nih.gov/28508338/

48. Sawka MN, Burke LM, Eichner ER, Maughan RJ, Montain SJ, Stachenfeld NS. American college of sports medicine position stand. Exercise and fluid replacement. *Med Sci Sports Exerc* [Internet]. 2007 Feb [cited 2017 Feb 14];39(2):377–390. Available from: https://www.ncbi.nlm.nih.gov/pubmed/17277604

49. Baker LB, Rollo I, Stein KW, Jeukendrup AE. Acute effects of carbohydrate supplementation on intermittent sports performance. *Nutrients* [Internet]. 2015 [cited 2020 Oct 1];7:5733–5763. Available from: https://pubmed.ncbi.nlm.nih.gov/26184303/

50. Russell M, Kingsley M. The efficacy of acute nutritional interventions on football skill performance. *Sports Medicine* [Internet]. 2014 [cited 2021 May 31];44:957–970. Available from: https://pubmed.ncbi.nlm.nih.gov/24728928/

51. Russell M, Benton D, Kingsley M. Influence of carbohydrate supplementation on skill performance during a football match simulation. *J Sci Med Sport* [Internet]. 2012 Jul [cited 2021 May 31];15(4):348–354. Available from: https://pubmed.ncbi.nlm.nih.gov/22230353/

52. Harper LD, Stevenson EJ, Rollo I, Russell M. The influence of a 12% carbohydrate-electrolyte beverage on self-paced football-specific exercise performance. *J Sci Med Sport* [Internet]. 2017 Dec 1 [cited 2021 May 31];20(12):1123–1129. Available from: https://pubmed.ncbi.nlm.nih.gov/28483560/

53. Rollo I, Homewood G, Williams C, Carter J, Goosey-Tolfrey VL. The influence of carbohydrate mouth rinse on self-selected intermittent running performance. *Int J Sport Nutr Exerc Metab* [Internet]. 2015 Dec 1 [cited 2021 May 31];25(6):550–558. Available from: https://pubmed.ncbi.nlm.nih.gov/26061762/

54. Carter JM, Jeukendrup AE, Jones DA. The effect of carbohydrate mouth rinse on 1-h cycle time trial performance. *Med Sci Sports Exerc* 2004;36(12):2107–2111.

55. Dorling JL, Earnest CP. Effect of carbohydrate mouth rinsing on multiple sprint performance. *J Int Soc Sports Nutr* [Internet]. 2013 Dec [cited 2021 May 31];10(1):41. Available from: https://pubmed.ncbi.nlm.nih.gov/24066731/

56. Duffield R, McCall A, Coutts AJ, Peiffer JJ. Hydration, sweat and thermoregulatory responses to professional football training in the heat. *J Sports Sci* [Internet]. 2012 Jun [cited 2021 May 31];30(10):957–965. Available from: https://pubmed.ncbi.nlm.nih.gov/22620496/

57. Maughan RJ, Shirreffs SM, Merson SJ, Horswill CA. Fluid and electrolyte balance in elite male football (football) players training in a cool environment. *J Sports Sci* [Internet]. 2005 Jan [cited 2021 May 31];23(1):73–79. Available from: https://pubmed.ncbi.nlm.nih.gov/15841597/

58. Kilding AE, Tunstall H, Wraith E, Good M, Gammon C, Smith C. Sweat rate and sweat electrolyte composition in international female football players during game specific training. *Int J Sports Med* [Internet]. 2009 [cited 2021 May 31];30(6):443–447. Available from: https://pubmed.ncbi.nlm.nih.gov/19288391/

59. McDermott BP, Anderson SA, Armstrong LE, Casa DJ, Cheuvront SN, Cooper L, et al. National athletic trainers' association position statement: Fluid replacement for the physically active. *J Athletic Training* [Internet]; 2017 [cited 2021 May 31];52:877–895. Available from: https://pubmed.ncbi.nlm.nih.gov/28985128/

60. Nédélec M, McCall A, Carling C, Legall F, Berthoin S, Dupont G. Recovery in football: Part II-recovery strategies. *Sports Med.* 2013;43:9–22.

61. Burke LM, van Loon LJC, Hawley JA. Postexercise muscle glycogen resynthesis in humans. *J Appl Physiol* [Internet]. 2017;122(5):1055–1067. Available from: https://jap.physiology.org/lookup/doi/10.1152/japplphysiol.00860.2016

62. Morton RW, McGlory C, Phillips SM. Nutritional interventions to augment resistance training-induced skeletal muscle hypertrophy. *Front Physiol.* 2015;6. Available from: https://doi.org/10.1136/bjsports-2017-097608

63. Van Loon LJC. Role of dietary protein in post-exercise muscle reconditioning. *Nestle Nutr Inst Workshop Ser* [Internet]. 2013 [cited 2021 May 31];75:73–83. Available from: https://pubmed.ncbi.nlm.nih.gov/23765352/

64. Evans GH, James LJ, Shirreffs SM, Maughan RJ. Optimizing the restoration and maintenance of fluid balance after exercise-induced dehydration. *J Appl Physiol* [Internet]. 2017;122(4):945–951. Available from: https://jap.physiology.org/lookup/doi/10.1152/japplphysiol.00745.2016

65. Barnes MJ. Alcohol: Impact on sports performance and recovery in male athletes. *Sport Med*. 2014;44(7):909–919.

66. Hobson RM, Maughan RJ. Hydration status and the diuretic action of a small dose of alcohol. *Alcohol Alcohol* [Internet]. 2010 May 24 [cited 2021 May 31];45(4):366–373. Available from: https://pubmed.ncbi.nlm.nih.gov/20497950/

67. Krustrup P, Mohr M, Steensberg A, Bencke J, Klær M, Bangsbo J. Muscle and blood metabolites during a football game: Implications for sprint performance. *Med Sci Sports Exerc* [Internet]. 2006 Jun [cited 2021 May 31];38(6):1165–1174. Available from: https://pubmed.ncbi.nlm.nih.gov/16775559/

68. Mata F, Valenzuela PL, Gimenez J, Tur C, Ferreria D, Domínguez R, et al. Carbohydrate availability and physical performance: Physiological overview and practical recommendations. *Nutrients*. 2019 May 1;11(5):1084.

69. Morton RW, Murphy KT, McKellar SR, Schoenfeld BJ, Henselmans M, Helms E, et al. A systematic review, meta-analysis and meta-regression of the effect of protein supplementation on resistance training-induced gains in muscle mass and strength in healthy adults. *Br J Sports Med* [Internet]. 2018 Mar 1 [cited 2021 May 31];52(6):376–384. Available from: https://pubmed.ncbi.nlm.nih.gov/28698222/

70. Phillips SM, Wernbom M, Augustsson J, Thomee R, Bamman MM, Petrella J, et al. The impact of protein quality on the promotion of resistance exercise-induced changes in muscle mass. *Nutr Metab (Lond)*. 2016;13(1):64.

71. Murphy CH, Hector AJ, Phillips SM. Considerations for protein intake in managing weight loss in athletes. *Eur J Sport Sci*. 2014;15(July):21–28.

72. Wall BT, Morton JP, van Loon LJ. Strategies to maintain skeletal muscle mass in the injured athlete: nutritional considerations and exercise mimetics. *Eur J Sport Sci*. 2015;15(1):27.

73. Volek JS, Noakes T, Phinney SD. Rethinking fat as a fuel for endurance exercise. *Eur J Sport Sci*. 2015;15(1):13–20.

2

EVALUATION OF MUSCLE STRUCTURE AND FUNCTION

Alejandro Muñoz-López and Manuel García-Sillero

2.1 Assessing the soccer player musculature

Muscle structure and function can be assessed to provide important information about a football player's fitness status. Many different methods and technologies can be used for this purpose. Because the literature shows several concepts and proposals related to this topic, in this chapter, we will present and explain what we understand, from a practical point of view, as interesting options to monitor the neuromuscular football player status directly related to the muscle function due to its muscle architecture.

The neuromuscular assessment can be approached from different options, as well as various definitions have been used. From the perspectives of chapter, we define the neuromuscular function as the ability to produce a certain expected force or power (e.g., for neuromuscular fatigue and the inability of the last) [1].

The muscle function, which is mainly represented by the muscle contraction, depends on several factors such as the fibre type distribution, the inter- and intra-muscular coordination, or the energy supply. That function can also be related to the peripheral or central structures of the human body. While the peripheral muscle function is more related to the isolated muscle, the central function is more likely depending on the superior brain centers and spinal cord. Following this division, assessment methods and technologies can be classified to provide information related to the muscle structure and function. The muscle structure is mostly related to the peripheral muscle function, and some tests will assess both peripheral and central function all at once.

In Figure 2.1, we present four technologies that are used for testing peripheral and central muscle function in football. Testing the central function without a peripheral function testing with those technologies is not possible. Electromyography

DOI: 10.4324/9781032637006-2

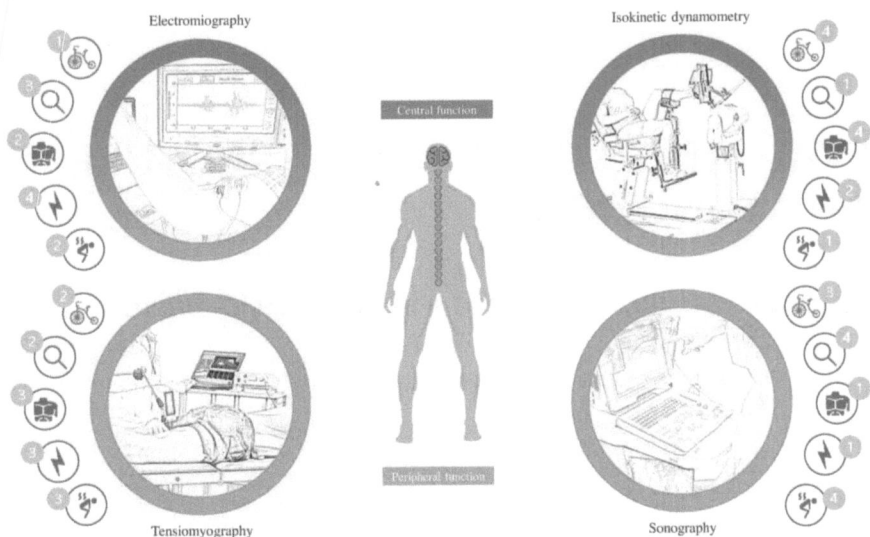

FIGURE 2.1 Technologies that can be used to monitor the muscle structure and function.

(EMG) and isokinetic dynamometry are used for testing both central and periph-eral functions all at once. In contrast, the isolated peripheral function can be tested using tensiomiography (TMG) or sonography. The decision on whether to use one or another could depend on many reasons, regardless of the economic cost. First, the portability plays an important role in football because football teams usually travel with all of those technologies. Regarding the presented ranking (based on our own experience and knowledge), it may be possible that different models of a same technology would alter the proposed ranking. However, it has been created to give a general idea. Besides portability, how fast the technician could assess a single muscle or movement is very important because usually more than one mus-cle and football player are being tested. In addition, the feasibility of a technology to detect the muscle fatigue, which may impair the muscle function [2], opens the door to use the specific variables as a training load marker. Furthermore, how selective is the technology that could isolate a single muscle function will allow to create an individual function mapping of the soccer player. Finally, the level of specialization required to implement and analyze the data provided is critical.

The areas on which we propose to use the four technologies are likely related to the detection of the muscle fatigue, the performance over specific or general sport tasks, and the reduction in the injury risk. In all those areas, the muscle structure and its function will have an important role. Current scientific evidence puts the incidence of injury in men's professional football at 8.1 injuries/1000 hours of exposure. Within these, the lower limb (6.8/1000 h) and competition (36/1000 h) show the highest rate. If we refer to the injured structure, the muscle/tendon is the area of greatest exposure (4.6/1000 h) [3]. These data, far from improving at a high level in recent years, show a worrying increase in the area of greatest demand for the player, such as the hamstring, with an increase of 4% [4]. These data should make football professionals reflect on the need to look for tools to assess the exact state of their players' muscle tissue.

Fatigue is behind many of the mechanisms of these muscle injuries. Aspects such as decreased stride length [5], loss of eccentric strength [6], and incomplete recovery after matches [7] are some of the multiple aspects surrounding the muscular injury. Understanding both acute and chronic fatigue processes is therefore a key factor in reducing the incidence of these injuries. Knowing and managing the technology that allows us to improve these processes is nowadays an obligation for physical trainers, physiotherapists, and doctors.

They are correlated to long rehabilitations and have a great tendency to recur. Therefore, the possibility of assessing the exact consequences of the injury, the process of selecting the most suitable exercises and tasks for each player, and the objectification of the Return to Play (RTP) process are a fundamental aspect in modern football.

2.1.1 Tensiomyography

TMG is a non-invasive technology, developed in Slovenia in the 1990s, to measure the neuromuscular status of the superficial muscles. It directly measures the relationship between muscle belly deformation and time. With the analysis of the muscle displacement (Dm) and time curve (Figure 2.2), several time-dependent variables are calculated to provide information about the muscle contractile properties, such as contraction time (Tc), delay time (Td), sustain time (Ts), and relaxation time (Tr). In addition, several research studies proposed the use of the contraction velocity $\left(Vc = \dfrac{Dm}{Td + Tc} \right)$ as another interesting variable.

The TMG is a mechanograph, variables of which are influenced by the muscle tone, the number or motor units recruited, the tissue density, and the muscle

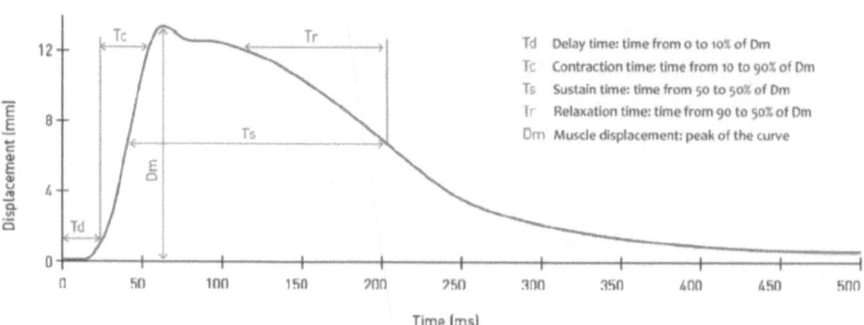

FIGURE 2.2 Displacement–time curve of a muscle measure with TMG. Muscle contractile properties are calculated using this relationship.

temperature [8]. It has been a direct relationship between the amount of type I fibres and the contraction time (the lower the percentage, the lower the contraction time) [9].

How to use it? TMG has been shown to be a reliable tool, even between observers [10, 11]. However, its reliability depends on following a standardized protocol. Thus, the following factors may contribute to the reliability of the measurements:

- Sensor location: the sensor may be placed on the point of visually higher muscle belly; despite that some research used the SENIAM standards.
- Electrodes size; the most effective size of the electrodes is 5 × 5 cm.
- Between stimulations time: leave about 10–15 seconds between stimulations to avoid excessive fatigue or a post-activation potentiation.
- Joints stabilization: use the manufacturers' pillows and supports to standardize the joint angles and stabilization during measurements.
- Look out for muscle temperature: important drop downs on muscle temperature may affect the results.

In relation to the protocol, the traditional approach is to start at a submaximal stimulation amplitude (i.e., 20–40 mA) and to increase by means of 10 mA until the stimulation that elicits the peak Dm. This method is used to elicit the maximal twitch muscle response. However, we have recently observed that a submaximal stimulation of 40 mA showed the best relationship with a repeated sprint protocol and the subsequent muscle fatigue (unpublished data). During an electrical stimulation, the Henneman's size principal is reversed [12] and, as such, the type II fibers are first recruited. Hence, our hypothesis is that high-speed sport tasks or fatigue can be better reflected with lower amplitudes. From a practical point of view, this approach can decrease the effective time for a TMG test on a single player, thus affecting the team assessment.

Specific fields of application and practical guidelines.

2.1.2 Muscle fatigue, acute and chronic

Fatigue, among other adverse effects, decreases the contractile capacity of the muscle during sport actions [13]. The use of TMG could help determine if the muscle function is restored from previous physical activity.

The composition of the fibers in a muscle determines its function. While fast-twitch fibers elicit a higher peak torque (REF) and activate faster (REF) compared to slow-twitch fibers, they are more likely to be fatigued after a physical effort (REF). TMG can be used to estimate which muscles have a higher composition of fast-twitch fibres (REF): the lower the Tc, the higher their percentage. What is more, Dm can also be used to detect fatigue, with some research showing a decrease in Dm associated to acute fatigue (REF). To detect muscle fatigue using TMG, we had recently shown that a lower stimulation amplitude (e.g., 20–40 mA) might be used instead of evoking the peak Dm. Using peak Dm, Sanchez-Sanchez et al. [14] showed that after repeated sprints (an action which often occurs during a football match), the Tc was decreased on the rectus femoris in both dominant and non-dominant legs, despite the biceps femoris not being affected. However, in a fatiguing leg extension protocol we showed that, after either concentric or eccentric actions, the biceps femoris showed reductions in Dm [15]. But after a simulated soccer match, TMG was not able to show changes in the muscle function, neither in the artificial turf nor natural grass surfaces [16]. In addition, TMG can be used to monitor an intensive training week. Raeder et al. [17] showed that a complex strength training protocol on team sports athletes reduced the contraction velocity of the vastus lateralis, while it was increased 4 days after the training session. Finally, the muscle contractile properties were not altered after a normal football training session, neither using passive or active recovery [18], which suggest that TMG can be performed after training. In conclusion, TMG can be used for assessing the fatigue of the muscle function, especially in the lower limbs of professional football players.

2.1.3   Performance

Knee is one of the main human body joints related to football performance, due to the relationship with specific sport tasks such as jumping, sprinting, kicking, or changing of direction. One of the biggest handicaps related to the use of TMG is that its analysis depend on which data are used as reference. For example, we found important differences on the lower limb muscles between the manufacturer software reference data, some reference data published (REF), and our own data from the teams where we used the technology (Table 2.1). Thus, we propose to individualize reference data as much as possible before proceeding with any TMG analyses. For purpose, if no individual data exist, published or manufacturer reference data can be used instead.

In addition to establish a reference (i.e., normal) data, a range may be used. We use percentile p40 and p60 to establish that range. However, this range can be varied in relation to the muscle structure (e.g., phasic or tonic muscle) or the playing position [19]. In addition, the reference data can be used to predict the performance of the muscle function, especially if the Vc measured at 40 mA is used on the rectus femoris (i.e., the higher the Vc, the better jump or sprint performance) [20]. García-García et al. [21] provided reference values for professional soccer players along a season.

2.1.4   Injury risk reduction

TMG can be implemented to detect muscle weaknesses of each player and avoid injuries, or even detect if they have occurred or not [22]. An important key factor in this area is that TMG is a non-invasive measurement and that no physical effort

CHAINS ANALYSIS

EXTENSION CHAIN	RIGHT			LEFT			SYMMETRIES
M.	Tc	Dm	Int.	Tc	Dm	Int.	
m.ES							
m.GT	40.2	14.2	U	39.7	18.5	U	93.42
m.RF	40	12.2	U	37.5	13.8	U	98.39
m.SO							
m.VM	37.3	13.4	U	30.8	9.79	U	80.09
m.VL	29	7.94	T	29.2	5.56	U	94.10
m.GM	21	4.46	T	20.4	3.07	T	91.97
m.GL	20.6	2.95	K	23.1	4.52	R	85.19

FLEXION CHAIN	RIGHT			LEFT			SYMMETRIES
M.	Tc	Dm	Int.	Tc	Dm	Int.	
m.RA							
m.OB							
m.TA							
m.ST	41.9	17.3	U	42.2	13.2	U	93.52
m.BF	38.6	11	U	36.2	11.3	U	95.84

CLOSE CHAIN	RIGHT			LEFT			SYMMETRIES
M.	Tc	Dm	Int.	Tc	Dm	Int.	
m.AL							
m.ST	41.9	17.3	U	42.2	13.2	U	93.52
m.VM	37.3	13.4	U	30.8	9.79	U	80.09
m.GL	20.6	2.95	R	23.1	4.52	K	85.19
m.PL							

OPEN CHAIN	RIGHT			LEFT			SYMMETRIES
M.	Tc	Dm	Int.	Tc	Dm	Int.	
m.GT	40.2	14.2	U	39.7	18.5	U	93.42
m.VL	29	7.94	T	29.2	5.56	U	94.10
m.BF	38.6	11	U	36.2	11.3	U	95.84
m.TA							
m.GM	21	4.46	T	20.4	3.07	T	91.97

FIGURE 2.3 TMG muscle chain custom report. Column "Int" shows the intervention for the muscle based on a combination of low, normal, or high Tc or Dm values for each muscle.

is required from the player. Hence, injured muscles or limbs can be tested. For example, Alvarez-Diaz et al. [23] showed that, after a year of ACL reconstruction, the contractile properties improved and also the bilateral symmetry. In relation to symmetry, the TMG provides the bilateral [24] and functional symmetry [19], which are automatically calculated using specific formulae to assess muscle balance and performance. More specifically, the bilateral symmetry is calculated using the following formulae:

$$Bilateral\ symmetry = 0.1 \times \frac{\min(TDr\ TDl)}{\max(TDr\ TDl)} + 0.6 \times \frac{\min(TCr\ TCl)}{\max(TCr\ TCl)}$$
$$+ 0.1 \times \frac{\min(TSr\ TSl)}{\max(TSr\ TSl)} + 0.2 \times \frac{\min(DMr\ DMl)}{\max(DMr\ DMl)}$$

i.e, the functional symmetry is calculated for different groups of muscles such as elbow, Achilles tendon, patellae ligament, knee, ankle, and leg, using the following formulae (in case of right (r) Knee – 4 muscles):

$$Functional\ symmetry = 0.1 \times \frac{\min(average(TDr1, TDr2)\ average(TDr3, TDr4))}{\max(average(TDr1, TDr2)\ average(TDr3, TDr4))}$$
$$+ 0.8 * \frac{\min(average(TCr1, TCr2)\ average(TCr3, TCr4))}{\max(average(TCr1, TCr2)\ average(TCr3, TCr4))}$$
$$+ 0.1 * \frac{\min(average(TSr1, TSr2)\ average(TSr3, TSr4))}{\max(average(TSr1, TSr2)\ average(TSr3, TSr4))}$$

where 1 = vastus lateralis, 2 = vastus medialis, 3 = rectus femoris, and 4 = biceps femoris.

Finally, because TMG allows to selectively test superficial muscles, a testing report can be organized to provide information related to how a whole muscle chain or weak structures are distributed. Figure 2.3 shows information of a custom report organizing muscles in muscle chains. With this view, the technician can have a clearer idea of each muscle chain weaknesses.

2.1.5 Isokinetic dynamometers

The first research using an isokinetic dynamometer was published in the 1970s, to our knowledge [25]. Since then, there has been an extensive use in both research and the field of isokinetic dynamometers.

An isokinetic dynamometer is a technology that primarily measures the time–torque curve to analyze the in vivo force–velocity relationships and other mechanical outcomes that may determine the soccer player performance. Despite being named "isokinetic," they also allow to measure under "isoinertial" or "isometric" conditions. In this chapter, we will only focus on the isokinetic loading condition.

They are primarily used as a method for assessing muscle function and imbalance in clinical, research, and sports environment [26]. In addition, they are considered the gold standard criterion for mechanical outcomes such as torque, work, or power in performance testing [27]. Indeed, they have the ability to detect injuries or discriminate between player level or training status. However, isokinetic dynamometers are expensive, and they are not portable (Figure 2.1).

Compared to the rest of the technologies in this chapter, they cannot be used to measure an isolated muscle. In contrast, this does not imply that it lacks utility entirely, as they measure a group of muscles (e.g., muscle chains) involved in a specific joint movement (i.e., the knee flexion). That result on the most famous application for this technology: the calculation of the hamstring to quadriceps ratio (ratio H:Q) [28–30].

2.1.5.1 How to use it

One of the most studied topics about isokinetic dynamometers is related to its reproducibility. Therefore, caution should be taken when protocols are implemented. It has been suggested that there are several competing demands on the design of the measurement protocol, which may affect the assessment and data interpretation [26].

Some of the factors that may affect the measurement are presented in Table 2.1. Those factors may consequently affect the data reproducibility. Research studies that studied the isokinetic dynamometer reproducibility are focused primarily on knee or hip muscles [31, 32]. It is shown that both isokinetic strength and muscular

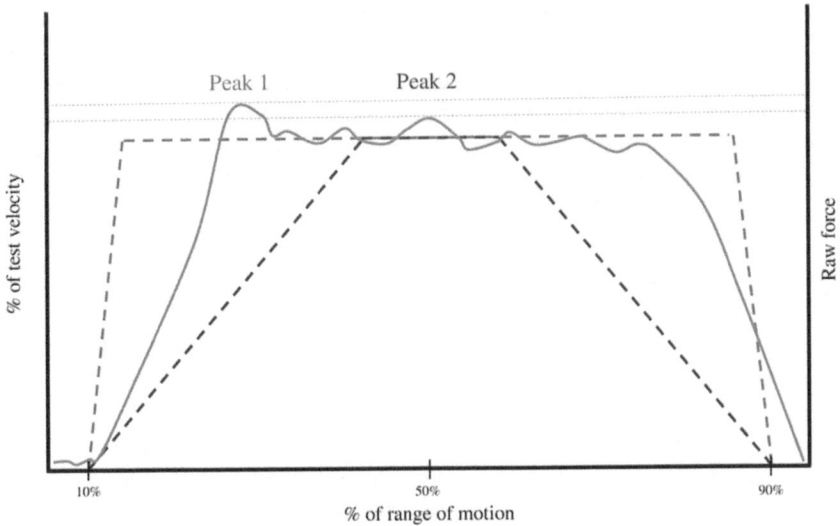

FIGURE 2.4   Load range concept.

endurance for quadriceps and hamstrings muscles are reproducible at common speeds of 60°/s or 180°/s [32], being constantly high either during concentric or eccentric muscle activations [31]. Finally, the eccentric peak hip adductor torque, but not the hip flexors, resulted in high reliability [31].

Another factor that affects the isokinetic measurements is the load range. During isokinetic exercises, the device involves three primary components: acceleration, sustained velocity, and deceleration [33] (Figure 2.4). Thus, sometimes the value obtained as, for example, peak torque could be achieved during the acceleration phase, especially at high speeds (i.e., > 180°/s). Therefore, practitioners must be aware of only analyzing the load range part of the repetition to avoid measurement errors.

In general, the following considerations have been proposed as basic principles of administration for isokinetic tests [34]:

- Perform a proper warm-up before the testing. Probably include more than one set for the testing because the second will result in higher outcomes.
- Isolate the muscle group to be tested. This may not result in difficulty because it is one of the main advantages of this technologies.
- Standardize the lever arm and range of motion.
- Align the center of rotation of the joint with that of the mechanical device.
- Subtract the weight of the limb from the calculation of the force movement.
- Even if a peak calculation is desired, consider calculating a mean over a small data window around that peak.
- Consider testing at different speeds to understand if the performance or disbalance is dependent to a given torque.

Specific fields of application and practical guidelines

2.1.6 Muscle fatigue, acute and chronic

Changes in muscle function can be attributed to altered muscle contractions by a transient or chronic fatigue. It has been shown that isokinetic repetitions on the leg extension and knee flexion impair the muscle contractile properties [15] at high speeds in a different manner. Those high speeds (i.e., > 180°/s) have been found to be highly reproducible during fatiguing isokinetic testing [35].

To assess the endurance to fatigue, Bosquet et al. [36] designed a high-intensity isokinetic fatigue test, consisted of 30 consecutive concentric knee extensions and flexions at 180°/s. They determined muscle fatigue as the slope of the curve after plotting peak torque or total work for each repetition across the set. Interestingly, they found associations between that slope and the anaerobic performance in typical physiological testing, which are determinants of football performance.

2.1.7 Performance

Performance measurements using isokinetic dynamometers are mostly related to normative data. Dias Scoz et al. [37] did a great research focused on normative data at different ages and positions over 10 years in football players. They found differences across ages and positions in the isokinetic peak torque on the knee extension at concentric activations. In addition, they showed a small difference between playing positions and a moderate effect of age in healthy professional football players. Finally, they observed that midfielders and goalkeepers showed the greatest reduction by age, after 29 years of age. These data may help predict the end of a career for a football player.

As it is shown on any physiological or performance measurement, there is a substantial intraindividual variability in isokinetic measurements, across seasons and irrespective to injury [38]. That opens the door to an effective monitoring using individual performance assessment tests, using variability markers such as the smallest worthwhile change [39].

2.1.8 Injury risk reduction

Most of the applications and studies involving isokinetic dynamometers are included in the attempt to reduce the injury risk and its usage during rehabilitation programs. The wider index studies are related to the strength-level differences between lateral limbs (bilateral deficit) or the hamstrings versus quadriceps strength levels (H:Q-ratio).

Isokinetic dynamometers offer the possibility to monitor unilateral exercises. Therefore, they are considered practical instruments for bilateral testing, of particular for the lower limbs. To avoid the residual effect of fatigue, testing would be randomized by legs order, and enough recovery time (i.e., < 5 min.) might be used. In addition, several ranges of speed may be tested to understand the limb imbalance because it might be possible that a football player would present a bilateral deficit at low speeds, but not at high speeds, or vice versa.

One of the most common and important football injuries is hamstring strains, and the imbalance between the knee extensors and flexors in the muscle function is considered a hamstring injury risk factor. Thus, the H:Q-ratio is used under isokinetic exercises to monitor the injury risk in football players. Typically, it can be calculated as the peak concentric knee flexion strength divided by the maximal concentric knee extension strength at the same angular velocity. This velocity is typically 60°/s. However, an alternative index (functional ratio and eccentric hamstring:concentric quadriceps) is another interesting alternative and shown to be at higher speeds [29], useful to prevent football injuries [30]. Despite those indexes being considered into official testing recommendations to prevent muscle injuries in football [34], caution should be taken to use those ratios as a magical standard to prevent injuries. In relation, it has been recently shown that isokinetic strength levels do not change from preinjury to return to sport levels after hamstring injuries [40].

2.1.9 Surface Electromyography

By EMG, an insight into the understanding of intentional and unconscious movement behaviour has been gained [41]. This technology can detect and analyze EMG, the electric potential generated during muscle contraction. EMG can be detected directly or indirectly by inserting electrodes into muscle tissue surface electrodes on the skin area directly above the muscle tissue. Surface EMG (sEMG) usually conveys information about muscle activation, such as muscle contraction strength, EMG performance of muscle fatigue, and motor unit (MU) recruitment [42].

The motor unit is the functional unit of the neuromuscular system. Each MU contains a motor neuron and muscle fiber provided by its axon branch [43]. After the motor neuron is fired, the action potential is generated at the neuromuscular junction and then spreads along all the muscle fibers to the tendon area. The sum of these potentials is called the motor unit action potential (MUAP), which is responsible for muscle contraction [42].

But EMG does not provide direct information about muscle power. For example, at the same activation level, defined as maximum isometric voluntary contraction (MIVC), muscles with greater cross-sectional area will generate more force than a smaller one.

In addition, because of the well-known force–length and force–velocity relationships, if muscles are moved at a more optimized length and/or speed, higher muscle force can be generated at the same activation level.

Therefore, inferring muscle strength from EMG amplitude during dynamic movements is even more problematic compared to isometric movements. In addition, there is an electromechanical delay between muscle activation and force generation. Considered together, it is obvious that a comprehensive understanding of force sharing between muscles cannot be based on EMG alone but requires a more direct estimation of the forces generated by individual muscles or muscle regions. Although the limitations associated with EMG inferring power as well known, they have received little attention in clinical research [44].

2.1.9.1   How to use it

There are many detection systems for recording surface EMG, which are developed based on different detection materials [45]. Generally, the electrodes are made of silver/silver chloride (Ag/AgCl), which promotes the impedance of the electrode skin resistance rather than capacitance. Therefore, the surface potential is less sensitive to the relative movement between the electrode surface and the skin. In addition, these electrodes provide a highly stable interface. When the electrolyte solution (gel) is inserted between the skin and the electrode, the skin comes into contact with the skin.

The main aspects to be considered when installing and correctly using EMG are as follows:

- The proper preparation of the skin ensures the elimination of hair, oils, and layers of skin scales.
- Shaving, wetting, and rubbing with alcohol, acetone, or ether are usually considered for cleaning the skin.

Figure 2.5 shows a schematic representation of the positioning of the surface electrodes including the observed surface EMG. Two electrodes are placed within the skin locations immediately over the muscle tissue, while the reference electrode is found near the bone areas on the skin.

Installing the electrode is another necessary drawback for sEMG detection. The devices could have a monopolar (a potential drop that is detected on the surface of the skin like a shot higher than the muscle tissue) or higher than the bipolar configuration that considerably reduces disturbance development [46].

Although tips for the positioning of surface electrodes were projected within the SENIAM project [47].

Specific fields of application and practical guidelines:

2.1.10   Muscle fatigue, acute and chronic

EMG is used to monitor fatigue by measuring the decrease in the maximum capacity to generate force, which is generally expressed as a deterioration in the MVIC [48]. Football is characterized by high-intensity, complex, and intermittent exercises that simultaneously demand various aspects of strength, speed, and endurance [49].

The use of EMG as an indicator of neuromuscular fatigue can provide important information for coaches. Rampini and cols. [50] demonstrated how the RMS

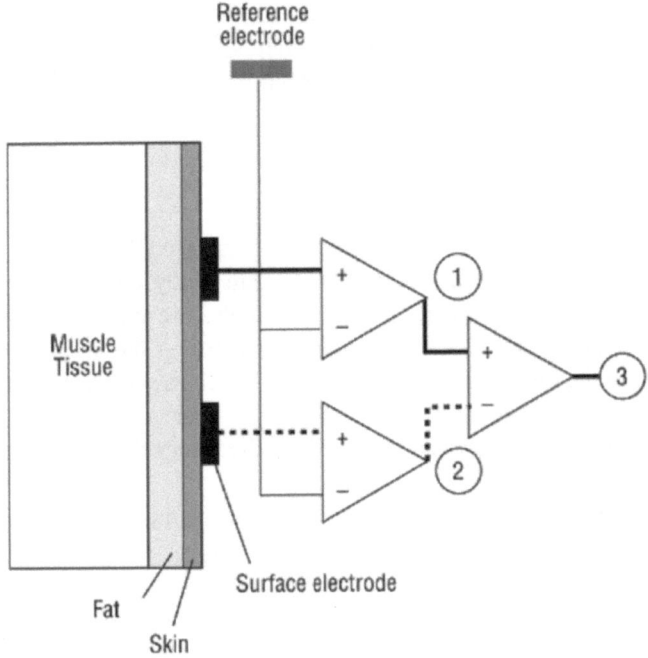

FIGURE 2.5 Conventional electrode montages (extracted from Cavalcanti Garcia and Vieira [43]).

values measured in the vastus medialis did not recover until 48 hours after the match, showing decreases of up to 12% in the post-match signal.

In order to gain a better understanding of fatigue from the point of view of the central nervous system, EMG signal monitoring has been combined with transcranial magnetic stimulation (TMS) activation to monitor fatigue post 24, 48, and 72 hours after a football match [7]. The voluntary activation (VA) decreases from 7.1% (post-match) to 4.7% (24 h) before recovering by 48 hours. These measures suggest that football professionals should use a range of subjective and objective items by monitoring fatigue and recovery, including sEMG.

Even the neuromuscular acute fatigue response has been studied through the performance of the hamstring muscles during a match using EMG [51]. This investigation (Figure 2.6) shows the distribution of the RMS signal in the two parts of a match.

Individualizing and measuring this parameter in the musculature with the highest injury rate in football [52] can be a very useful tool in the field of injury prevention.

2.1.11 Performance

Neuromuscular activity could be a good indicator of performance in football players. Not only during specific tasks, even looking for general strategies to improve

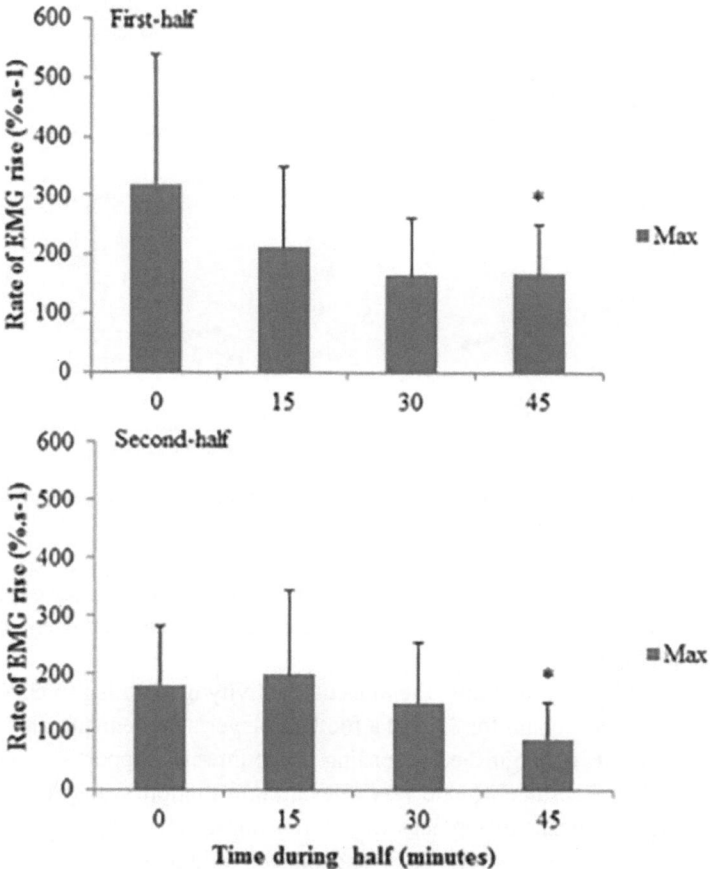

FIGURE 2.6 Biceps femoris EMG signal evolution during a soccer match (extracted from Marshall et al. [51]).

during the game or training situations. The lack of change in EMG activity and the V-wave amplitude suggests a better post-performance after activation exercises. The magnitude of the post-activation potentiation enhancement (PAPE) has been controlled applying different protocols [53] using sEMG control.

The possibility of analyzing the neuromuscular response during the sport itself is undoubtedly the greatest contribution of the sEMG to the analysis of a football player's performance. Probably, the kicking task has been the most studied in the literature. Scurr et al. [54] examined that EMG activation in three muscles of the quadriceps (vastus lateralis, vastus medialis, and rectus femoris) of the kicking leg was normalized and averaged across all participants to compare between muscles, targets (four goal's corner), and the phase of the kick.

When all targets were averaged, the normalized EMG value during the kicking contact phase of the rectus femoris muscle (RF 77%), vastus lateralis (VL 89%),

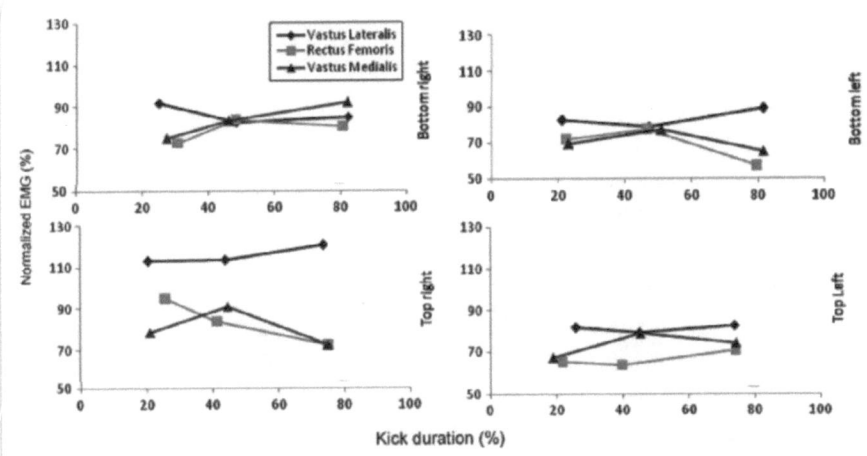

FIGURE 2.7 Quadriceps EMG during soccer instep kicking to each target area (adapted from Scurr et al. [54]).

and vastus medialis (VM 83%) were identified. It showed that the peak activation of the VL is higher and the distribution of muscle activity can vary depending on the type of kicking.

Through EMG, we even know the muscular activity of each leg in curved running actions, which account for 85% of a football player's movements. In this case, muscle activity was distinguished according to the internal support on strong and weak legs [49]. The results provide very relevant information, with greater activations showing significant differences ($p \leq 0.05$) during curve sprinting between outside, higher in biceps femoris (BF) and gluteus medius (Gm), and inside leg higher in semitendinosus (ST) and adductor (AD) during 17-m sprint actions, confirming that each leg plays a different role in curved running actions, which needs to be properly addressed by practitioners. The specific work on the weak leg and on the change of direction in curved actions will be of special interest for player development, derived from the EMG analysis.

2.1.12 Injury risk reduction

EMG is one of the most commonly used methods to examine muscle activity. In conventional EMG studies, electrodes are paced over the mid-belly of the studied muscle. It is widely used to measure muscle activation in both isometric and dynamic actions, although it provides valuable information about neural control movement [48].

Exercise programs are used to prevent and treat injuries in football, and exercise selection is one of the most special uses of the sEMG. In order to evaluate exercise intensity, many studies have been conducted recently for the purpose of using sEMG to measure muscle activity during exercises, which is often used to prevent and treat common football injuries.

Serner and cols. evaluated the neuromuscular activity of eight hip adduction exercises, normalizing them with the MVIC [55]. They found significant differences (14–108%; $p < 0.0001$) in the normalized peak EMG signal (nEMG). Therefore, the use of EMG can be decisive when individualizing and ordering exercises in the different phases and stages of an injury prevention process in football teams.

The action of this muscle has also been analyzed during the kicking action at various intensities (50–75–100% of maximum kicking speed [56]). For this purpose, the muscle activity was assessed using sEMG of the adductor magnus (AM) and adductor longus (AL). The kicking showed an increase in the EMG signal ($p < 0.016$) with the increase in the ball velocity. This muscle activity analysis is of great importance for football professionals for daily use for groin injury prevention.

In this line, the hamstring muscle (HAM) has possibly been the most studied due to the related incidence of injury. Those who have previously suffered hamstring muscle injuries, reduced strength, and EMG activation within the extended range indicated changes in neuromuscular control. The extended range assessment of isometric eccentric flexor torque may be useful for assessing football players who have previously been injured [57].

Trying to find the best time (before or after training) to implement HAM prevention exercises through the EMG signal has also been the subject of study [58]. Strength gains and increases in the BF sEMG signal are important reasons for the placement of this stimulus prior to training, with the necessary fatigue control and risk that this would entail.

The presence of previous injury history in HAMs can be a key factor in the footballer's training process. In case of previous injury, an increased sEMG signal in the gluteus maximus (GM) and medial HAM is often the usual measure [59].

The analysis of movement patterns through EMG activity provides an opportunity to identify the most involved muscle groups in a particular movement and determine the range of deficits between the limbs. The synergy of the gluteal and femoral musculature is shown to be an important factor in injury prevention. Recent studies have analyzed lower limb asymmetry (left–right) during sprinting (30 m) [60]. Left/right asymmetries were found between hamstring (LH/RH) muscles (5 m speed tests; $p = 0.044$ / 30 m $p = 0.045$) and in left and right glutes (LG/RG) (5 m speed test $p = 0.044$ / 30 m $p = 0.043$). This information indicates that during resistance training of football players, the HAM and gluteal muscles should be selectively and additionally activated to prevent injuries and improve sprint performance and how the use of EMG can help professionals to reach these goals.

In the area of HAM exercise selection, we find contradictions in the scientific literature, especially when compared to MRI results [6, 56, 61], mainly due to the cross-talk effect.

In an attempt to clarify this situation, Bourne and colleagues analyzed the activation of the hamstring musculature in ten of the most commonly used exercises:

(1) bilateral stiff-leg deadlift (SDL), (2) hip hinge (HH), (3) unilateral stiff-leg deadlift (USDL), (4) lunge (L), (5) unilateral bent-knee bridge (bKB), (6) unilateral straight knee bridge (SKB), (7) leg curl (LC), (8) 45° hip extension (HE), (9) glute-ham raise (GHR), and (10) Nordic hamstring exercise (NHE).

As can be observed in Figure 2.8, the average BF activation changed from 21.4% (L) to 99.3% (SKB) MVIC during the concentric phase and 10.7% (HH) to 71.9% (NHE) during the eccentric phase. Average MH muscle activity ranged from 18.1% (L) to 120.7% (LC) during the concentric phase and 11.6% (HH) to 101.8% (NHE) during the eccentric phase.

While high levels of EMG are fundamental for rising strength and voluntary activation, exercise selection is basic during rehabilitation or in secondary injury prevention. It is well known nowadays that BF suffers inhibition some months after injury [62]. This inhibition could explain the deficit in the eccentric knee flexor strength, the BF long head atrophy, and the shortening of BF long head fascicles [63].

2.1.13   Ultrasonography

Ultrasound (US) imaging has been widely utilized in analysis and clinical settings to assess the morphology and mechanical properties of muscles and tendons. Within the elite sports, like football, the regular analysis of such attributes has good potential [70]:

• Testing responses to coaching
• Detecting athletes at higher risk of injury
• Screening for structural abnormalities associated with current or future system diseases
• Monitoring the recovery process of athletes after musculoskeletal injury.

2.1.14   How to use it

The use of the US would be the subject of an entire book, so we will summarize the most important recommendations for practical application in the field of elite sport:
Specific fields of application and practical guidelines:

2.1.15   Muscle architecture

Muscle architecture has been previously thought to be one of the main determinants of muscle function. Architectural characteristics will affect the relationships between muscle force length and force speed [64]. Some authors [42] tried to

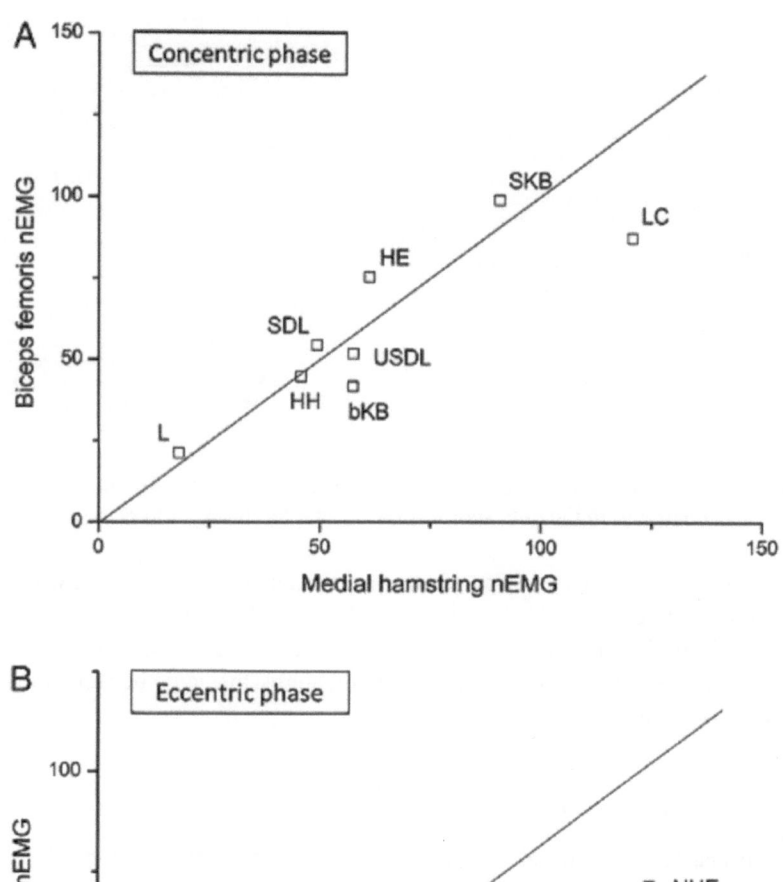

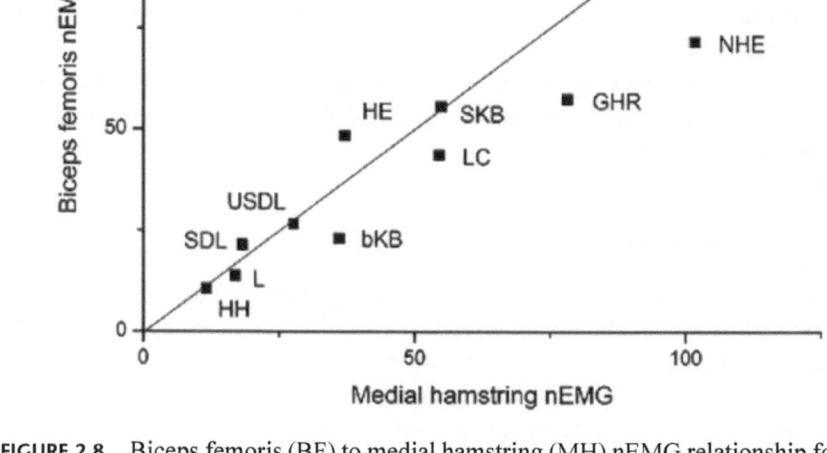

FIGURE 2.8 Biceps femoris (BF) to medial hamstring (MH) nEMG relationship for the (A) concentric and (B) eccentric phases of each exercise (adapted from Bourne, et al. [65]).

DOs	Better think twice
✓ Use an ultrasound system that fits your necessities – ask yourself "what do i need?"	• Avoid applying excessive compresión with the trnasducer on the muscle acquiring your scans – absolutely no pressure!
✓ Operator training is required before starting the acquisition of data – expertise is needed	
✓ Calculate your ICC, Cv, and minimal detectable change on repeated measures along with data collection – repeatability is key!	• Try to avoid a single scan site, small field of view, and trigonometric extrapolations for muscles with longer fascicle lenght – what you don't see may not be what you get
✓ Aling the transducer with muscle fascicles plane – know what you see	• Refrain from implementing dynamic ultrasound scans i ftime and equipment are limited – keep it short and simple
✓ Choose your transducer wisely: shape, field of view and temporal resolution – know what you need	• Do not misuse your panoramic ultrasound: keep full muscle reconstructions to a minimum to avoid out-of-plane errors, instead choose tailored regions of interest to follow few entire fascicles in the right plane – EFOV is not the solution to everything
✓ Use panoramic ultrasound for muscle with longer fascicles – larger field of view, different picture	

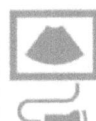

FIGURE 2.9   Practical recommendations for the implementation of ultrasound-based imaging in the elite sports context (adapted from Sarto et al. [71]).

explain that shorter fibers exhibit a lower maximum shortening speed, which may affect the contraction at the entire muscle level [64]. In contrast, the maximum force produced by muscles is proportional to the number of parallel sarcomeres, and therefore, proportional to their penetration angle (the angle between the longitudinal axis of the entire muscle and its fibers).

2.1.16   Muscle dimensions

The advantage of using muscle volume (MV) is that it can explain regional differences in muscle size, which is particularly important for detecting changes in muscle mass caused by resistance training [66]. Assessment of muscle size may play a key role in sports performance. Indeed, CSA is closely related to the joint torque production and isokinetic muscle strength of different muscle groups in football players [67].

2.1.17   Muscle quality

In addition to measurement muscle morphology, quantitative musculus ultrasound can even be wont to estimate muscle mass (based on tissue composition). Echo strength (or "echogenicity") could be a metric of the reflectivity of sound waves mirrored by tissue. Echogenicity is an indicator of muscle composition and muscle mass [68]. Connective tissue and fat are additionally reflective than muscle tissue and thus are visible as light-weight gray within the image. Low-echo intensity values are thought to be associated with higher muscle mass. In distinction, high-echo intensity values are thought to be associated with muscle degeneration [69]. Facts have established that ultrasound could be a reliable tool for evaluating the muscle mass of young athletes [70].

2.1.18 Tendon dimensions

Tendon size is usually expressed by tendon thickness and ACSA. The size of the tendon is related to the stress distribution in the tendon itself. Therefore, a larger tendon ACSA can distribute the stress in a larger area, which in turn enables greater force to be transmitted through the tissue [71].

2.1.19 Tendon mechanical properties

The combination of ancient B-type US and isometric force measuring will live sinew deformation (elongation) and therefore the force generated throughout isometric contraction. In addition to sinew stiffness (or "elasticity"), alternative sinew mechanical properties like strain, stress, Young's modulus, and physical phenomenon may be obtained [72].

2.1.20 Muscle and tendon stiffness measured with elastography (SWE)

The recent introduction of SWE US for evaluating the mechanical properties of muscle-associated tendons permits for an alternate quantitative assessment of stiffness within the style of an elastogram [73]. In short, the fundamental principle of SWE is to come up with a displacement of acoustic radiation force pulses within the underlying tissue, which results in the propagation of transient shear waves. The obtained instant shear wave speed (that is, the speed at which the wave returns to the transducer) is directly associated with the elastic properties of the tissue (that is, the shear modulus) and might be mapped to associate elastic map, which might be or superimposed on the B-mode US scan; similar to several yank technologies, SWE could be a technique that depends on operators. However, once utilized by skilled operators, it is a reliable tool for evaluating the mechanical properties of various muscles throughout static and passive stretching [74]. Similarly, smart responsibleness was found once evaluating connective tissue characteristics.

References

1. Place N, Millet GY. Quantification of neuromuscular fatigue: What do we do wrong and why? *Sport Med* [Internet]. 2020;50(3):439–447. Available from: https://doi.org/10.1007/s40279-019-01203-9
2. Gibson H, Edwards RHT. Muscular exercise and fatigue. *Sport Med An Int J Appl Med Sci Sport Exerc.* 1985;2(2):120–132.
3. López-Valenciano A, Ruiz-Pérez I, Garcia-Gómez A, Vera-Garcia FJ, De Ste Croix M, Myer GD, et al. Epidemiology of injuries in professional football: A systematic review and meta-analysis. *Br J Sports Med.* 2020;54(12):711–718.
4. Ekstrand J, Waldén M, Hägglund M. Hamstring injuries have increased by 4% annually in men's professional football, since 2001: A 13-year longitudinal analysis of the UEFA Elite Club injury study. *Br J Sports Med.* 2016;50(12):731–737.

5. Small K, McNaughton LR, Greig M, Lohkamp M, Lovell R. Soccer fatigue, sprinting and hamstring injury risk. *Int J Sports Med.* 2009;30(8):573–578.
6. Mendiguchia J, Garrubes MA, Cronin JB, Bret C, de los Arcos A, Malliarpoulos N, Maffulli N, Idoate F. Nonuniform changes in MRI measurements of the thigh muscles after two hamstring strengthening exercises. *J Strength Cond Res.* 2013;27(3):574–581.
7. Brownstein CG, Dent JP, Parker P, Hicks KM, Howatson G, Goodall S, Thomas K. Etiology and recovery of neuromuscular fatigue following competitive soccer match-play. *Front Physiol.* 2017 Oct 275;8:831.
8. Šimunič B. *Model of longitudinal contractions and transverse deformations in skeletal muscles.* Ljubljana:.University of Ljubljana; 2003.
9. Dahmane R, Djordjevič S, Šimunič B, Valenčič V. Spatial fiber type distribution in normal human muscle: Histochemical and tensiomyographical evaluation. *J Biomech.* 2005;38(12):2451–2459.
10. Rodriguez-Matoso D, Rodríguez-Ruiz D, Sarmiento S, Vaamonde D, Da Silva-Grigoletto ME. Reproducibility of muscle response measurements using tensiomyography in a range of positions. *Rev Andaluza Med del Deport.* 2010;3(3):81–86.
11. Lohr C, Schmid T, Medina Porqueres I, Braumann KM, Reer R, Porthun J. Diagnostic accuracy, validity, and reliability of tensiomyography to assess muscle function and exercise-induced fatigue in healthy participants. *A Systematic Review with Meta-Analysis. J Electromyogr Kinesiol.* 2019;47:65–87.
12. Knaflitz M, Merletti R, De Luca CJ. Inference of motor unit recruitment order in voluntary and electrically elicited contractions. *J Appl Physiol.* 1990;68:1657–1667.
13. Nédélec M, Mccaliy A, Carling C, Legally F, Berthoin S, Nedelec M, et al. Recovery in soccer (Part I) post-match fatigue and time course of recovery. *Sport Med.* 2012 Dec;42(12):997–1015.
14. Sánchez-Sánchez J, Bishop D, García-Unanue J, Ubago-Guisado E, Hernando E, López-Fernández J, et al. Effect of a repeated sprint ability test on the muscle contractile properties in elite futsal players. *Sci Rep.* 2018;8(1):1–8.
15. Muñoz-López A, De Hoyo M, Nuñez FJ, Sañudo B. Using tensiomyography to assess changes in knee muscle contraction properties after concentric and eccentric fatiguing muscle actions. *J Strength Cond Res.* 2020 Mar;Epub ahead(February);4(1):37–41.
16. López-Fernández J, García-Unanue J, Sánchez-Sánchez J, León M, Hernando E, Gallardo L. Neuromuscular responses and physiological patterns during a soccer simulation protocol. Artificial turf versus natural grass. *J Sports Med Phys Fitness* [Internet]. 2018;58(11):1602–1610. Available from: https://www.minervamedica.it/index2.php?show=R40Y2018N11A1602
17. Raeder C, Wiewelhove T, De Paula Simola RÁ, Kellmann M, Meyer T, Pfeiffer M, et al. Assessment of fatigue and recovery in male and female athletes following days of intensified strength training. *J Strength Cond Res* [Internet]. 2016 Dec [cited 2019 May 7];30(12):3412–3427. Available from: https://www.ncbi.nlm.nih.gov/pubmed/27093538
18. Rey E, Lago-Penas C, Lago-Ballesteros J, Casáis L. The effect of recovery strategies on contractile properties using tensiomyography and perceived muscle soreness in professional soccer players. *J Strength Cond Res.* 2012;26(11):3081–3088.
19. García-García O, Serrano-Gómez V, Hernández-Mendo A, Morales-Sánchez V. Baseline mechanical and neuromuscular profile of knee extensor and flexor muscles in professional soccer players at the start of the pre-season. *J Hum Kinet.* 2017;58(1):23–34.
20. Loturco I, Kobal R, Kitamura K, Fernandes V, Moura N, Siqueira F, et al. Predictive factors of elite sprint performance: Influences of muscle mechanical properties and functional parameters. *J Strength Cond Res.* 2019;33(4):974–986.

21. García-García O, Serrano-Gómez V, Hernández-Mendo A, Tapia-Flores A. Assessment of the in-season changes in mechanical and neuromuscular characteristics in professional soccer players. *J Sports Med Phys Fitness*. 2016;56(6):714–723.

22. Dias PS, Fort JS, Marinho DA, Santos A, Marques MC. Tensiomyography in physical rehabilitation of high level athletes. *Open Sports Sci J*. 2010;3(1):47–48.

23. Alvarez-Diaz P, Alentorn-Geli E, Ramon S, Marin M, Steinbacher G, Rius M, et al. Effects of anterior cruciate ligament reconstruction on neuromuscular tensiomyographic characteristics of the lower extremity in competitive male soccer players. *Knee Surgery, Sport Traumatol Arthrosc*. 2015;23(11):3407–3413.

24. López-Fernández J, García-Unanue J, Sánchez-Sánchez J, Colino E, Hernando E, Gallardo L. Bilateral asymmetries assessment in elite and sub-elite male futsal players. *Int J Environ Res Public Health*. 2020;17(9):3169.

25. Katch FI, McArdle WD, Pechar GS, Perrine JJ. Measuring leg force-output capacity with an isokinetic dynamometer-bicycle ergometer. *Res Q Am Alliance Heal Phys Educ Recreat*. 1974;45(1):86–91.

26. Gleeson NP, Mercer TH. The utility of isokinetic dynamometry in the assessment of human muscle function. *Sport Med*. 1996;21(1):18–34.

27. Paul DJ, Nassis GP. Testing strength and power in soccer players: The application of conventional and traditional methods of assessment. *J Strength Cond Res*. 2015;29(6):1748–1758.

28. Tatlıcıoğlu E, Atalağ O, Kırmızıgil B, Kurt C, Acar MF. Side-to-side asymmetry in lower limb strength and hamstring-quadriceps strength ratio among collegiate american football players. *J Phys Ther Sci*. 2019;31(11):884–888.

29. Correia P, Santos P, Mil-Homens P, Gomes M, Dias A, Valamatos MJ. Rapid hamstrings to quadriceps ratio at long muscle lengths in professional football players with previous hamstring strain injury. *Eur J Sport Sci* [Internet]. 2020;20(10):1405–1413. Available from: https://doi.org/10.1080/17461391.2020.1714741

30. Delextrat A, Gregory J, Cohen D. The use of the functional H:Q ratio to assess fatigue in soccer. *Int J Sports Med* [Internet]. 2010 Mar;31(3):192–197. Available from: https://www.ncbi.nlm.nih.gov/pubmed/20157872

31. Sole G, Hamrén J, Milosavljevic S, Nicholson H, Sullivan SJ. Test-retest reliability of isokinetic knee extension and flexion. *Arch Phys Med Rehabil*. 2007;88(5):626–631.

32. Pincivero DM, Lephart SM, Karunakara RA. Reliability and precision of isokinetic strength and muscular endurance for the quadriceps and hamstrings. *Int J Sports Med*. 1997;18(2):113–117.

33. Brown LE, Whitehurst M, Gilbert R, Buchalter DN. The effect of velocity and gender on load range during knee extension and flexion exercise on an isokinetic device. *J Orthop Sports Phys Ther*. 1995;21(2):107–112.

34. Bisciotti GN, Volpi P, Alberti G, Aprato A, Artina M, Auci A, et al. Italian consensus statement (2020) on return to play after lower limb muscle injury in football (soccer). *BMJ Open Sport Exerc Med*. 2019;5(1):e000505.

35. Saenz A, Avellanet M, Hijos E, Chaler J, Garreta R, Pujol E, et al. Knee isokinetic test-retest: A multicentre knee isokinetic test-retest study of a fatigue protocol. *Eur J Phys Rehabil Med*. 2010;46(1):81–88.

36. Bosquet L, Gouadec K, Berryman N, Duclos C, Gremeaux V, Croisier JL. Physiological interpretation of the slope during an isokinetic fatigue test. *Int J Sports Med*. 2015;36(8):680–683.

37. Scoz RD, Alves BMO, Burigo RL, Vieira ER, Ferreira LMA, Da Silva RA, et al. Strength development according with age and position: A 10-year study of 570 soccer players. *BMJ Open Sport Exerc Med*. 2021;7(1):e000927.

38. van Dyk N, Witvrouw E, Bahr R. Interseason variability in isokinetic strength and poor correlation with nordic hamstring eccentric strength in football players. *Scand J Med Sci Sport*. 2018;28(8):1878–1887.

39. Muñoz-López A, Naranjo-Orellana J. Individual versus team heart rate variability responsiveness analyses in a national soccer team during training camps. *Sci Rep* [Internet]. 2020;10(1):1–10. Available from: https://doi.org/10.1038/s41598-020-68698-5

40. Van Dyk N, Wangensteen A, Vermeulen R, Whiteley ROD, Bahr R, Tol JL, et al. Similar isokinetic strength preinjury and at return to sport after hamstring injury. *Med Sci Sports Exerc*. 2019;51(6):1091–1098.

41. De Luca CJ. The use of surface electromyography in biomechanics. *J Appl Biomech*. 1997;13(2):135–163.

42. Roberto Merletti PJP. *Electromyography: physiology, engineering and noninvasive applications*. Hoboken, NJ: IEEE Press; 2004. 520 p.

43. Garcia MA, Cavalcanti TMMV. Medicina del deporte. *Rev Andaluza Med del Deport*. 2010;43(2S):17–28.

44. Hug F, Hodges PW, Tucker K. Muscle force cannot be directly inferred from muscle activation: Illustrated by the proposed imbalance of force between the vastus medialis and vastus lateralis in people with patellofemoral pain. *J Orthop Sports Phys Ther*. 2015;45(5):360–365.

45. Christie A, Kamen G, Greig Inglis J, Gabriel DA. Relationships between surface EMG variables and motor unit firing rates. *Eur J Appl Physiol*. 2009;107(2):177–185.

46. Roeleveld K, Stegeman DF, Falck B, Stålberg EV. Motor unit size estimation: Confrontation of surface EMG with macro EMG. *Electroencephalogr Clin Neurophysiol - Electromyogr Mot Control*. 1997;105(3):181–188.

47. Hermens HJ, Freriks B, Disselhorst-Klug C, Rau G. Development of recommendations for SEMG sensors and sensor placement procedures. *J Electromyogr Kinesiol*. 2000 Oct;10(5):361–374.

48. Hegyi A, Csala D, Péter A, Finni T, Cronin NJ. High-density electromyography activity in various hamstring exercises. *Scand J Med Sci Sport*. 2019;29(1):34–43.

49. Filter A, Olivares-Jabalera J, Santalla A, Morente-Sánchez J, Robles-Rodríguez J, Requena B, et al. Curve sprinting in soccer: Kinematic and neuromuscular analysis. *Int J Sports Med*. 2020;41(11):744–750.

50. Rampinini E, Bosio A, Ferraresi I, Petruolo A, Morelli A, Sassi A. Match-related fatigue in soccer players. *Med Sci Sports Exerc*. 2011 Nov;43(11):2161–2170.

51. Marshall PWM, Lovell R, Jeppesen GK, Andersen K, Siegler JC. Hamstring muscle fatigue and central motor output during a simulated soccer match. *PLoS One*. 2014;9(7):1–11.

52. Bengtsson H, Ekstrand J, Waldén M, Hägglund M. Muscle injury rate in professional football is higher in matches played within 5 days since the previous match: A 14-year prospective study with more than 130 000 match observations. *Br J Sports Med*. 2018;52(17):1116–1122.

53. Bergmann J, Kramer A, Gruber M. Repetitive Hops Induce Postactivation Potentiation in Triceps Surae as well as an Increase in the Jump Height of Subsequent Maximal Drop Jumps. *PLoS One*. 2013;8(10):1–10.

54. Scurr JC, Abbott V, Ball N. Quadriceps EMG muscle activation during accurate soccer instep kicking. *J Sports Sci*. 2011;29(3):247–251.

55. Serner A, Jakobsen MD, Andersen LL, Hölmich P, Sundstrup E, Thorborg K. EMG evaluation of hip adduction exercises for soccer players: Implications for exercise selection in prevention and treatment of groin injuries. *Br J Sports Med*. 2014;48(14):1108–1114.

56. Watanabe K, Nunome H, Inoue K, Iga T, Akima H. Electromyographic analysis of hip adductor muscles in soccer instep and side-foot kicking. *Sport Biomech* [Internet]. 2020;19(3):295–306. Available from: https://doi.org/10.1080/14763141.2018.1499800

57. Sole G, Milosavljevic S, Nicholson H, Sullivan SJ. Selective strength loss and decreased muscle activity in hamstring injury. *J Orthop Sports Phys Ther*. 2011;41(5):354–363.

58. Lovell R, Knox M, Weston M, Siegler JC, Brennan S, Marshall PWM. Hamstring injury prevention in soccer: Before or after training? *Scand J Med Sci Sport*. 2018;28(2):658–666.

59. Emami M, Arab AM, Ghamkhar L. The activity pattern of the lumbo-pelvic muscles during prone hip extension in athletes with and without hamstring strain injury. *Int J Sports Phys Ther*. 2014 May;9(3):312–319.

60. Pietraszewski P, Gołaś A, Matusiński A, Mrzygłód S, Mostowik A, Maszczyk A. Section III-sports training muscle activity asymmetry of the lower limbs during sprinting in elite soccer players. *J Hum Kinet* [Internet]. 2020 [cited 2021 Apr 30];75(2020):239–245. Available from: https://www.johk.pl

61. Zebis MK, Skotte J, Andersen CH, Mortensen P, Petersen HH, Viskær TC, et al. Kettlebell swing targets semitendinosus and supine leg curl targets biceps femoris: An EMG study with rehabilitation implications. *Br J Sports Med*. 2013;47(18):1192–118.

62. David AO, Morgan DW, Timmins RG, Dear NM, Shield AJ. Rate of torque and EMG development during anticipated eccentric contraction is lower in previously strained hamstrings. *Am J Sports Med*. 2012;41:116–125.

63. Timmins RG, Shield AJ, Williams MD, Lorenzen C, Opar DA. Biceps femoris long head architecture: A reliability and retrospective injury study. *Med Sci Sports Exerc*. 2015;47(5):905–913.

64. Narici M, Franchi M, Maganaris C. Muscle structural assembly and functional consequences. *J Exp Biol*. 219(2), 276–284.

65. Bourne MN, Williams MD, Opar DA, Al Najjar A, Kerr GK, Shield AJ. Impact of exercise selection on hamstring muscle activation. *Br J Sports Med*. 2017;51(13): 1021–1028. doi:10.1136/bjsports-2015-095739.

66. Franchi MV, Longo S, Mallinson J, Quinlan JI, Taylor T, Greenhaff PL, et al. Muscle thickness correlates to muscle cross-sectional area in the assessment of strength training-induced hypertrophy. *Scand J Med Sci Sport*. 2018;28(3):846–853.

67. Masuda K, Kikuhara N, Takahashi H, Yamanaka K. The relationship between muscle cross-sectional area and strength in various isokinetic movements among soccer players. *J Sports Sci*. 2003;21(10):851–858.

68. Stock MS, Thompson BJ. Echo intensity as an indicator of skeletal muscle quality: applications, methodology, and future directions. *Eur J Appl Physiol* [Internet]. 2021;121(2):369–380. Available from: https://doi.org/10.1007/s00421-020-04556-6

69. Matt SS, Thompson BJ. Echo intensity as an indicator of skeletal muscle quality: applications, methodology, and future directions. *Eur J Appl Physiol*. 2020;121(2): 369–380.

70. Mangine GT, Fukuda DH, LaMonica MB, Gonzalez AM, Wells AJ, Townsend JR, et al. Influence of gender and muscle architecture asymmetry on jump and sprint performance. *J Sport Sci Med*. 2014;13(4):904–911.

71. Sarto F, Spörri J, Fitze DP, Quinlan JI, Narici MV., Franchi MV. Implementing ultrasound imaging for the assessment of muscle and tendon properties in elite sports: Practical aspects, methodological considerations and future directions. *Sports Med*. 2021;51: 1151–1170.

72. Seynnes OR, Bojsen-Møller J, Albracht K, Arndt A, Cronin NJ, Finni T, et al. Ultrasound-based testing of tendon mechanical properties: a critical evaluation. *J Appl Physiol* [Internet]. 2015 Jan 15 [cited 2021 May 3];118(2):133–141. Available from: https://www.physiology.org/doi/10.1152/japplphysiol.00849.2014

73. E Lima KMM, Costa Júnior JFS, Pereira WCdeA, De Oliveira LF. Assessment of the mechanical properties of the muscle-tendon unit by supersonic shear wave imaging elastography: A review. *Ultrasonography [Internet]*. 2018 [cited 2021 May 3]; 37:3–15. Available from: https://pubmed.ncbi.nlm.nih.gov/28607322/

74. Dubois G, Kheireddine W, Vergari C, Bonneau D, Thoreux P, Rouch P, et al. Reliable protocol for shear wave elastography of lower limb muscles at rest and dur-ing passive stretching. *Ultrasound Med Biol* [Internet]. 2015 [cited 2021 May 3];41(9):2284–2291. Available from: https://hal.archives-ouvertes.fr/hal-02494020

3

CARDIORESPIRATORY FITNESS TESTING

José Naranjo Orellana

3.1 Introduction

Football may be the most popular sport in the world, in which the performance depends on technical, physical, tactical, and physiological factors, among others [1].

There are a large number of publications and great reviews about physiology in football [2], from which we know, for example, that distances covered by top-level field players are 10–12 km, with midfield players running the longest distances [3, 4] and that the distance covered in the second half is reduced about 5–10% [4, 5].

Currently, we know much about the physiological demands of a highly competitive football match: number and frequency of high-intensity actions, of involvements with the ball or of passes [4, 6], as well as the differences in these demands in function of position in field [7, 8]. Although strength and power are equally as important as endurance in football, cardiovascular fitness is one of the most important aspects of physical fitness conditioning in football [2].

Because of the game duration, the effort made is mainly dependent of aerobic metabolism [2]. However, the reality of a match indicates that there exists an alternation of high-intensity actions with more leisurely actions that allow recovery from the effort made. Therefore, it would be very important to know how the oxygen uptake (VO_2) evolves throughout a competitive match.

In this sense, given that in an incremental effort there is a linear relationship between VO_2 and heart rate (HR), this relationship becomes an interesting tool since VO_2 values can be deduced from those of HR [1, 9]. For this reason, the equation governing this relationship is an information that should always be provided to technicians when stress tests are performed on football players in the laboratory.

In football, there is a growing tendency to carry out functional evaluations through field tests. Although it is true that these tests present ideal mechanical

DOI: 10.4324/9781032637006-3

conditions, that they are easier to perform, and that they are easier to fit into the training routine, it is also true that there are basic data on the players' capabilities that can only be accurately obtained in the laboratory. Therefore, the cardiopulmonary stress test should be part of the football players' evaluation routine and should provide information on those variables that cannot be accurately evaluated by field tests. We dedicate the following sections to these aspects.

3.2 Maximal oxygen uptake (VO_{2max}) and maximal aerobic speed

Cardiovascular fitness is one of the most important aspects of physical fitness conditioning in football [2]. In this context, well-developed aerobic fitness helps the football players to maintain repetitive high-intensity actions within a match, accelerate the recovery process, and maintain their physical condition at a good level until the end of the match. Aerobic fitness in football players is usually established by measuring VO_{2max} during a continuous graded exercise test using a treadmill in the laboratory.

Among the various reasons why it is necessary to perform laboratory stress tests on football players is the fact that aerobic endurance performance depends on VO_{2max}, ventilatory thresholds, and running economy [10] and these variables are most accurately assessed with laboratory protocols. The coefficient of variation of these tests does not exceed 3% [11].

VO_{2max} is the highest amount of oxygen that the body can utilize during exhaustive exercise while breathing air at sea level [12], and it is considered the gold standard of aerobic ability.

From the work of Shephard [13], the primary criterion for attainment of VO_{2max} is a plateau in VO_2 [13]. Several secondary criteria exist in the case of a plateau in VO_2 not being reached, which include a rise in the respiratory exchange ratio (RER) above 1.15, blood lactate concentration above 8 mmol l^{-1}, and increase in heart rate to age-predicted maximum [12].

It is true that these criteria have been questioned on occasions [11], beginning with the existence of the plateau itself or requiring that alternative criteria (RER, blood lactate, and maximal heart rate) be given simultaneously [14]. Among these alternative criteria, the most criticized is the application of HR to age-predicted maximum as an indicator of maximum effort [15]. However, their usefulness makes these criteria that are still used in daily practice to decide whether an incremental test has been maximum or not.

On the other hand, there are things that we have known for some years, like the players with high VO_{2max} levels also have high levels of muscle glycogen required to perform high-intensity actions throughout the game. Smaros [16] described that the players with the highest VO_{2max} were also those who developed a greater number of sprints and were the ones who were most often involved in decisive actions in the match. In addition, the better use of fat as an energy source at the same intensities makes these players able to "save" glycogen for decisive actions [17]. Therefore, it seems clear that the information on VO_{2max} is useful for technicians.

Regarding the VO_{2max} values that we can take as a reference in football, we know that these differ with the position on the field [18] and with the competitive level [19, 20]. However, according to a recent meta-analysis [21], the ranges found in the literature do not differ too much, reporting values from 59.2 to 63.2 ml/kg/min for elite male players and from 57.8 to 61.7 ml/kg/min for amateurs.

3.2.1 What about protocols?

There is considerable agreement regarding the ergometer, considering mostly the treadmill as the most suitable ergometer for evaluating football players, but the same is not the case with the protocols. We can find a great variety of different protocols in the literature, and this makes the reproducibility of the data and the possibilities of comparisons scarce. For example, there are works that use protocols with increments of 1.2 km/h every 2 minutes and a fixed slope of 3% [22]; others use ramps or short increments (1 km/h every minute) with a fixed slope of 1 % [23], and there are even works with steps of 3 min increasing 3 km/h and with variable slope [24].

Therefore, there are many protocols that vary not only in the stage duration and increment but also in the total test duration [25], and this seems to be a key point. In the 1970s, Froelicher et al. [26] and Pollock et al. [27] reported that the longer the protocol duration, the lower the VO_{2max}. Since then, most studies report that protocol durations around 10 min may support higher VO_{2max} values [28, 29, 25].

As a summary, and that is also our experience, there is currently considerable consensus in using protocols with increments of 1 km/h every minute or 0.5 km/h every 30 seconds, with a constant slope between 1 and 2% [23, 30].

Maximal aerobic speed (MAS) can be simply defined as the lowest running velocity at which maximal oxygen uptake occurs [31]. Research suggests that MAS can be used as an important tool for studying aerobic capacities in football.

In football, it is much more common to measure MAS through field tests than in the laboratory, even in professional players [32, 33]. However, the values provided in the different studies show very similar data, although there is a certain tendency to find higher values in field tests. It is logical that this is the case since in the laboratory the MAS is determined based on the recorded VO_2 data, while in the field, it is estimated from the maximum speed that the player can maintain in certain circumstances. Thus, in field tests, data are provided for professional players around 17.4 [33] and 17.7 [32] km/h, while in the few published studies with MAS values obtained in the laboratory, data are reported between 17.14 [30] and 17.4 km/h [34].

Concerning other categories, we know that MAS values are higher with age. In 2019, a work was published in which the MAS was measured in the different ranks of a professional football team, reporting values of 14.7 km/h in U-13 players, 14.9 km/h in U-14, 15.8 km/h in U-15, and 16.6 km/h for U-16 [35].

3.3 First and second ventilatory thresholds (VT1 and VT2)

The first ventilatory threshold (VT1) was described by Hollmann during the Third Pan American Congress of Sports Medicine held in Chicago in 1959 [36], although the concept was later consolidated and developed by Wasserman and McIlroy in 1964 [37]. The technique that we use today was definitively described by Reinhardt, Müller, and Schmülling in 1979 [38]. This technique is based on using the ventilatory equivalents of oxygen (VE/VO$_2$) and carbon dioxide (VE/VCO$_2$) to more reliably detect the changes that occur in ventilation when reaching the first and second thresholds. Thus, the first threshold (VT1) is manifested by the fact that VE/VO$_2$ (which decreases from the beginning of the test) reaches its minimum value and begins to increases. The second threshold (VT2) is defined by the moment in which the same occurs with VE/VCO$_2$, that is, it reaches its minimum value and begins to increase.

From these pioneering works, we know that the metabolic significance of the first ventilatory threshold lies precisely in the fact that it is the intensity of exercise from which glycolysis is activated (and therefore the accumulation of lactate in the blood begins) due to a decrease in the rate of fat oxidation.

In 1980, Skinner and MacLellan described a model to explain the transition from aerobic to anaerobic metabolism in incremental exercise [39]. This model consists of three phases and is based on the observed changes in the ventilatory response as a result of the predominance of different metabolic situations and taking into account that the ventilatory response precedes any chemical change in the composition of the blood.

In the first phase, while the load is of low intensity, large amounts of fatty acids are released into the circulation and diffuse into the muscle cell, becoming the main source of energy used during this phase. This high availability of fatty acids has a profound depressant effect on glycolysis [40], thus reducing the amount of lactic acid produced with respect to the resting state. In this phase, ventilation increases in proportion to the intensity of the exercise due to the action of the central nervous system from stimuli originating in the exercising and respiratory muscles.

In the second phase, there is a greater increase in ventilation due to the additional increase in CO$_2$ from the anaerobic phase of glycolysis, but the acidosis that occurs is fundamentally buffered by bicarbonate, keeping the partial pressure of CO$_2$ in arterial blood constant (PaCO$_2$). For this reason, this phase is known as the "Isocapnic Buffering phase."

In the third phase, lactic acid production increases a lot because the energy begins to be produced mainly without incorporating pyruvate into the mitochondria. In this way, the acid–base balance is broken and the pH of the blood tends to decrease. This metabolic acidosis cannot be compensated by bicarbonate and other chemical buffers, so the stimulation of the respiratory centers causes an increase in ventilation in order to evacuate CO_2 and thus try to keep the blood pH constant. This increase constitutes a true hyperventilation (with a marked decrease in $PaCO_2$) compensating for acidosis. For all these reasons, this phase is also known as the "Respiratory Compensation phase" or the "Hyperventilation phase." The moment of change between phase I and phase II and between phase II and phase III is called the first and second ventilatory thresholds (VT1 and VT2) respectively.

The determination of VT1 and VT2 requires the use of protocols in ramp or with very short steps in order to be able to detect accurately the changes of linearity of the ventilation. Currently, the determination of ventilatory thresholds is considered the best method to assess the aerobic endurance of an athlete.

The VT1 reflects the intensity of effort at which the athlete begins to use glycolysis due to the inhibition of fatty acid oxidation [40]. Therefore, in a sport whose base is fundamentally aerobic, a high VT1 position must be linked to performance since the higher the intensity at which glycolysis is activated, the greater the glycogen reserves. In fact, over the course of a season, changes in VT1 position well reflect the fitness of football players, even without changes in VO_{2max} or MAS [41].

In professional players, mean values of VT1 and VT2 have been reported at 64 and 79% of VO_{2max}, respectively [42]. The VT2, and particularly the speed achieved in the VT2, has been considered very important factors in football to program and control workloads [43]. VT2 speed values between 14 and 16 km/h have been described in professional players.

According to Broich et al. [44], conventional field-level tests yield insufficient information on underlying physiological and metabolic mechanisms of endurance performance capacity. Taking result of spiroergometric tests into account is critical for designing and evaluating player-specific training programs aimed at optimizing each player's performance.

3.4 Mechanical efficiency

A useful piece of information to extract from a cardiopulmonary stress test is mechanical efficiency, although it is rare to see its use in football. However, in our experience in evaluating elite football players, this variable has enormous application possibilities.

Mechanical efficiency indicates the proportion of metabolic energy that is transformed into mechanical work [45]. Its calculation is based on the relationship between mechanical work and energy cost, which in incremental protocols is expressed by the slope of the relationship between VO_2 and workload.

When competing at more or less constant speeds, the running economy concept is used. It is the ratio between work intensity and oxygen consumption (VO_2), and it is expressed as VO_2 at a standardized workload (liters of O_2 consumed per kilometer during running to a given speed). However, in football, the global concept of mechanical efficiency measured in an incremental test is more useful since it better represents the reality of a football match in which different speeds are

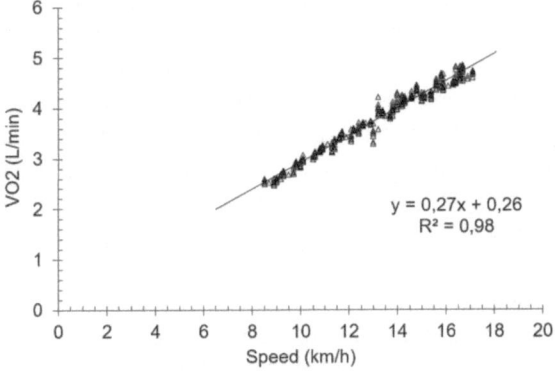

FIGURE 3.1   Mechanical efficiency of an elite soccer player in an incremental test. The slope of the line indicates that 0.27 L/min of O2 are consumed for every km/h that speed increases. By equating the units of time (in hours) and eliminating them, we obtain that the efficiency is 16.2 L (author's data).

continuously combined (Figure 3.1). In this sense, the units would also be liters of oxygen per kilometer, but in this case as an average of all speeds.

Improvements in running economy or mechanical efficiency elicited changes in aerobic performance without accompanying changes in VO_{2max} or lactate threshold, so it should be considered when implementing training regimes in football [46, 47]. On the other hand, the knowledge of the mechanical efficiency of the components of a team can provide information of great interest regarding the energy expenditure made in a match. In our experience, we observe mechanical efficiency values in football players that range between 10 and 18 L/km (unpublished data) according to the field position and time of the season. If we use the data of distances traveled in a match, we can easily estimate the total liters of oxygen that have been consumed and, through the thermal equivalent (4.8 kcal per liter of oxygen), the total energy expenditure in kcal.

3.5   Heart rate assessment. Relationship with VO_2

The determination of the HR during a cardiopulmonary stress test is of great interest for the football player's training since it can facilitate the determination of intensities, knowing, for example, at what HR the ventilatory thresholds are.

But perhaps, the most interesting information that HR can provide in an incremental test is its relationship with VO_2. Since the late 1980s, we have known that HR and VO_2 present a linear relationship that can be very useful for training [48–50].

Figure 3.2 shows the HR–VO_2 relationship obtained from an incremental test in a professional football player. Through the equation for this player ($y = 0.47 \times -32.41$), it will be possible to know the VO_2 that corresponds to the work done with

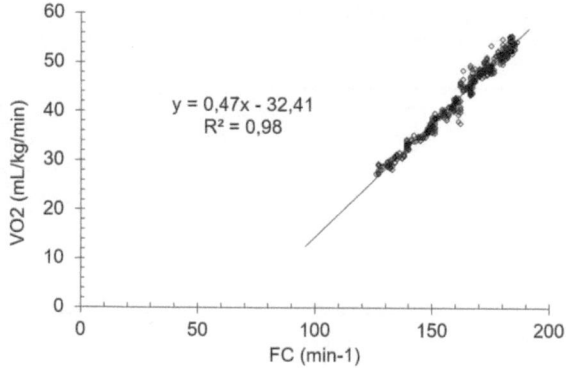

FIGURE 3.2 HR–VO$_2$ relationship of an elite soccer player in an incremental test (author's data).

any known HR. By also knowing the player's VO$_{2max}$, we can have fairly accurate information on the intensity of the work being done. For example, if this player's VO$_{2max}$ is 55 mL/kg/min, we know that when he works with a HR of 165 min^{-1}, he has a VO$_2$ of 45.14 mL/kg/min, which means an intensity of 82%.

On the contrary, if we want a group of players to carry out work with a certain intensity, from the equation of each one, we can determine which HR each of them should work at to satisfy that intensity.

3.6 Practical applications. Usefulness for training

The appropriate protocols to perform an effort test to a football player will be incremental in ramp or steps of 1 minute, starting at 7–8 km/h with increments of 1 km/h every minute, until exhaustion.

At least the following measurements will be extracted from the test and provided to the technicians:

- VO$_{2max}$ and MAS as measures of maximum aerobic power.
- VT1 (HR, speed, and %VO$_{2max}$) as a measure of the utilization of fatty acids and the ability to save muscle glycogen.
- VT2 (HR, speed, and %VO$_{2max}$) as a measure of aerobic endurance.
- Mechanical efficiency of the player. This measurement will allow us to know how efficient the aerobic metabolism is and make predictions regarding energy expenditure.
- VO$_2$–HR equation, to be able to safely establish work intensities.

For the evaluation of the test, the position in field will be taken into account as well as the physical performance expected of the player. As a general rule, the following references will be used:

TABLE 3.1 Results of a stress test performed on a treadmill by a professional football player

	VT1	VT2	MAX
Speed (km/h)	12	17	19
FC (min-1)	157	181	192
VO$_2$ (mL/kg/min)	36.8	49.5	60.4
%VO$_{2max}$	61%	82%	

Mechanical efficiency: 12.8 L/km
Relationship between VO$_2$ (y) and HR (x):
Y = 0.56 × −51.87

- VO$_{2max}$ greater than 57 mL/kg/min
- MAS higher than 17 km/h
- VT1 above 60% of VO$_{2max}$
- VT2 above 75% of VO$_{2max}$ and with a speed greater than 14 km/h
- Mechanical efficiency between 10 and 18 L/km, although it is desirable that the value be as low as possible, which indicates greater efficiency.

Table 3.1 shows an example with the main data of a stress test performed on a 26-year-old professional footballer on a treadmill, with a ramp protocol starting at 7 km/h and with increments of 1 km/h every minute.

The maximum aerobic power of this player is very good, with an MAS of 19 km/h and a VO$_{2max}$ of 60.4 mL/kg/min. The VT1 is in an acceptable position (61% of the VO$_{2max}$), which indicates a good utilization of fatty acids at speeds below 12 km/h. VT2 is at 82% of VO$_{2max}$, indicating very good aerobic endurance (confirmed by a speed of 17 km/h at this threshold). Its mechanical efficiency is quite good, being in the lower zone of the range observed in football players. Finally, the equation relating VO$_2$ and HR will allow us to make accurate estimates of the work intensity based on HR measurements.

References

1. Bangsbo J. The physiology of football: with special reference to intense intermittent exercise. *Acta Physiol Scand. 1994*; 15 Suppl. 619:1–156
2. Stølen T, Chamari K, Castagna C, Wisløff U. Physiology of Football. an Update. *Sports Med.* 2005; 35(6):501–536
3. Ekblom B. Applied physiology of football. *Sports Med.* 1986; 3(1):50–60
4. Mohr M, Krustrup P, Bangsbo J. Match performance of high-standard football players with special reference to development of fatigue. *J Sports Sci. 2003* July; 21(7):519–528
5. Bangsbo J, Nørregaard L, Thorsøe F. Activity profile of competition football. *Can J Sports Sci.* 1991 June; 16(2):110–116
6. Withers RT, Maricic Z, Wasilewski S, et al. Match analysis of Australian professional football players. *J Hum Mov Stud.* 1982; 8:159–176
7. Reilly T, Thomas V. A motion analysis of work-rate in different positional roles in professional football match-play. *J Hum Mov Stud.* 1976; 2:87–97

8. Mayhew SR, Wenger HA. Time motion analysis of professional football. *J Hum Mov Stud.* 1985; 11:49–52

9. Hoff J, Wisløff U, Engen LC, et al. Football specific aerobic endurance training. *Br J Sports Med.* 2002 June; 36(3):218–221

10. Pate RR, Kriska A. Physiological basis of the sex difference in cardiorespiratory endurance. *Sports Med.* 1984; 1:87–98

11. Howley ET, Bassett DR, Jr, Welch HG. Criteria for maximal oxygen uptake: review and commentary. *Med Sci Sports Exerc.* 1995; 27:1292–1301

12. Astrand PO, Rodahl K. *Textbook of work physiology: physiological bases of exercise.* New York: McGraw Hill; 1986

13. Shephard RJ. Tests of maximum oxygen intake a critical review. *Sports Med.* 1984; 1(2):99–124

14. Midgley AW, McNaughton LR, Polman R, Marchant D. Criteria for determination of maximal oxygen uptake: a brief critique and recommendations for future research. *Sports Med.* 2007; 37(12):1019–1028

15. Svensson M, Drust B. Testing football players. *J Sports Sci.* 2004; 23:601–618

16. Smaros G. Energy usage during a football match. In: Vecchiet L, editor. *Proceedings of the 1st international congress on sports medicine applied to football.* Rome: D. Guanello; 1980. pp. 795–801

17. Reilly T, Thomas V. A motion analysis of work-rate in different positional roles in professional football match-play. *J Hum Mov Stud.* 1976; 2:87–89

18. Da Silva CD, Bloomfield J, Bouzas Marins JC. A review of stature, body mass and maximal oxygen uptake profiles of U-17, U-20 and first division players in Brazilian football. *J Sport Sci Med.* 2008; 7:309–319

19. Arnason A, Sigurdsson SB, Gudmundsson A, Holme I, Engebretsen L, Bahr R.Physical fitness, injuries, and team performance in football. *Med Sci Sports Exerc.* 2004; 36: 278–285

20. Slimani M, Nikolaidis PT. Anthropometric and physiological characteristics of male football players according to their competitive level, playing position and age group: a systematic review. *J Sports Med Phys Fitness.* 2019 Jan; 59(1):141–163

21. Slimani M, Znazen H, Miarka B, Bragazzi NL. Maximum oxygen uptake of male football players according to their competitive level, playing position and age group: implication from a network meta-analysis. *J Hum Kinet.* 2019; 66:233–245

22. Santos-Silva PR, Fonseca AJ, Weigand de Castro A, D'Andréa Greve JM, Hernandez AJ. Reproducibility of maximum aerobic power (VO_{2max}) among football players using a modified heck protocol. *Clinics* (Sao Paulo). 2007 Aug; 62(4):391–396

23. Alvero Cruz JR, Ronconi M, Garcia Romero J, Naranjo Orellana J. Effects of detraining on breathing pattern and ventilatory efficiency in young football players. *Int J Sports Med Phys Fitness.* 2019; 59(1):71–75

24. Metaxas TI, Koutlianos NA, Kouidi EJ, Deligiannis AP. Comparative study of field and laboratory tests for the evaluation of aerobic capacity in football players. *J Strength Condition Res.* 2005; 19(1):79–84

25. Yoon B-K, Kravitz L, Robergs R. VO_{2max}, protocol duration and the VO_2 Plateau. *Med Sci Sports Exerc.* 2007; 39(7):1186–1192

26. Froelicher V, Brammell H, Davis G, Noguera I, Stewart A, Lancaster MC. A comparison of three maximal treadmill exercise protocols. *J Appl Physiol.* 1974; 36:720–725

27. Pollock ML, RL. Bohannon RL, KH. Cooper KH, Ayres JJ, Ward A, White SR, Linnerud AC. A comparative analysis of four protocols for maximal treadmill stress testing. *Am Heart J.* 1976; 92:39–46

28. Buchfuhrer MJ, Hansen JE, Robinson TE, Sue DY, Wasserman K, Whipp BJ. Optimizing the exercise protocol for cardiopulmonary assessment. *J Appl Physiol.* 1983; 55:1558–1564
29. Astorino TA, Rietschel JC, Tam PA, Taylor K, Johnson SM, Freedman TP, Sakarya CE. Reinvestigation of optimal duration of VO_{2max} testing. *JEPonline.* 2004; 7(6):1–8
30. Clemente FM, Clark C, Castillo D, Sarmento H, Nikolaidis PT, Rosemann T, Knechtle B. Variations of training load, monotony, and strain and dose-response relationships with maximal aerobic speed, maximal oxygen uptake, and isokinetic strength in professional football players. *PLoS ONE.* 2019; 14(12):e0225522
31. Billat LV, Koralsztein JP. Significance of the velocity at VO_{2max} and time to exhaustion at this velocity. *Sport Med.* 1996; 22(2):90–108
32. Rago V, Brito J, Figueiredo P, Krustrup P, Rebelo A. Application of individualized speed zones to quantify external training load. *J Hum Kinet.* 2020; 72:279–289
33. Requena B, García I, Suárez-Arrones L, Sáez de Villarreal E, Naranjo Orellana J, Santalla A. Off-season effects on functional performance, body composition, and blood parameters in top-level professional football players. *J Strength Cond Res.* 2017; 31(4):939–946
34. Labsy Z, Collomp K, Frey A, De Ceaurriz J. Assessment of maximal aerobic velocity in football players by means of an adapted Probst field test. *J Sports Med Phys Fitness.* 2004; 44(4):375–382
35. Rowan A, Atkins S, Comfort P. A comparison of maximal aerobic speed and maximal sprint speed in elite youth football players. *Professional Strength & Conditioning.* 2019; 53:24–29
36. Hollmann W. 42 years ago-development of the concepts of ventilatory and lactate threshold. *Sports Med.* 2001; 31:315–320
37. Wasserman K, McIlroy MB. Detecting the threshold of anaerobic metabolism in cardiac patients during exercise. *Am J Cardiol.* 1964; 14:844–852
38. Reinhardt U, Müller PH, Schmülling RM. Determination of anaerobic threshold by the ventilation equivalent in normal individuals. *Respiration.* 1979; 38:36–42
39. Skinner JS, Mclellan TH. The transition from aerobic to anaerobic metabolism. *Research Quarterly for Exercise and Sport.* 1980; 51(1):234–248
40. Newsholme E. The regulation of intracelular and extracelular fuel supply during sustained exercise. *Ann NY Acad Sci.* 1977; 301:81–91
41. Edwards AM, Clark N, Macfadyen AM. Lactate and ventilatory thresholds reflect the training status of professional football players where maximum aerobic power is unchanged. *J Sports Sci Med.* 2003; 2:23–29
42. Algrøy EA, Hetlelid KJ, Seiler S, Pedersen JIS. Quantifying training intensity distribution in a group of Norwegian professional football players. *Int J Sports Physiol Perform.* 2011; 6(1):70–81
43. Abt G, Lovell R. The use of individualized speed and intensity thresholds for determining the distance run at high-intensity in professional football. *J Sports Sci.* 2009; 27(9):893–898
44. Broich H, Sperlich B, Buitrago S, Mathes S, Mester J. Performance assessment in elite football players: field level test versus spiroergometry. *J Hum Sport Exerc.* 2012; 7(1):287–295
45. Ito A, Komi PV, Sjödin B, Bosco C, Karlsson J. Mechanical efficiency of positive work in running at different speeds. *Med Sci Sports Exerc.* 1983; 15(4):299–308
46. Helgerud J, Engen LC, Wisloff U, Hoff J. Aerobic endurance training improves football performance. *Med Sci Sports Exerc.* 2001; 33:1925–1931

47. Hoff J. Training and testing physical capacities for elite football players. *J Sports Sci.* 2005; 23(6):573–582
48. Meijer GA, Westerterp KR, Koper H, Hoor FT. Assessment of energy expenditure by recording heart rate and body acceleration. *Med Sci Sports Exerc.* 1989; 21:343–347
49. Schulz S, Westerterp KR, Brück K. Comparison of energy expenditure by the doubly labeled technique with energy intake, heart rate, and activity recording in man. *Am J Clin Nutr.* 1989; 49:1146–1154
50. Bernard T, Gavarry O, Bermon S, Giacomoni M, Marconnet P, Falgairette G. Relationships between oxygen consumption and heart rate in transitory and steady states of exercise and during recovery: influence of type of exercise. *Eur J Appl Physiol.* 1997; 75:170–176

4

ASSESSMENT OF RANGE OF MOTION IN FOOTBALL PLAYERS

Sergio Hernández-Sánchez, José Luis Hernández-Davó and Víctor Moreno-Pérez

4.1 Relationships between flexibility and injury

The complex and multifactorial nature of sport injuries is widely accepted. Within this multifactorial nature, flexibility is usually evaluated with the aim to determine injury risk in soccer players [1–4]. Despite some controversial results [5, 6], lower flexibility values have been linked to increased injury incidence [2, 7–9]. In support of the usefulness of flexibility assessment as an injury monitoring tool, Ayala et al. [10] showed that hip flexion ROM was consistently included in the preventive model that better predicts hamstring muscle injury. A limited capacity to store and release the high energy required during high-intensity actions has been proposed as a mechanism predisposing to hamstring injury in soccer players with reduced ROM [9].

Although hamstring strains have received the greatest attention, groin injuries, including adductor muscles strains, have also been investigated. Similarly, to hamstring flexibility, the relationships between a decreased hip ROM with an increased injury risk in soccer players are somehow controversial. However, compared to healthy individuals, soccer players are characterized by lower values of hip abduction ROM [11]. Further, some prospective studies have reported decreased hip abduction ROM as a risk factor for sustaining adductor strains [12]. Although speculative, muscular tightness, vascular deprivation, and concomitant groin factors (e.g., tendon pathologies) have been proposed as underpinning mechanisms leading to adductor strains in soccer players with a reduced hip ROM [3, 12].

Other specific deficits in flexibility have been proposed as risk factors in soccer players. Witvrouw et al. [9] reported that a decreased quadriceps flexibility at preseason was related to the incidence of quadriceps strains during the season. In addition, in the last few years, several studies have suggested a reduced ankle

DOI: 10.4324/9781032637006-4

dorsiflexion ROM as a risk factor not only for ankle sprains and Achilles' tendinopathy but also for hamstring strains [13–15].

4.1.1 Ankle dorsiflexion range of motion and lower limb injuries

Ankle joint mobility is essential for gait biomechanics as well as to perform common movement actions in soccer, such as sprinting and running that require 20–30° of ankle dorsiflexion [16].

After the thigh, the ankle is the most common injury location (19% and 7% of match injuries, respectively) in professional soccer players during competition, reaching an incidence of 39 injuries per 1000 hours of competition [17]. With sprain being the most frequent acute injury, other chronic conditions such as ankle osteoarthritis or Achilles tendinopathy have also a higher rate in soccer players than the general population [18]. All these injuries can potentially cause a limitation of ankle joint mobility as a sequelae.

Restricted ankle dorsiflexion, either constitutionally or secondary to an injury as pointed, has been associated with changes in the lower limb biomechanics that can negatively influence the player's physical performance [19] and increase the risk of injury [20]. In fact, some soccer-related injuries in the lower limb such as anterior cruciate ligament tears, Achilles or patellar tendinopathies, and hamstring strain injuries have been associated with a limited ankle dorsiflexion in the scientific literature [14, 15].

In professional soccer players, Moreno-Perez et al. [21] found a progressive decrease in the ankle dorsiflexion ROM throughout a competitive season, being greater in pre-season compared to mid-season (dominant, −8.1%; non-dominant, −12.5%) and post-season (dominant, −9.6%; non-dominant, −13.8%).

Therefore, it is important to include the ankle mobility assessment as a preparticipation screening in soccer players [22] and monitor their evolution throughout the competitive season since the reduced ankle dorsiflexion is a modifiable risk factor for lower limb injuries [23, 24].

In the literature, there are several methods and tools to measure ankle dorsiflexion ROM. Weight-bearing measures, despite not measuring motion at a specific joint (talocrural, subtalar, and tarsal) are more indicative of the functional ankle dorsiflexion ROM (i.e., for walking and running) and may be more reliable (ICC = 0.93–0.96) than measures obtained in a non-weight-bearing position (ICC = 0.32–0.72) [25]. For this reason, the weight-bearing lunge test is a reference test for ankle dorsiflexion ROM measurement [26].

4.1.1.1 Weight-bearing lunge test [27]

The test starts with the subject in a standing position, face to the wall. The tested foot must be on a tape line, perpendicular to the wall, the knee in line with the second toe and the heel in contact with the ground, and the great toe 10 cm away from the wall. The subject can contact with the wall using only two fingers from each hand to maintain a stable position and the leg not being tested can rest on the floor.

The player then lunges forward trying to touch a vertical line on the wall with his/her knee while maintaining the heel in contact with the ground. If this happens, the subject moves the foot away from the wall until the knee touches the wall lightly always without lifting the heel from the ground. This puts the ankle joint in maximal dorsiflexion (Figure 4.1)

When the participant reaches the final lunge position, measurement techniques for ankle dorsiflexion ROM in this test including the use of a standard goniometer, an inclinometer, or a tape measure have been carried out. All of these have shown

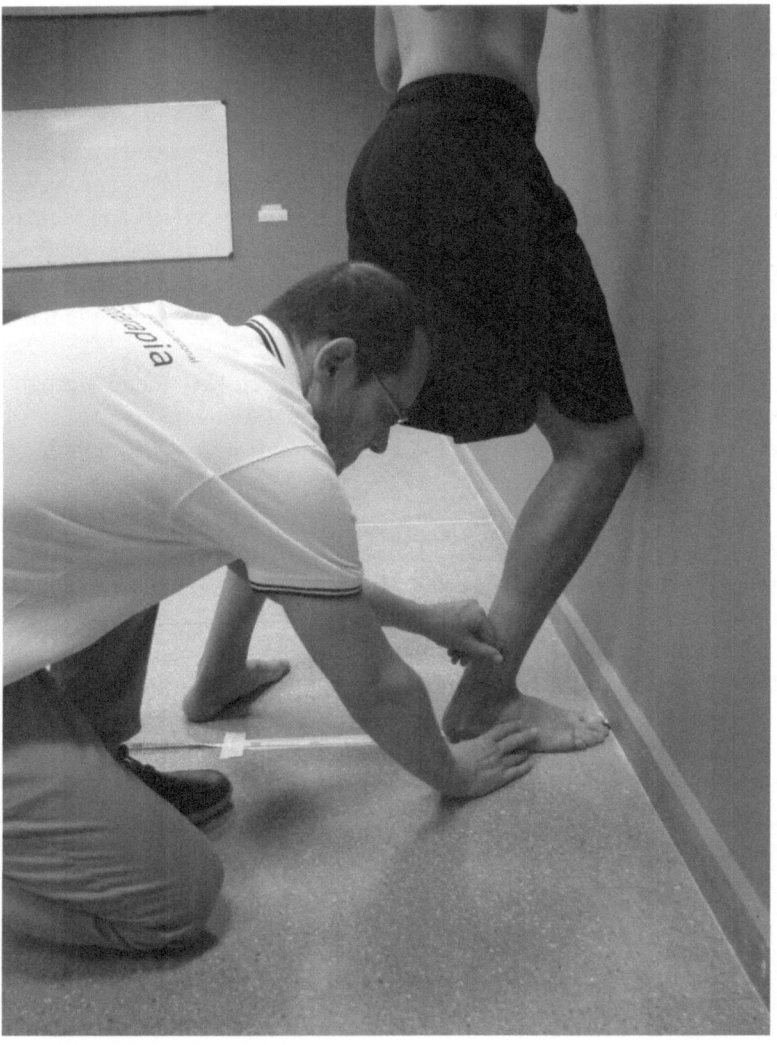

FIGURE 4.1   Weight-bearing lunge test [27].

good reliability (ICC = 0.85–0.99); low measurement error, even in novice evalua-tors [26, 28]; and strong evidence of its inter-rater reliability (ICC = 0.80–0.99) as well as intra-rater reliability (ICC = 0.65–0.99) [29].

4.1.1.2 Inclinometer

The device is placed at the tibial tuberosity, and the angle of the tibia relative to the ground is measured (Figure 4.2). Cejudo et al. [30] described a new simplified version of the weight-bearing lunge test (Figure 4.3) to assess ankle dorsiflexion ROM and reported high relative reliability scores (ICC > 0.9). Using this variation,

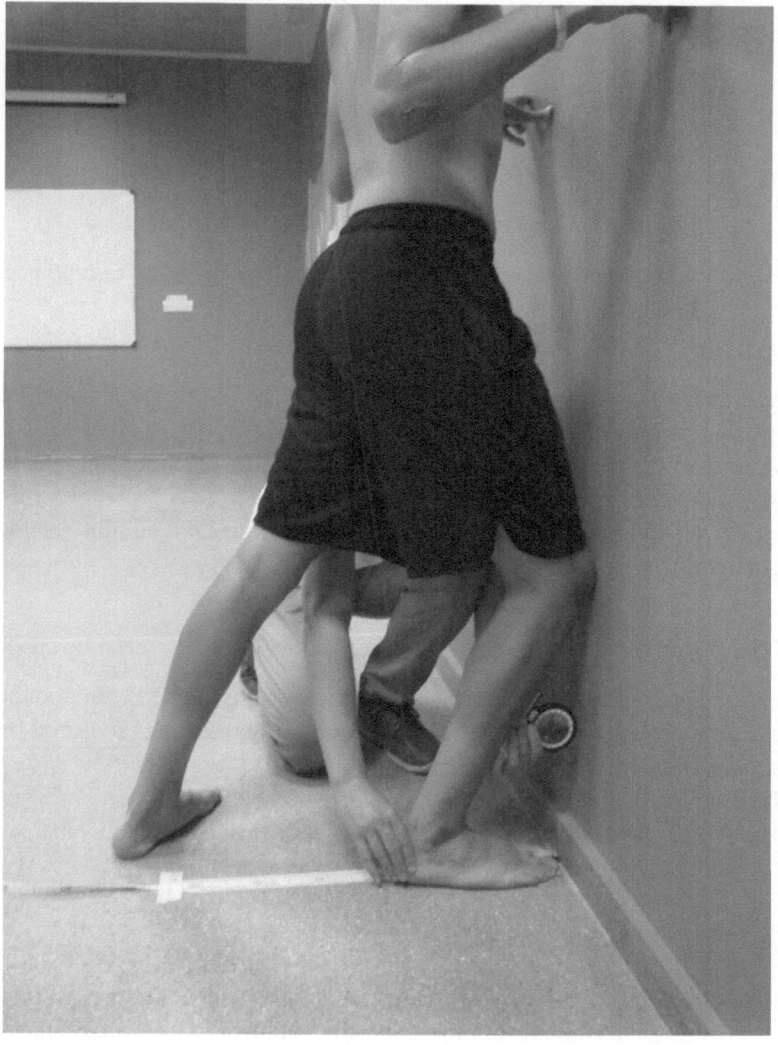

FIGURE 4.2 The use of inclinometer during the weight-bearing lunge test.

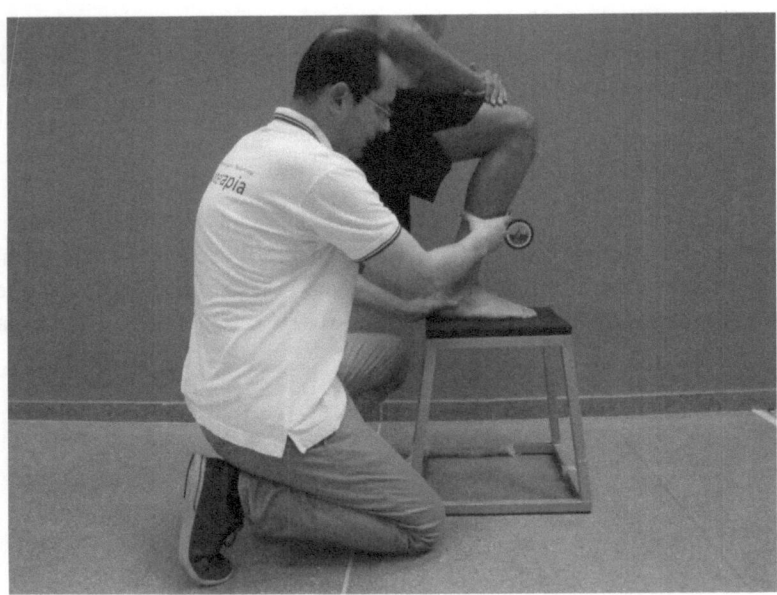

FIGURE 4.3 The simplified version of the weight-bearing lunge test proposed by Cejudo et al. [30].

changes larger than 3.8° from baseline scores after an intervention would indicate that a real change in ankle dorsiflexion ROM was likely.

More recently, the smartphone technology allows to measure joint ranges (Figure 4.4); for example, the Dorsiflex mobile application [31] has shown adequate levels of reliability for the measurement of this range of mobility during the weight-bearing test.

4.1.1.3 Goniometer

In case of using a standard goniometer, the stable arm is aligned with floor and the mobile arm through the shaft of the fibula by visually bisecting the lateral malleolus and the fibular head [32] (Figure 4.5).

Reported normative values for both goniometer and inclinometer measures are within 30°–50°, and the minimal detectable change (MDC) for inclinometer measures is within the range 1.5°–6.4° [33].

4.1.1.4 Tape measure

The use of a tape measure is easy, quick, and inexpensive alternative that does not require prior technical training from the evaluator as it is associated with

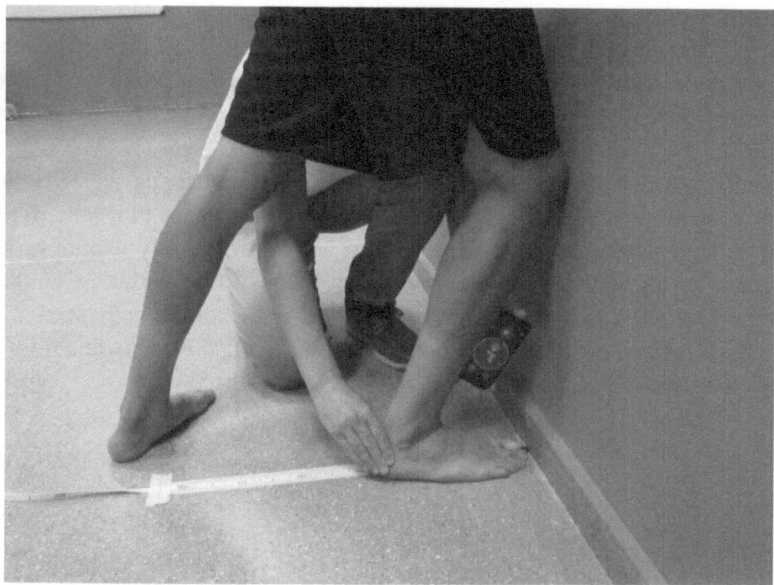

FIGURE 4.4   Ankle dorsiflexion range of motion measurement using smartphone technology during the weight-bearing lunge test.

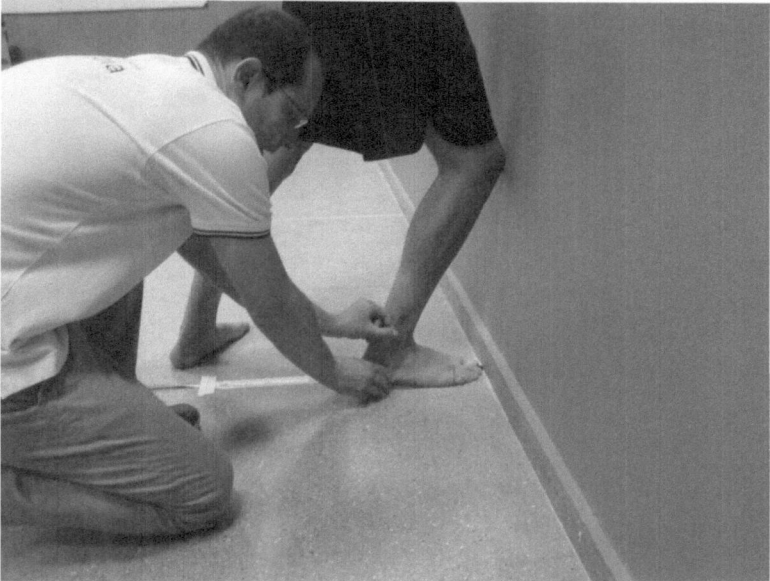

FIGURE 4.5   Goniometric assessment of ankle dorsiflexion ROM.

a goniometer or inclinometer [32]. When the maximal ankle dorsiflexion is reached, the distance between the big toe and the wall is then measured (in centimetres), with each centimeter corresponding to approximately 3.6° of ankle dorsiflexion. The MDC for the tape measure method is between 0.4 and 1.6 cm [23].

Finally, the use of complements such as the leg motion device (LegMotion, Check your Motion, Albacete, Spain) enables the performance of a weight-bearing lunge test in standardized conditions, allowing to control some potential variations that occur during testing that need to be controlled, such as variations in the subtalar and foot position, the visual reference for the knee or the maintenance of the foot alignment during the performance of the test (Figure 4.6). The reliability of the leg motion System test was very high (ICC = 0.96–0.98) [34].

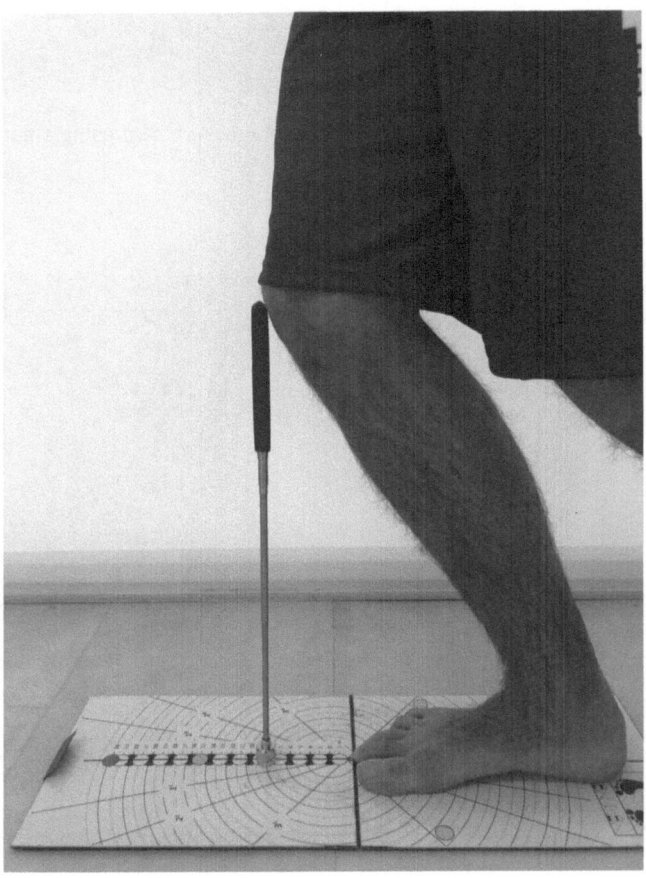

FIGURE 4.6   Leg motion device.

4.1.2 Hamstring injuries

Hamstring muscle injuries are the most common noncontact muscle injuries in male soccer players and are associated with significant time loss, decreased performance, significant re-injury rates, and the high costs [35]. The incidence of acute hamstring injury in soccer varies between 0.3 and 1.9/1000 exposure hours, and the recurrence rate is 4–68% [36].

Considering the high incidence of hamstring injuries in soccer and its consequences for the players and the clubs, identification of risk factors is essential for injury and re-injury prevention [37]. Traditionally, reduced hamstring flexibility has been considered a risk factor for hamstring tears [9]. However, previous hamstring injury is the most strongly risk factor related to hamstring injury in the literature, and conflicting evidence exists for hamstring flexibility or tightness as risk factor for hamstring tears [6, 38].

Hamstring tightness, defined as a lack of hip flexion and/or knee extension ROM with a concomitant feeling of restriction in the posterior thigh, can cause a dysfunctional or restricted movement of the hip [39]. However, this perceived tightness is actually considered a multidimensional condition that may include musculoskeletal imbalance, neural tension, and lumbopelvic dysfunction [40]. Extensibility of neural structures has been described as a relevant contributor to musculoskeletal flexibility, [41], and hamstring flexibility could be, in part, a reflection of neural tissue mechano-sensitivity, that should be considered during hip flexion ROM assessment.

Several clinical examination tests have been proposed to assess the hamstring tightness. The active knee extension (AKE) and the passive straight leg raise (PSLR) tests have been considered the gold standard in research settings [42].

4.1.2.1 Active Knee Extension (AKE) test

The AKE test [43] assesses the range of active knee extension in a position of hip flexion (90°). For the assessment, the subject lies supine on a firm table with their arms folded across the chest and head resting on the stretcher (without a pillow underneath the head). The participant left the hip of the tested side to 90°, keeping the thigh in the vertical position throughout the test, controlled by an assistant. The opposite leg is placed in a fully extended position on the table. The foot of the leg being tested should be kept relaxed.

The leg being tested is actively straightened until the subject feels the first stretch sensation or when the thigh begins to move from the vertical position. The contralateral limb is secured by a second examiner, fully extended on the stretcher and in neutral rotation. At this point, the inclinometer is placed at the tibia, and the angle respect to the vertical line is recorded (Figure 4.7).

The test has showed excellent inter-rater (ICC = 0.81–0.87) and intra-rater (ICC = 0.75–0.94) reliability values for assessing hamstring flexibility in healthy adults [10, 44].

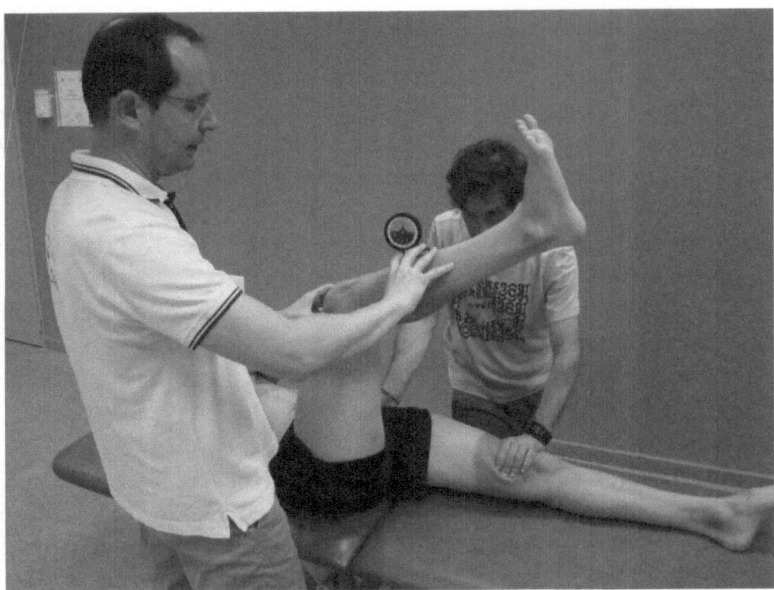

FIGURE 4.7   Active Knee Extension test [43].

Normative data suggest that a knee flexion angle of 40° is the average range across ages and sexes, and a knee flexion angle of 20° or less is considered normal ROM on the AKE test [45, 46].

This test can also be performed passively, when the aim is to examine the "end feel" of the joint movement and the tightness of the hamstring muscles. In this case, from the initial test position, the tester passively extends the knee to the end of range, at which point, the knee flexion angle is measured. The intra- and inter-rater reliability have been reported as very high (ICC=0.98–0.99) and has been recommended as the most reliable measure of hamstring length [39, 42]. Normative data are limited, but a rough guide for males is a knee flexion angle of 38° and females 28° across all ages. The movement stops when the tester feels a strong resistance or when pelvic rotation or a posterior pelvic tilt movement is observed. If the participant being tested feels an intolerable sensation of tension or pain, the test must also be stopped.

Whiteley et al. [47] recently proposed the development of this test but with maximal hip flexion (Maximal Hip Flexion Active Knee Extension) considering that it is a good associated indicator with rehabilitation progression and perceived running effort (Figure 4.8).

4.1.2.2   Passive Straight Leg Raise test

The PSLR is performed with the subject supine. The examiner slowly flexed the participant's hip passively while maintaining knee extension until the point of

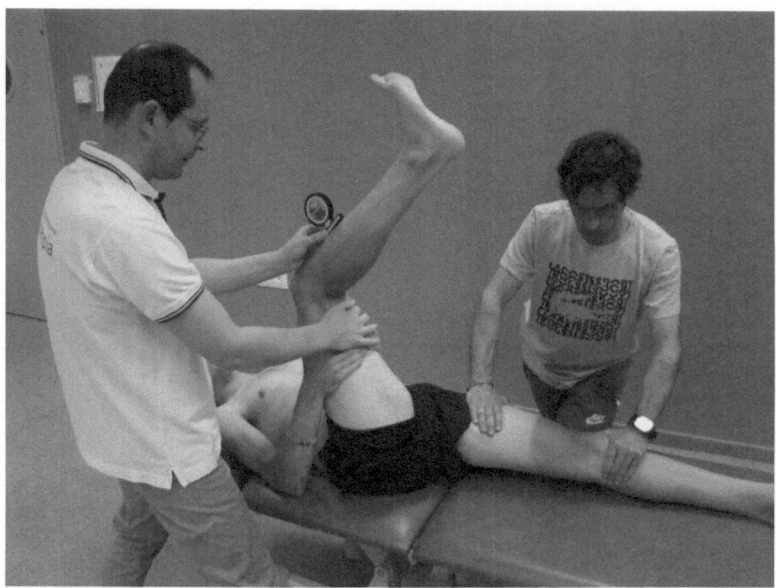

FIGURE 4.8 Maximal Hip Flexion Active Knee Extension proposed by Whiteley et al. [47].

discomfort is reached. Care should be taken to avoid rotation of the pelvis or flexion of the uninvolved leg and to avoid hamstring involuntary contractions that can affect negatively the results [48]. The ROM measurement is recorded with an inclinometer placed at the frontal thigh or by placing the arm of the inclinometer in the longitudinal axis of the mobilized segment through the imaginary bisector line [49] (Figure 4.9).

The normal ROM for the PSLR has been reported as 80° of hip flexion [45]. The PSLR has been reported to have high intra-rater ($r = 0.91$) and inter-rater ($r = 0.93$) reliability [50]. Besides, the PSLR has been reported to be moderately correlated with the AKE test ($r = 0.72$) [51].

However, caution should be exercised when interpreting results with some of the tests described, since, for example, PSLR does not measure hamstring muscle extensibility in isolation. PSLR is strongly influenced by factors other than hamstring stiffness, such as mechanosensivity of the sciatic nerve, and therefore might not always accurately evaluate hamstring stiffness. Foo et al. [48] warned that less activity of involuntary hamstring muscles can reduce passive hip ROM during the PSLR test in healthy people.

The standard error of measurement (SEM) values for PSLR and AKE test (2.2° and 2.9°, respectively) indicate a high precision in the individual scores, which reduces bias in measurement [52].

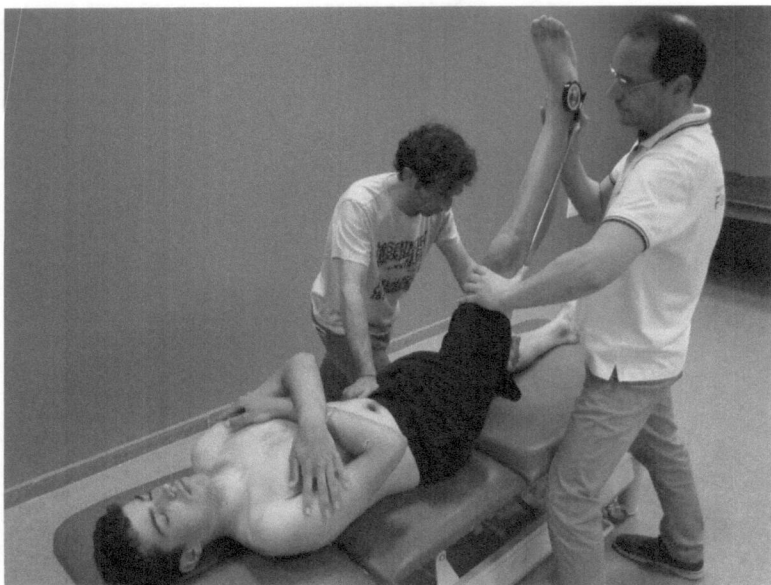

FIGURE 4.9   Passive straight leg raise test.

Finally, other global tests as the Sit and reach, V-Sit and Reach, or the toe touch tests can be appropriate measures to determine the spine ROM but not to evaluate the hamstring muscle flexibility [53].

4.1.3   Groin injuries

Groin injuries are one of the most frequent types of lower limb injury in soccer with values ranging from 7% to 18% of the total amount of injuries [54–56] with an incidence of 0.2–2.1/1000 h [55]. Furthermore, long-term symptoms and a high risk of re-injury are also other major problems of the groin injury in soccer players [57, 58].

Multiple pathologies (e.g., hernia, pubic bone or edema/avulsion fractures, adductor strains, adductor tendinopathies, external oblique or rectus abdominis tear, nerve entrapment, as well as hip joint pathology) may cause similar symptoms and can refer pain to the groin region [56]. However, the literature indicates that adductor is one of the most common injuries in soccer players [59]. These injuries usually result from sudden changes in direction or repetitive sprinting and kicking actions during practices and competition [60, 61].

According to Walden et al. [55], impaired pelvic movement could negatively affect the player's performance and induce a higher risk of recurrence and chronicity of groin injury. Particularly, previous studies have identified a hip decreased ROM in the abduction [3], total hip [62], internal rotation [12], and extension ROM related to an increased risk of groin injuries. However, some results from different studies are contradictory regarding the evidence of reduced ROM being a risk factor [57, 63].

To evaluate the hips of the players, we can use the following tests:

4.1.3.1   Bent knee fall out test

The bent knee fallout test demonstrated stronger association with cam and pincer morphology in a previous study with a 9% increased chance of having a cam for each 1 cm of the lower range [58]. The referred test demonstrated excellent inter-tester reliability in a study involving elite soccer players, (ICC = 0.91) for the bent knee fallout test on the right side and on the left (ICC = 0.92) [64]. Based on Malliaras et al. [65], players will lay supine on a bench with the hips in 45° of hip flexion and knees at 90° of flexion (Figure 4.10). They will be instructed to allow their knees to fall outward while keeping their feet together, and the examiner uses gentle overpressure to check that the player had relaxed at the limit of movement. The distance between the head of the fibula and the supporting surface is measured; therefore, a higher score represents lower hip ROM.

4.1.3.2   Hip rotation ROM test

Regarding the restricted total hip rotation, previous authors hypothesized that restricted hip rotations induce increased stress over the symphysis and surrounding

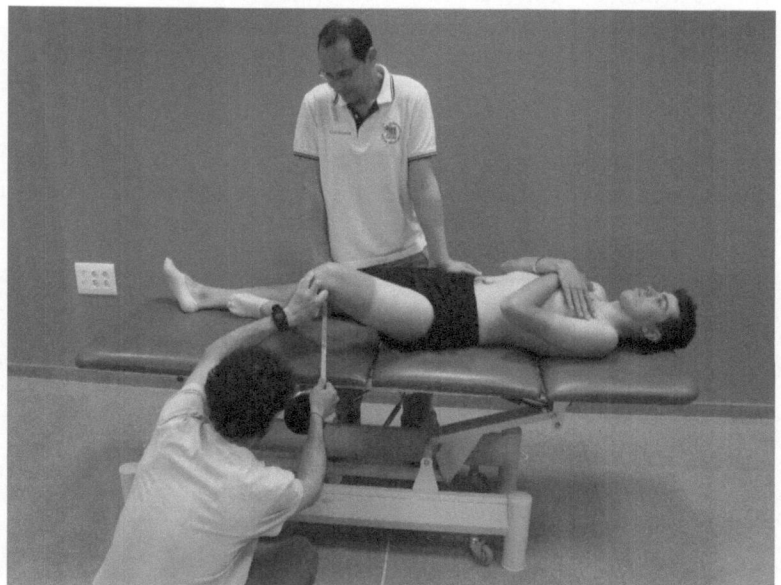

FIGURE 4.10   Bent knee fallout test.

soft tissues [66, 67]. In this line, a systematic review and meta-analysis showed that smaller (< 85°) total hip internal rotational ROM (with the hips and knees 90° flexed) is the most consistent risk factor for development of groin pain between athletes with groin pain from those without [62]. In addition, recently, van Klij et al. [68] showed that cam morphology size and duration were associated with limited hip internal rotation. The player will be positioned in a supine position with their knees flexed to 90° (zero starting position), after the internal rotation and external rotation are measured as the deviation from the zero-starting position, in which the longitudinal axis of the leg is perpendicular to the transverse line across the anterior superior iliac spines (Figure 4.11) [69]. Regarding the ICC, the previous study showed a good reliability (ICC = 0.91–0.95) using the hip rotation ROM test.

4.1.3.3 Hip flexion ROM test

Significant associations between cam morphology presence and limited passive hip flexion were observed and influenced by cam morphology size in comparison with hips without cam. The average flexion was lower in hips with cam morphology [68]. According to Lopez-Valenciano [22], the previous normalized values in hip flexion ROM in soccer players were around 80°. Usually, hip flexion had been measured in passive with the player in the supine position with inclinometer. The inclinometer is placed approximately on the external malleolus, and the distal arm was aligned parallel to an imaginary bisecting line of the limb [70]. The examiner performs a maximal flexion of the evaluated limb slowly and progressively, avoiding the knee flexion and external rotation of the limb. The referred test has shown good reliability (ICC = 0.94) in a previous study [71].

4.1.3.4 Hip abduction ROM test

In a previous study, Arnason et al. [3] showed that soccer players with less ROM for hip abduction are at increased risk of groin strains. The normal profiles in the

(a)   (b)

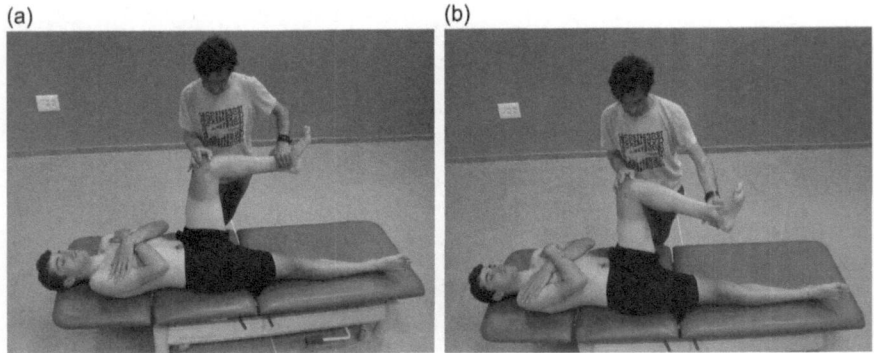

FIGURE 4.11 Hip internal and external rotation test.

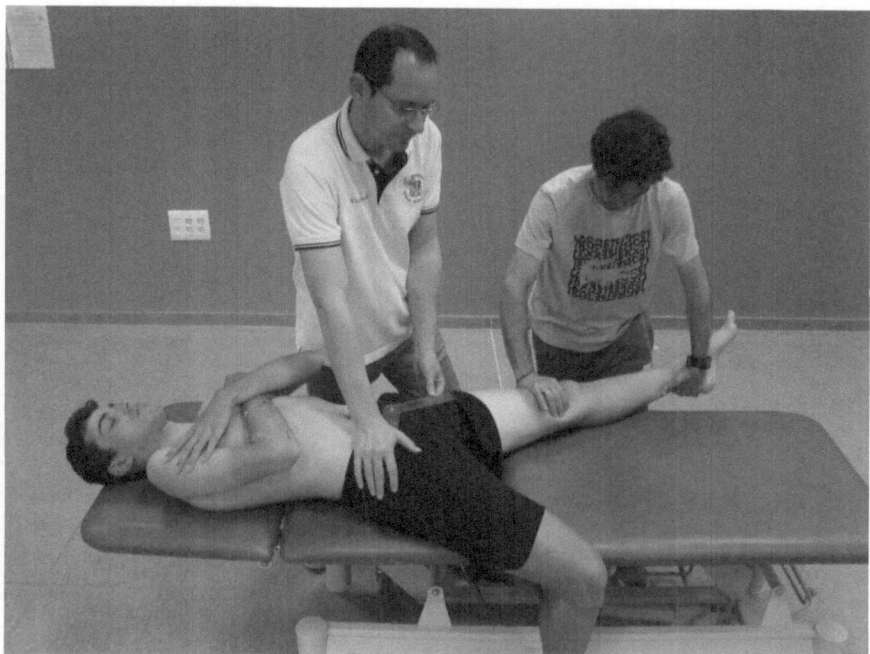

FIGURE 4.12   Hip abduction ROM test.

hip abduction ROM are around 60°–63° in professional soccer players [22]. For the assessment of hip passive abduction ROM test, the player is placed in the supine position with one leg fixed in slight abduction outside the examination table (Figure 4.12). The other limb is placed on a sliding board and passively abducted. The extent of abduction was measured using a double-armed goniometer, with the axis 5 cm below the anterior iliac spine, one arm pointing horizontally 5 cm below the other anterior iliac spine, and the other arm to the midpoint of the patella. The findings from the hip passive abduction ROM test show good relative intra-tester (ICC = 0.95) reliability in futsal players [71].

4.1.3.5   New device for assessment of the sagittal plane tilt

Active pelvic tilt, defining the ability of an individual to actively tilt the pelvis anteriorly and posteriorly over a frontal axis, and hip ROM parameters [72]. Previous studies identified a reduced of the active anterior (degree of rotation around a medial–lateral axis through the anterior–superior spine iliac in the sagittal plane) and total pelvic tilt on injured sides in 17 athletes with groin injury compared with 27 healthy control assessment with the inclinometer properties of the smartphone device [72] with an intra-class reliability of ICC = 0.89–0.93 [73] (Figure 4.13). The referred study showed 10.2° of anterior pelvic tilt in the injured sides and 13.7°

(a)   (b)

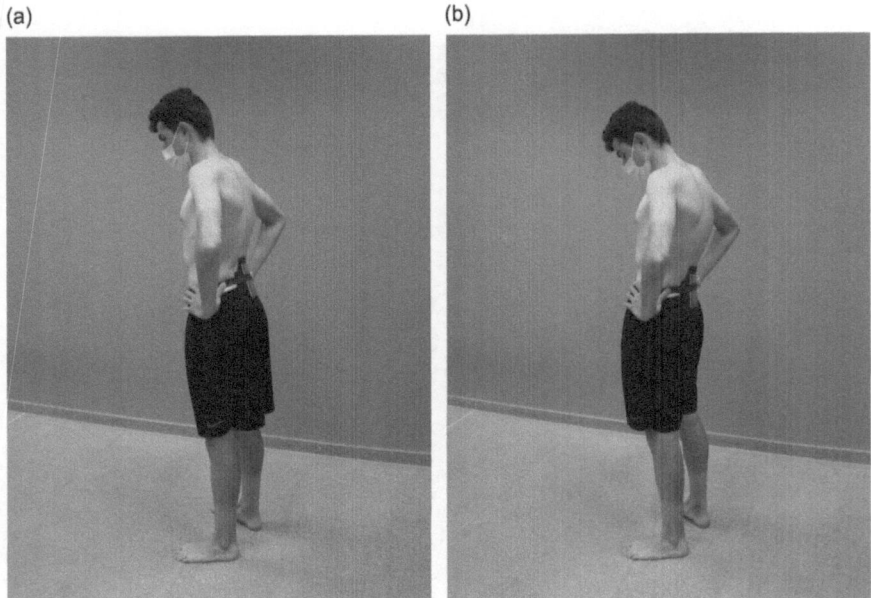

FIGURE 4.13 New device for assessment of the sagittal plane tilt.

in the non-injured sides, while the total pelvic tilt in the injured sides is 21.1° and 27.2° in the non-injured side [72].

4.1.4 Shoulder injuries

The upper limb injuries are less frequent than lower injuries in soccer [74]. In this regard, the percentage of soccer injuries is approximately 67.7% in the lower limb and 13.4% in the upper limb [74]. However, in the last years, shoulder injuries have represented an increasing health problem in soccer players [75]. Previous studies reported that the goalkeepers are more exposed to shoulder disorders than other field players [76]. Shoulder injuries in soccer players but particularly in goalkeepers have been reported to have an impact on the athletes' performance and training activities. In this sense, 28% of shoulder injuries in soccer players are severe because of which participation in training and games is stopped for > 28 days [77]. Although the majority of shoulder injuries affect the glenoid labrum in soccer players, the rotator cuff injuries can represent one of the most frequent injuries in goalkeepers [78].

Regarding the risk factors in shoulder injuries, a glenohumeral internal rotation deficit (GIRD) of the dominant shoulder compared to the non-dominant shoulder is considered a major risk factor for glenohumeral joint injury in overhead athletes as it causes an imbalance in the soft tissues and could lead to shoulder instability [79], resulting in subacromial impingement syndromes and labral tears [80].

(a)   (b)

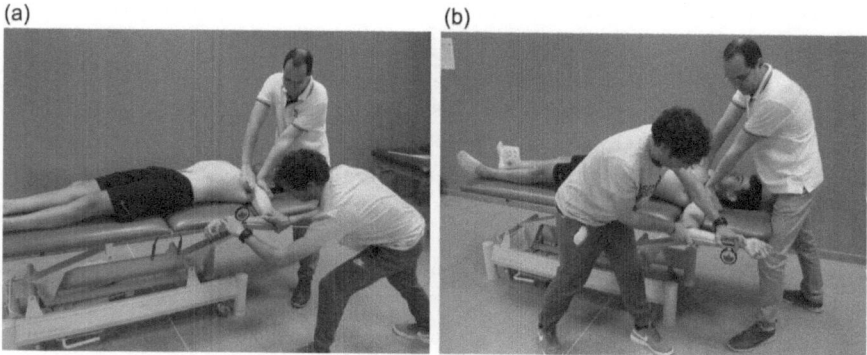

FIGURE 4.14 Assessment of the shoulder rotation range of motion: testing for gleno-humeral internal rotation position and for glenohumeral external rotation position.

Specifically, several studies showed that shoulder internal rotation problems are identified when there is a loss of rotation greater than 18°–20° in the dominant shoulder and with a corresponding more than 5° loss of total arc motion when compared to the non-dominant shoulder [79].

Usually, shoulder internal and external ROM is measured with a manual incli-nometer (Figure 4.14) [81, 82], goniometers [83], or with photograph and soft-ware for calculation angles [84]. Each participant lay supine on a bench, with the shoulder in 90° of abduction and the elbow flexed to 90° (forearm perpendicular to the bench). From this starting position, an examiner held the participant's proxi-mal shoulder region (i.e., clavicle and scapula) against the bench to stabilize the scapula, while another examiner rotated the humerus in the glenohumeral joint to produce maximum passive external rotation and internal rotation in dominant and non-dominant sides. The ICC for this test ranged from 0.88 to 0.93.

4.2 Range of motion during specific soccer actions

Despite not being a sport with extremely high flexibility requirements, some spe-cific soccer actions during play are benefitted from greater ROMs. One example is the sprint, which is considered the most important action in goal situations [85]. ROM for the lower limb joints increases as the velocity of displacement increases. Thus, sprinting performance is increased as longest stride lengths are used, which is linked to a higher degree of knee extension and a greater ROM in hip flexion exten-sion [86, 87]. This is of particular interest as most hamstring strain injuries take place during high-intensity accelerations and sprints [88], and especially, during the late swing phase, when the muscles are at a greater length [89]. Consequently, it can be suggested that a combination of an adequate hamstring flexibility together with the ability to produce great forces at greater muscle lengths may prevent from hamstring strains. This could explain the effectiveness of the Nordic hamstring exercises on reducing hamstring strains as it achieves concomitant increases in eccentric strength and muscle fascicle length [90].

Apart from sprinting, kicking actions also require substantial flexibility values. Specifically, a high hip extension ROM is requested during the back swing of the kick [91]. Interestingly, Takahashi et al. [92] showed that soccer players with a history of groin pain showed a smaller hip extension ROM in the back swing. In addition, although scarcely studied, ankle ROM may play a role in soccer kicking. This is supported by the extreme ankle plantar flexion taking place during the previous moments before ball contact [93].

4.3 Flexibility in youth soccer players

The incidence of muscular strain injuries is lower in young than in adult soccer players. However, increases in training volume and intensity due to early specialization have led to an increased risk of lower limb injuries in young soccer players [94], with the greatest injury incidence at the ages of 15 and 17 years [95]. Cejudo et al. [96] reported progressive decreases in different measures of hip, knee, and ankle ROM from U-10 to U-19 soccer players. Similarly, Sanz et al. [8] showed significant lower values in the active straight leg rise test in U-11 and U-13 players compared with U-9 players. Interestingly, although not reaching statistical significance, young soccer players who suffered from hamstring strain showed a tendency for lower hamstring flexibility. Considering that a reduction in hip ROM may be linked to muscular tightness [11], which is a risk factor for muscle injuries [89], the maintenance of hip mobility during soccer players' growth is worthy. Training programs aiming at increasing/maintaining flexibility could be especially relevant in periods of rapid growth, which is matched with U-15 players, where recent studies have reported the higher and more severe injury rates [8, 97].

References

1. García-Pinillos F, Ruiz-Ariza A, Moreno del Castillo R, Latorre-Román PÁ. Impact of limited hamstring flexibility on vertical jump, kicking speed, sprint, and agility in young football players. *J Sports Sci.* 2015; 33(12):1293–1297. doi:10.1080/02640414.2015.1022577

2. Bradley PS, Portas MD. The relationship between preseason range of motion and muscle strain injury in elite soccer players. *J Strength Cond Res.* 2007; 21(4):1155–1159. doi:10.1519/R-20416.1

3. Arnason A, Sigurdsson SB, Gudmundsson A, Holme I, Engebretsen L, Bahr R. Risk factors for injuries in football. *Am J Sports Med.* 2004; 32(1):5–16. doi:10.1177/0363546503258912

4. Bittencourt N, Ocarino J, Sorrentino F, Jales F, Gabriel S, Mendonça L, Fonseca S. Normative data for muscle flexibility in male soccer players. *Br J Sports Med.* 2014; 48:568–569. doi:10.1136/bjsports-2014-093494.24

5. Rolls A, George K. The relationship between hamstring muscle injuries and hamstring muscle length in young elite footballers. *Phys Ther Sport.* 2004; 5(4):179–187. doi:10.1016/j.ptsp.2004.08.005

6. van Doormaal MC, van der Horst N, Backx FJ, Smits DW, Huisstede BM. No relationship between hamstring flexibility and hamstring injuries in male amateur soccer players: A prospective study. *Am J Sports Med.* 2017; 45(1):121–126. doi:10.1177/0363546516664162

7. Henderson G, Barnes CA, Portas MD. Factors associated with increased propensity for hamstring injury in English Premier League soccer players. *J Sci Med Sport.* 2010; 13(4):397–402. doi:10.1016/j.jsams.2009.08.003

8. Sanz A, Pablos C, Ballester R, Sánchez-Alarcos JV, Huertas F. Range of motion and injury occurrence in elite Spanish Soccer Academies. Not only a hamstring shortening-related problem. *J Strength Cond Res.* 2020; 34(7):1924–1932. doi:10.1519/JSC.0000000000003302

9. Witvrouw E, Danneels L, Asselman P, D'Have T, Cambier D. Muscle flexibility as a risk factor for developing muscle injuries in male professional soccer players. A prospective study. *Am J Sports Med.* 2003; 31(1):41–46.

10. Ayala F, López-Valenciano A, Gámez Martín JA, De Ste Croix M, Vera-Garcia FJ, García-Vaquero MDP, Ruiz-Pérez I, Myer GD. A preventive model for hamstring injuries in professional soccer: Learning algorithms. *Int J Sports Med.* 2019; 40(5):344–353. doi:10.1055/a-0826-1955

11. Ekstrand J, Gillquist J. The frequency of muscle tightness and injuries in soccer players. *Am J Sports Med.* 1982;10(2):75–78. doi:10.1177/036354658201000202

12. Ibrahim A, Murrell GA, Knapman P. Adductor strain and hip range of movement in male professional soccer players. *J Orthop Surg.* 2007; 15(1):46–49. doi:10.1177/230949900701500111

13. Gabbe BJ, Bennell KL, Finch CF, Wajswelner H, Orchard JW. Predictors of hamstring injury at the elite level of Australian football. *Scand J Med Sci Sports.* 2006; 16(1):7–13. doi:10.1111/j.1600-0838.2005.00441.x

14. Wahlstedt C, Rasmussen-Barr E. Anterior cruciate ligament injury and ankle dorsiflexion. *Knee Surg Sports Traumatol Arthrosc.* 2015; 23(11):3202–3207. doi:10.1007/s00167-014-3123-1

15. Whitting JW, Steele JR, McGhee DE, Munro BJ. Dorsiflexion capacity affects achilles tendon loading during drop landings. *Med Sci Sports Exerc.* 2011; 43(4):706–713. doi:10.1249/MSS.0b013e3181f474dd

16. Pink M, Perry J, Houglum PA, Devine DJ. Lower extremity range of motion in the recreational sport runner. *Am J Sports Med.* 1994; 22(4):541–549. doi:10.1177/036354659402200418

17. Pfirrmann D, Herbst M, Ingelfinger P, Simon P, Tug S. Analysis of injury incidences in male professional adult and elite youth soccer players: A systematic review. *J Athl Train.* 2016; 51(5):410–424.

18. Cloke DJ, Spencer S, Hodson A, Deehan D. The epidemiology of ankle injuries occurring in English Football Association academies. *Br J Sports Med.* 2009; 43(14):1119–1125. doi:10.1136/bjsm.2008.052050

19. Macrum E, Bell DR, Boling M, Lewek M, Padua D. Effect of limiting ankle-dorsiflexion range of motion on lower extremity kinematics and muscle-activation patterns during a squat. *J Sport Rehabil.* 2012; 21(2):144–150.

20. Mason-Mackay AR, Whatman C, Reid D. The effect of reduced ankle dorsiflexion on lower extremity mechanics during landing: A systematic review. *J Sci Med Sport.* 2017; 20(5):451–458. doi:10.1016/j.jsams.2015.06.006

21. Moreno-Pérez V, Soler A, Ansa A, López-Samanes Á, Madruga-Parera M, Beato M, Romero-Rodríguez D. Acute and chronic effects of competition on ankle dorsiflexion

ROM in professional football players. *Eur J Sport Sci*. 2020; 20(1):51–60. doi:10.1080/17461391.2019.1611930

22. López-Valenciano A, Ayala F, Vera-García FJ, de Ste Croix M, Hernández-Sánchez S, Ruiz-Pérez I, Cejudo A, Santonja F. Comprehensive profile of hip, knee and ankle ranges of motion in professional football players. *J Sports Med Phys Fitness*. 2019; 59(1):102–109. doi:10.23736/S0022-4707.17.07910-5

23. Hoch MC, McKeon PO. Normative range of weight-bearing lunge test performance asymmetry in healthy adults. *Man Ther*. 2011; 16(5):516–519.

24. Rabin A, Portnoy S, Kozol Z. The association of ankle dorsiflexion range of motion with hip and knee kinematics during the lateral step-down test. *J Orthop Sports Phys Ther*. 2016; 46(11):1002–1009. doi:10.2519/jospt.2016.6621

25. Venturini C, Ituassu NT, Teixeira LM, Deus C. Intrarater and interrater reliability of two methods for measuring the active range of motion for ankle dorsiflexion in healthy subjects. *Rev Bras Fisioter*. 2006; 10:407–411.

26. Hall EA, Docherty CL. Validity of clinical outcome measures to evaluate ankle range of motion during the weight-bearing lunge test. *J Sci Med Sport*. 2017; 20(7):618–621. doi:10.1016/j.jsams.2016.11.001

27. Bennell KL, Talbot RC, Wajswelner H, Techovanich W, Kelly DH, Hall AJ. Intra-rater and inter-rater reliability of a weight-bearing lunge measure of ankle dorsiflexion. *Aust J Physiother*. 1998; 44(3):175–180.

28. Konor MM, Morton S, Eckerson JM, Grindstaff TL. Reliability of three measures of ankle dorsiflexion range of motion. Int *J Sports Phys Ther*. 2012; 7(3):279–287.

29. Powden CJ, Hoch JM, Hoch MC. Reliability and minimal detectable change of the weight-bearing lunge test: A systematic review. *Man Ther*. 2015; 20(4):524–532. doi:10.1016/j.math.2015.01.004

30. Cejudo A, Sainz de Baranda P, Ayala F, Santonja F. A simplified version of the weight-bearing ankle lunge test: Description and test-retest reliability. *Man Ther*. 2014; 19(4):355–359. doi:10.1016/j.math.2014.03.008

31. Balsalobre-Fernández C, Romero-Franco N, Jiménez-Reyes P. Concurrent validity and reliability of an iPhone app for the measurement of ankle dorsiflexion and inter-limb asymmetries. *J Sports Sci*. 2019; 37(3):249–253. doi:10.1080/02640414.2018.1494908

32. Munteanu SE, Strawhorn AB, Landorf KB, Bird AR, Murley GS. A weightbearing technique for the measurement of ankle joint dorsiflexion with the knee extended is reliable. *J Sci Med Sport*. 2009; 12(1):54–59.

33. Cosby NL, Hertel J. Relationships between measures of posterior talar glide and ankle dorsiflexion range of motion. *Athl Train Sports Health Care*. 2011; 3(2):76–85.

34. Calatayud J, Martin F, Gargallo P, García-Redondo J, Colado JC, Marín PJ. The validity and reliability of a new instrumented device for measuring ankle dorsiflexion range of motion. *Int J Sports Phys Ther*. 2015; 10(2):197–202.

35. Ekstrand J, Waldén M, Hägglund M. Hamstring injuries have increased by 4% annually in men's professional football, since 2001: A 13-year longitudinal analysis of the UEFA Elite Club injury study. *Br J Sports Med*. 2016; 50(12):731–737. doi:10.1136/bjsports-2015-095359

36. Diemer WM, Winters M, Tol JL, Pas HIMFL, Moen MH. Incidence of acute hamstring injuries in soccer: A systematic review of 13 studies involving more than 3800 athletes with 2 million sport exposure hours. *J Orthop Sports Phys Ther*. 2021; 51(1):27–36.

37. van Beijsterveldt AM, van de Port IG, Vereijken AJ, Backx FJ. Risk factors for hamstring injuries in male soccer players: A systematic review of prospective studies. *Scand J Med Sci Sports*. 2013; 23(3):253–262. doi:10.1111/j.1600-0838.2012.01487.x

38. van Dyk N, Farooq A, Bahr R, Witvrouw E. Hamstring and ankle flexibility deficits are weak risk factors for hamstring injury in professional soccer players: A prospective cohort study of 438 players including 78 injuries. *Am J Sports Med.* 2018; 46(9):2203–2210. doi:10.1177/0363546518773057

39. Youdas JW, Krause DA, Hollman JH, Harmsen WS, Laskowski E. The influence of gender and age on hamstring muscle length in healthy adults. *J Orthop Sports Phys Ther.* 2005; 35(4):246–252.

40. Hansberger BL, Loutsch R, Hancock C, Bonser R, Zeigel A, Baker RT. evaluating the relationship between clinical assessments of apparent hamstring tightness: A correlational analysis. Int *J Sports Phys Ther.* 2019; 14(2):253–263.

41. McHugh MP, Johnson CD, Morrison RH. The role of neural tension in hamstring flexibility. *Scand J Med Sci Sports.* 2012; 22(2):164–169. doi:10.1111/j.1600-0838.2010.01180.x

42. Davis DS, Quinn RO, Whiteman CT, Williams JD, Young CR. Concurrent validity of four clinical tests used to measure hamstring flexibility. *J Strength Cond Res.* 2008; 22(2):583–588.

43. Gajdosik R, Lusin G. Hamstring muscle tightness reliability of an active-knee-extension test. *Phys Ther.* 1983; 63(7):1085–1088.

44. Reurink G, Goudswaard GJ, Oomen HG, et al. Reliability of the active and passive knee extension test in acute hamstring injuries. *Am J Sports Med.* 2013; 41(8):1757–1761.

45. Cook G. *Movement: Functional movement systems: Screening, assessment, and corrective strategies.* Santa Cruz, CA: On Target Publications; 2010.

46. Malliaropoulos N, Kakoura L, Tsitas K, Christodoulou D, Siozos A, Malliaras P, Maffulli N. Active knee range of motion assessment in elite track and field athletes: Normative values. *Muscles Ligaments Tendons J.* 2015; 5(3):203–207. doi:10.11138/mltj/2015.5.3.203

47. Whiteley R, van Dyk N, Wangensteen A, Hansen C. Clinical implications from daily physiotherapy examination of 131 acute hamstring injuries and their association with running speed and rehabilitation progression. *Br J Sports Med.* 2018; 52(5):303–310.

48. Foo Y, Héroux ME, Chia L, Diong J. Involuntary hamstring muscle activity reduces passive hip range of motion during the straight leg raise test: A stimulation study in healthy people. *BMC Musculoskelet Disord.* 2019; 20(1):130.

49. Cejudo A, Sainz de Baranda P, Ayala F, De Ste Croix M, Santonja-Medina F. Assessment of the range of movement of the lower limb in sport: Advantages of the ROM-SPORT I battery. *Int J Environ Res Public Health.* 2020; 17(20):7606. doi:10.3390/ijerph17207606

50. Gabbe BJ, Bennell KL, Wajswelner H, Finch CF. Reliability of common lower extremity musculoskeletal screening tests. *Phys Ther Sport.* 2004; 5(2):90–97.

51. Cameron DM, Bohannon RW. Relationship between active knee extension and active straight leg raise test measurements. *J Orthop Sports Phys Ther.* 1993; 17(5):257–260.

52. Neto T, Jacobsohn L, Carita AI, Oliveira R. Reliability of the active-knee-extension and straight-leg-raise tests in subjects with flexibility deficits. *J Sport Rehabil.* 2015; 24(4):2014–2020. doi:10.1123/jsr.2014-0220

53. Muyor JM, Vaquero-Cristóbal R, Alacid F, López-Miñarro PA. Criterion-related validity of sit-and-reach and toe-touch tests as a measure of hamstring extensibility in athletes. *J Strength Cond Res.* 2014; 28(2):546–555. doi:10.1519/JSC.0b013e31829b54fb

54. Mosler AB, Weir A, Eirale C, Farooq A, Thorborg K, Whiteley RJ, Hölmich P, Crossley KM. Epidemiology of time loss groin injuries in a men's professional football league: A 2-year prospective study of 17 clubs and 606 players. *Br J Sports Med.* 2018; 52(5):292–297.

55. Waldén M, Hägglund M, Ekstrand J. The epidemiology of groin injury in senior football: A systematic review of prospective studies. *Br J Sports Med.* 2015; 49(12):792–797. doi:10.1136/bjsports-2015-094705

56. Werner J, Hägglund M, Waldén M, Ekstrand J. UEFA injury study: A prospective study of hip and groin injuries in professional football over seven consecutive seasons. *Br J Sports Med.* 2009; 43(13):1036–1040.

57. Engebretsen AH, Myklebust G, Holme I, Engebretsen L, Bahr R. Intrinsic risk factors for groin injuries among male soccer players: A prospective cohort study. *Am J Sports Med.* 2010; 38(10):2051–2057.

58. Mosler AB, Agricola R, Thorborg K, Weir A, Whiteley RJ, Crossley KM, Hölmich P. Is bony hip morphology associated with range of motion and strength in asymptomatic male soccer players? *J Orthop Sports Phys Ther.* 2018; 48(4):250–259.

59. Hölmich P, Thorborg K, Dehlendorff C, Krogsgaard K, Gluud C. Incidence and clinical presentation of groin injuries in sub-elite male soccer. *Br J Sports Med.* 2014; 48(16):1245–1250.

60. Delahunt E, Kennelly C, McEntee BL, Coughlan GF, Green BS. The thigh adductor squeeze test: 45° of hip flexion as the optimal test position for eliciting adductor muscle activity and maximum pressure values. *Man Ther.* 2011; 16(5):476–480.

61. Machotka Z, Kumar S, Perraton LG. A systematic review of the literature on the effectiveness of exercise therapy for groin pain in athletes. *BMC Sports Sci Med Rehabil.* 2009; 1(1):5.

62. Tak I, Engelaar L, Gouttebarge V, Barendrecht M, Van Den Heuvel S, Kerkhoffs G, Langhout R, Stubbe J, Weir A. Is lower hip range of motion a risk factor for groin pain in athletes? A systematic review with clinical applications. *Br J Sports Med.* 2017; 51(22):1611–1621. doi:10.1136/bjsports-2016-096619

63. Tyler TF, Nicholas SJ, Campbell RJ, McHugh MP. The association of hip strength and flexibility with the incidence of adductor muscle strains in professional ice hockey players. *Am J Sports Med.* 2001; 29(2):124–128.

64. O'Brien J, Santner E, Finch CF. The inter-tester reliability of the squeeze and bent-knee-fall-out tests in elite academy football players. *Phys Ther Sport.* 2018; 34:8–13.

65. Malliaras P, Hogan A, Nawrocki A, Crossley K, Schache A. Hip flexibility and strength measures: Reliability and association with athletic groin pain. *Br J Sports Med.* 2009; 43(10):739–744.

66. Fricker PA. Management of groin pain in athletes. *Br J Sports Med.* 1997; 31(2):97–101. doi:10.1136/bjsm.31.2.97

67. Verrall GM, Hamilton IA, Slavotinek JP, Oakeshott RD, Spriggins AJ, Barnes PG, Fon GT. Hip joint range of motion reduction in sports-related chronic groin injury diagnosed as pubic bone stress injury. *J Sci Med Sport.* 2005; 8(1):77–84.

68. van Klij P, Ginai AZ, Heijboer MP, Verhaar JAN, Waarsing JH, Agricola R. The relationship between cam morphology and hip and groin symptoms and signs in young male football players. *Scand J Med Sci Sport.* 2020; 30(7):1221–1231.

69. Nussbaumer S, Leunig M, Glatthorn JF, Stauffacher S, Gerber H, Maffiuletti NA. Validity and test-retest reliability of manual goniometers for measuring passive hip range of motion in femoroacetabular impingement patients. *BMC Musculoskelet Disord.* 2010; 11:194. doi:10.1186/1471-2474-11-194

70. Moreno-Pérez V, Ayala F, Fernandez-Fernandez J, Vera-Garcia FJ. Descriptive profile of hip range of motion in elite tennis players. *Phys Ther Sport.* 2016; 19:43–48.

71. Cejudo A, Sainz de Baranda P, Ayala F, Santonja F. Test-retest reliability of seven common clinical tests for assessing lower extremity muscle flexibility in futsal and handball players. *Phys Ther Sport.* 2015; 16(2):107–113.

72. Van Goeverden W, Langhout RFH, Barendrecht M, Tak IJR. Active pelvic tilt is reduced in athletes with groin injury; a case-controlled study. *Phys Ther Sport.* 2019; 36:14–21. doi:10.1016/j.ptsp.2018.12.011

73. Chaudhari AMW, et al. *Validation of a novel clinical tool to measure pelvic tilt.* Gait & Clinical Movement Analysis Society Annual Meeting, Vol. 3, 2013.

74. Kirkendall DT, Dvorak J. Effective injury prevention in soccer. *Phys Sportsmed.* 2010; 38(1):147–157. doi:10.3810/psm.2010.04.1772

75. Longo UG, Loppini M, Berton A, Martinelli N, Maffulli N, Denaro V. Shoulder injuries in soccer players. *Clin Cases Miner Bone Metab.* 2012; 9(3):138–141.

76. Terra BB, Ejnisman B, Figueiredo EA, Andreoli CV, Pochini AC, Cohen C, Arliani GG, Cohen M. Arthroscopic treatment of glenohumeral instability in soccer goalkeepers. *Int J Sports Med.* 2013; 34(6):473–476.

77. Ekstrand J, Hägglund M, Waldén M. Injury incidence and injury patterns in professional football: The UEFA injury study. *Br J Sports Med.* 2011; 45(7):553–558.

78. Goodman AD, Etzel C, Raducha JE, Owens BD. Shoulder and elbow injuries in soccer goalkeepers versus field players in the National Collegiate Athletic Association, 2009–2010 through 2013–2014. *Phys Sportsmed.* 2018; 46(3):304–311.

79. Wilk KE, MacRina LC, Fleisig GS, Porterfield R, Simpson CD, Harker P, Paparesta N, Andrews JR. Correlation of glenohumeral internal rotation deficit and total rotational motion to shoulder injuries in professional baseball pitchers. *Am J Sports Med.* 2011; 39(2):329–335.

80. Gerber C, Werner CML, Macy JC, Jacob HAC, Nyffeler RW. Effect of selective capsulorrhaphy on the passive range of motion of the glenohumeral joint. *J Bone Jt Surg - Ser A.* 2003; 85(1):48–55.

81. Cools AM, Johansson FR, Borms D, Maenhout A. Prevention of shoulder injuries in overhead athletes: A science-based approach. *Braz J Phys Ther.* 2015; 19(5):331–339. doi:10.1590/bjpt-rbf.2014.0109

82. Moreno-Pérez V, Elvira J, Fernandez-Fernandez J, Vera-Garcia F. A comparative study of passive shoulder rotation range of motion, isometric rotation strength and serve speed between elite tennis players with and without history of shoulder pain. *Int J Sports Phys Ther.* 2018; 13(1):39–49.

83. Hellem A, Shirley M, Schilaty N, Dahm D. Review of shoulder range of motion in the throwing athlete: Distinguishing normal adaptations from pathologic deficits. *Curr Rev Musculoskelet Med.* 2019; 12(3):346–355.

84. Moreno-Pérez V, Moreside J, Barbado D, Vera-Garcia FJ. Comparison of shoulder rotation range of motion in professional tennis players with and without history of shoulder pain. *Man Ther.* 2015; 20(2):313–318.

85. Faude O, Koch T, Meyer T. Straight sprinting is the most frequent action in goal situations in professional football. *J Sports Sci.* 2012; 30(7):625–631. doi:10.1080/02640414.2012.665940

86. Mero A, Komi PV, Gregor RJ. Biomechanics of sprint running. A review. *Sports Med.* 1992; 13(6):376–392. doi:10.2165/00007256-199213060-00002

87. Novacheck TF. The biomechanics of running. *Gait Posture.* 1998; 7(1):77–95. doi:10.1016/s0966-6362(97)00038-6

88. Huygaerts S, Cos F, Cohen DD, et al. Mechanisms of hamstring strain injury: Interactions between fatigue, muscle activation and function. *Sports* (Basel). 2020; 8(5):65. doi:10.3390/sports8050065

89. Chumanov ES, Heiderscheit BC, Thelen DG. Hamstring musculotendon dynamics during stance and swing phases of high-speed running. *Med Sci Sports Exerc*. 2011; 43(3):525–532. doi:10.1249/MSS.0b013e3181f23fe8

90. Presland JD, Timmins RG, Bourne MN, Williams MD, Opar DA. The effect of Nordic hamstring exercise training volume on biceps femoris long head architectural adaptation. *Scand J Med Sci Sports*. 2018; 28(7):1775–1783. doi:10.1111/sms.13085

91. Nunome H, Asai T, Ikegami Y, Sakurai S. Three-dimensional kinetic analysis of side-foot and instep soccer kicks. *Med Sci Sports Exerc*. 2002; 34(12):2028–2036. doi: 10.1097/00005768-200212000-00025

92. Takahashi S, Kawamoto R, Kato S, Saho Y, Hirose N, Fukubayashi T. *Hip kinematics and muscle activity during inside soccer kick in players with a history of groin pain*. 34th International Conference of Biomechanics in Sports (2016), Tsukuba, Japan, July 18-22, 2016.

93. Nunome H, Lake M, Georgakis A, Stergioulas LK. Impact phase kinematics of instep kicking in soccer. *J Sports Sci*. 2006; 24(1):11–22. doi:10.1080/02640410400021450

94. Bowen L, Gross AS, Gimpel M, Li FX. Accumulated workloads and the acute: Chronic workload ratio relate to injury risk in elite youth football players. *Br J Sports Med*. 2017; 51(5):452–459. doi:10.1136/bjsports-2015-095820

95. Valle X, Malliaropoulos N, Párraga Botero JD, et al. Hamstring and other thigh injuries in children and young athletes. *Scand J Med Sci Sports*. 2018; 28(12):2630–2637. doi:10.1111/sms.13282

96. Cejudo A, Robles-Palazón FJ, Ayala F, et al. Age-related differences in flexibility in soccer players 8-19 years old. *Peer J*. 2019; 7:e6236. doi:10.7717/peerj.6236

97. Read PJ, Oliver JL, De Ste Croix MBA, Myer GD, Lloyd RS. An audit of injuries in six English professional soccer academies. *J Sports Sci*. 2018; 36(13):1542–1548. doi:10. 1080/02640414.2017.1402535

5

STRENGTH AND MUSCLE POWER TESTING

Eduardo Sáez de Villarreal Sáez
and Rodrigo Ramírez-Campillo

5.1 Introduction

The purpose of this chapter is to provide strength and conditioning professionals with evidence-based information permitting the effective implementation of an appropriate test battery of football-specific strength and power tests. Initially, this chapter will deal with the rationale for strength and power testing and will be specifically aimed at laboratory and field-based tests.

Often these data are used as part of the selection criteria into professional teams, and it can be used to investigate the effectiveness of training programs and to answer the many research questions that arise in attempts to optimize football performance. As such, a high standard of quality control needs to be exhibited during testing situations.

It is considered essential that strength and power testing be administered before a player begins a strength and conditioning program and/or competitive season. Testing sessions using the same battery should be re-administered systematically throughout the training phases of the season in order to continually assess progress and make the necessary adjustments. To prevent fatigue affecting either the testing results or the game performance within the competitive season, it is advisable to conduct strength and power testing a day which does not fall within 2 days before or after a competition.

The assessment of strength and power is not as well developed as the other components of fitness in football, such as endurance, technique, and tactic performance. There is also a lack of consistency in terms of the rationale for and execution of strength and power testing protocols. This chapter contains guidelines for the assessment of strength and power for football players involved in training programs. Before proceeding into these protocols, it is important to realize that

DOI: 10.4324/9781032637006-5

this is a working document that outlines the desired protocols for the assessment of strength and power based on the current theory. It is to be expected that these protocols will be updated with the discovery of new and pertinent information and with the development and acquisition of new innovative testing equipment.

5.2 Objectives of strength and power testing

The assessment of strength and power in football players is of critical importance in exercise science to

- generate a profile of the players strengths, weaknesses, and potential problems,
- generate a profile of the football and the relevance of strength and power to it,
- monitor the effects of training, detraining, and rehabilitation,
- provide motivation and encouragement to the athlete using feedback and goal setting,
- increase the players' accountability by using testing to monitor their compliance to training, and
- monitor the football players' skill/technique acquisition under maximal load.

5.3 Why is testing so important?

Football researchers have examined the physical, physiological, and technical requirements of a range of training and testing methods. In modern football, the physiological and physical demands are essential to optimal performance at all levels (adults, youth, and juniors). These demands include high-intensity movements, such as sprinting, jumping, cutting, changing of directions, and ball-shooting; moderate intensity movements, such as jogging; and low-intensity movements, such as walking. These demands are influenced by different factors: these are players' position, skill level, style of play, and tactical strategies used by the team [1]. Careful inspection of a match reveals that during a typical game, a 2–4-second sprint occurs every 90 seconds [2, 3]; high-speed sprinting only contributes approximately 3% to the total distance covered in games [4], and the most crucial moments of the game, such as winning ball possession, scoring, or conceding goals, depend on the ability of the athlete to perform these high-speed movements [5].

Sprinting ability is an integral component of successful performance and the ability to accelerate in football underlies successful game play [6]. Straight-line sprinting can be broken down into three phases: acceleration, attainment of maximal speed, and lastly the maintenance of maximal speed or speed endurance [7, 8]. Football is also characterized by brief periods of intense activity, followed by periods of recovery, and players must be able to perform these intense tasks repeatedly [9]. Some 96% of sprints are shorter than 30 m, and 49% are over a distance of 10 m only [10]. Thus, the performance over distances of 10 m or less and the velocity attained during the first step are considered to be key indicators of player potential [11, 12]. These are distinct qualities of speed, and specific tests should be used to evaluate each component within an appropriate test battery.

It is generally accepted that high-intensity actions such as agility or change of directions are integral elements for success in football and therefore need to be trained and tested as part of a periodized training program [6]. Mirkov et al. [13] examined the reliability of football-specific field tests and reported that the most appropriate indicator of overall football performance may be agility testing. Agility is defined as the ability to change direction rapidly without losing balance and using a combination of strength, power, and neuromuscular coordination, which is further affected by the athlete's perceptual and decision-making skills [6, 14]. Agility constitutes around 11% of player movement [6], and on average, a player takes 50 turns during a single match [15]. Previous literature, although, suggests that a football player changes direction every 2–4 seconds [16] and makes 1,200–1,400 directional changes [17] during a game. Thus, the ability to produce fast-paced variable actions can impact performance and, therefore, a football player's agility must be assessed.

The sport of football requires athletes to become more athletic, and short-term muscle power becomes more crucial in many game situations. Jumping ability and strength make important contributions to the performance potential of football players [18]. Football requires repeated powerful movements like kicking, tackling, and jumping [19, 20]. Measures of power generation, including jumping height and distance, have been shown to be positively correlated to performance in football [21, 22]. It is therefore of vital importance to measure a player's power generation capacity and reactive strength ability or stretch shortening cycle (SSC) augmentation. For example, significant correlations have been found between 1 repetition maximum (1RM) squat relative to body mass and countermovement jump (CMJ) peak power, CMJ peak velocity, and CMJ height [23]. In summation, a player's reactive strength and power ability are therefore essential to many key movements within football, and thus these parameters should also be assessed as part of an appropriate test battery.

All these training strategies suggest that the inclusion of a more football-specific laboratory and field-based testing, which are integrated into the normal football training program, has the potential to assess improvements. Those being in strength, jumping, agility, and sprinting performances and should be administered and re-administered systematically throughout the training phases of the season to assess progress and make program alterations where needed.

5.4 Player preparation

A primary objective of testing is to assess changes in performance as a result of prescribed training loads. Many physiological capacities can be influenced by variables such as diet, fatigue, medications, illness, injury, and environmental conditions. Players who present themselves for testing sessions should be in a similar state with regard to nutrition and fatigue for every testing session [24]. Therefore, a standardized test protocol is strongly recommended for reliable testing.

The following issues should be monitored and standardized as much as possible when performing tests over an extended training period.

5.4.1 Training

Players should have no training-induced severe physiological or neural fatigue in the 72 hours prior to testing [25]. This excludes players from participating in any maximal physiological testing or physical training prior to strength testing. No unaccustomed exercise should be performed 72 hours prior to strength testing, which may result in sarcomere damage and/or decreased activation of motor units. Unaccustomed exercises include a change in resistance exercise selection; increases in training volume (number of sets, exercises, or resistance sessions), or the performance of high-volume eccentric contractions [26].

To ensure task familiarization, the strength measures should be incorporated into the usual training routine prior to testing. An equivalent volume of training programs should be performed prior to all test sessions. At least 3 days prior to testing, there should be a decrease in strength training volume of up to 50% but with training intensity remaining the same.

5.4.2 Supplements

Alcohol. Based on ethical grounds, the consumption of alcohol prior to strength and power testing should be excluded.

Stimulants. Consumption of stimulants such as nicotine and caffeine should be controlled prior to high power neuromuscular assessments. From a practical perspective, habitual coffee drinkers are unlikely to report a marked improvement in test results and normal daily intakes can be maintained (caffeine content of retail coffee beverages ranges from 60 to 120 mg of caffeine per serve). The use of caffeinated sports or commercial beverages in amounts greater than 6 mg.kg-1 2 hours prior to testing should be discouraged.

Creatine Monohydrate. Creatine monohydrate (CM) may have short-term effects on maximal strength testing results. Maximal 1RM leg press strength has significantly increased up to 25.2% in young males [27]. Longer-term CM use over 12 weeks will result in greater strength gains in 1RM bench press and squat [28]. CM use to achieve greater rates in 1RM results should be noted in testing records. Stout [29] reports a reduced onset of neuromuscular fatigue. CM also significantly enhances repetitive power performance in squat and bench press measures [30]. This may indicate the need for caution when examining measures of explosive strength and power over a number of trials. Of more importance is the effect of CM on strength endurance (maximum repetition tests) [30]. CM use to boost strength endurance test results should be noted in testing records.

5.4.3 Frequency and scheduling of testing

A planned testing schedule should be outlined in an annual plan and should be reflective of the specific targets established for each phase of training. Annual planning of testing will enable the strength and conditioning coach to address issues as they occur. While feedback can be attained from each session based on training loads, the recommended minimum time period for scheduled testing to evaluate athlete progress is 6 weeks. Recognized significant improvements should be greater than the error of measurement (or variation in maximum results between testing trials).

Time of Testing. While strength has been reported to peak in the early evening (14:00–19:00 hours) [31], players should be tested at the same time of day in subsequent tests to avoid fluctuations in performance due to circadian rhythm [32]. Therefore, strength and power testing should occur at the same time of day as regular training.

Test Order. It is imperative that strength and power testing can be coordinated with other physiological assessments during the annual training cycle and within a given testing week. Testing power should be assessed at different time points to endurance and field testing due to the effects of potentiation. The time span needs to be greater than 1 hour to avoid this phenomenon. A weekly testing/training plan needs to be developed at the start of an annual cycle to ensure that physiological assessment of the athlete is coordinated with training. This ensures that testing conditions (day, time, etc.) are maintained throughout the year. This plan needs to be distributed to the player prior to their initial assessment and the player educated of the rationale and importance of adhering to this plan.

Tests should be completed in an order whereby fast and explosive power tests are completed prior to slower strength and strength endurance tests. Furthermore, multi-segment or multi-body part exercises should be completed prior to single segment exercises. Strength tests – complete more "explosive" tests prior to less "explosive" tests; complete "complex – whole body" tests prior to "simple – single" tests. The following is an example of suggested test order: Power test (vertical jump tests [countermovement jump, squat jump, drop jump], strength [snatch, power cleans, squats, leg press, bench press, bench pull, chins]), and strength endurance.

5.4.4 Warm-up

Physiologically, a "specific warm-up" results in a spectrum of advantages that include increases in the heart rate and blood circulation gradually; increases body core temperature and muscle temperature; permits freer movement in joints; prepares the joints and associated muscles to function through their full range of motion, improves the efficiency of muscular actions, reduces risk of injury, improves the transmission of nerve impulses, and aids psychological preparation [33]. Completing the combination of advantages of the specific warm-up is the psychological preparation for the activity to follow, which prepares the athlete mentally for a maximal effort while also enhancing the transmission of nerve impulses for the specific movement and or exertion [33].

The warm-up process should be broken into two sections. First, the "general warm-up" consisting of a light aerobic format (5 minutes minimum in an ergometer, footing, and treadmill). This should be then followed by a test "specific warm-up" in which the action of the test is mimicked at a gradual increase in weight and decrease of repetitions. Exercise specific warm-up: action duration $\leq$ 40–60% of specified RM $\leq$ 10 reps. with a recovery of $\geq$ 2 minutes; $\leq$ 60–80% of specified RM $\leq$ 5 reps. with a recovery of $\geq$ 2 minutes; 90% of specified RM $\leq$ 3 reps. with a recovery of $\geq$ 5 minutes.

The intensity and duration of the warm-up should be adjusted to the individual's level of strength/fitness and/or training age. This is to be known as the tester/coach's duty of care. It is at the player's discretion as to whether they utilize stretching of any form as part of a general warm-up and in recovery periods of the specific warm-up. As a minimum, all players are required to perform an initial trial at ~90% of specified repetition maximum for each test to be performed.

5.4.5 Planning

Before undertaking any strength or power test, a thorough plan should be in place regarding the type of data to be acquired. For example, in isokinetic testing, one may choose to record peak torque, peak or average power, or work performed by the specific muscle group of interest. An examiner must determine a priori why and what they are testing prior to the evaluation and what specific information is of interest. As noted below, strength and power testing are specialized and returns information based on precise anatomical configurations, muscle length–tension relationships, and velocities of muscle action. The practitioner must also be aware of data reduction techniques designed to eliminate extraneous information. If a clear understanding of the limitations of testing is established prior to interpretation, there will be little chance for erroneous conclusions.

5.4.6 Safety

Suitable safety measures should be in place prior to commencing any testing battery. These include, but are not limited to, inspection of equipment for broken or frayed components, appropriate lighting and temperature of the environment, as well as removal of all hazards near and around the testing site. Emergency procedures need to be formalized. All testing personnel need to be familiar with these procedures and be certified in basic life support. Most importantly, all testing procedures should be conducted under the diligent supervision of individuals experienced in physiological testing and measurement (i.e., an exercise physiologist with certification or accredited strength and conditioning coach/scientist). Attention to these simple safety measures will help ensure the protection of both the examiner and examinee.

5.4.7 Familiarization

Many of the players who will undergo strength and power testing may have little or no experience in performing the strength testing maneuvers. While strength testing has generally been shown to be reliable [25], novice players will likely improve strength scores on subsequent testing simply due to increased familiarity and comfort with the testing [34]. This is especially true for strength tests that require relatively higher levels of motor skill such as isotonic testing with free weights. If possible, novice players should be given a familiarization session prior to actual testing. This should involve having the player proceed through the entire test protocol while giving maximal effort. The subsequent testing session should occur at a time in which residual muscle soreness is over (e.g., 2–3 days).

5.4.8 Specificity

It is well established that various aspects of strength are associated with high levels of specificity. For example, many testing devices on the market today are designed to test and exercise muscles using the open kinetic chain. That is, only the isolated muscles of one joint are being examined. The information gathered from this type of testing will lead the examiner to specific conclusions regarding that single joint. Different results and conclusions may occur with multi-joint testing. Similarly, strength data derived from one type of contraction mode may correlate poorly with data from another mode. Throughout, it should be kept in mind that testing should be as specific as possible to the setting in which the information will be applied.

5.5 What should be tested?

A number of laboratory and field tests have been developed to evaluate players' abilities, determine individual strengths and weaknesses, and assess the effect of various training and other procedures expected to improve football performance. In general, the tests have provided valuable results due to their high reproducibility, standardized testing conditions, as well as reliable and precise equipment [35]. However, laboratory measurements are less accessible and often too expensive for routine use. Furthermore, these tests are time-consuming, and as a result, laboratory testing is rarely used throughout the season [36]. Also, logistically, it is very difficult to get an athlete or a team of athletes to a testing laboratory. Laboratory tests are often very expensive, thus making them inaccessible for regular use even for clubs with sound financial backing.

These inhibitory factors have led to the design of valid and reliable field tests. In further support, coaches have less than a month of preseason in some cases before the season officially begins. It is important that assessments are administered in a timely manner without compromising reliability and validity and ensuring each player has undergone sufficient recovery between each test. On the other hand, the sport-specific field tests are popular among both coaches and players due to their simplicity, validity, and minimal use of equipment.

5.5.1 General recommendations for strength and power test

All of the following tests must be supervised by an accredited strength and conditioning coach/scientist. All exercises need to be performed in a controlled manner. Any noted technical violations will result in the trial being invalid, and second attempt at the same weight will be provided.

The following general guidelines must be adhered to for all tests:

- Ensure that the player has performed appropriate warm-up. As a minimum, all players are required to perform a trial at ~90% of specified repetition maximum for each test. In the first test, player should perform an initial trial at ~90% of weight lifted in training.
- Lowering and lifting actions must be performed in a continuous manner. A single rest of no more than 2 seconds is allowed between repetitions.
- A maximum of 5-minutes recovery between trials is allowed.
- Minimum weight increments of 2.5 kg should be used between trials. However, increments should be guided by ease of each trial.
- Ideally, the specified RM test should be completed within four trials (not including the warm-up).
- If the player is unable to complete tests as per protocol, then this should be noted on testing result information, and values should not be included in any mathematical calculations.
- It is recommended that a spotter, other than supervising coach, should be used where possible.
- If a player is unable to adequately complete one rep within a set, then set/test should be recorded as a failure. If the tester is unsure as to successful completion, or the player believes that they can complete successfully, allow the player a second attempt with 2–3 minutes of the initial trial.
- Player body mass for each test session should be recorded as body mass including clothes and shoes.

5.5.2 Laboratory testing

5.5.2.1 Power tests

Vertical Jump Test (Sargent Jump, Vertical Leap).

The player stands side on to a wall and reaches up with the hand closest to the wall. Keeping the feet flat on the ground, the point of the fingertips is marked or recorded. This is called the standing reach height. The athlete then stands away from the wall and leaps vertically as high as possible using both arms and legs to assist

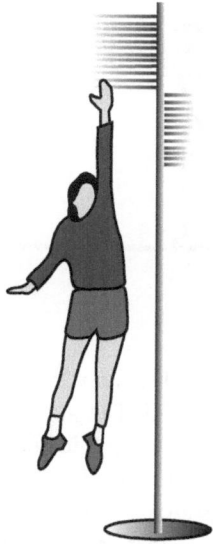

FIGURE 5.1 Vertec vertical jump tester.

in projecting the body upward. An attempt was made to touch the wall at the highest point of the jump. The difference in distance between the standing reach height and the jump height is the score. The best of three attempts is recorded. The vertical jump test can also be performed using a specialized apparatus called the Vertec. The procedure when using the Vertec is very similar to as described in Figure 5.1.

5.5.2.2 Vertical Jump Measurements (using flight time)

These methods measure the jump airtime using an electrical contact-operated system and from that calculate jump height. Similarly, a force platform can also be used to calculate jump height (plus other measures), or jump height can be calculated from video. Equipment required is an electronic timing mat, infrared laser system, or wearable devices. Jump height can be calculated using a timing mat or laser system which measures the time the feet are off the mat. Examples of different types of vertical jump test:

Squat Jump (SJ) Test. In this test, no arm swinging or countermovement is allowed. Not moving the arms isolates leg muscles and reduces the effect of variations in coordination of the arm movements. The player stands in socks or bare feet on the mat with weight evenly distributed over both feet. Hands are placed on the hips and stay there throughout the test. The player squats down until the knees are bent at 90 degrees, keeping the trunk straight. Once the mat is reset, the player jumps vertically as high as possible and lands back on the mat with both feet hitting the ground at the same time. The best score of at least three attempts is recorded. Both the take-off and landing must be from both feet, with no initial steps or

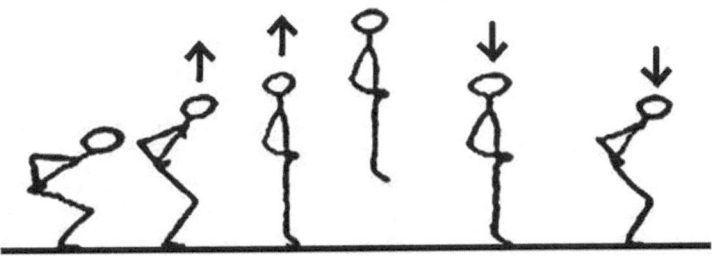

FIGURE 5.2 Squat Jump test.

shuffling. The timing mat may give a score of the time in the air, and the calculated vertical jump height can be calculated. The jump height is affected by how much you bend your knees, so the test can be invalidated if the subject does not bend the knees to the required 90 degrees each time. The best result of at least three attempts is recorded. One minute of rest is allocated between each trial (Figure 5.2) [37].

Countermovement Jump (CMJ) Test. Jump height is calculated using a timing mat which measures the time the feet are off the mat. The player stands upright in socks or bare feet, as still as possible on the mat with weight evenly distributed over both feet. Hands are placed on the hips and stay there throughout the test. When all is ready, the player squats down until the knees are bent at 90 degrees, then immediately jumps vertically as high as possible, landing back on the mat on both feet at the same time. The take-off must be from both feet, with no initial steps or shuffling. They also must not pause at the base of the squat. The best result of at least three attempts is recorded. One minute of rest is allocated between each trial (Figure 5.3) [38].

Loaded Countermovement Jump. The load that maximizes power output during CMJ loaded is also determined by adjusting the added loads until the highest power output is obtained. Warm-ups consist of a set of five repetitions with the weight of the Olympic bar (20 kg). The Olympic bar is then progressively increased in 10-kg increments for each set (i.e., bar only; bar + 10 kg; bar + 20 kg; bar + 30 kg) with two trials executed with each weight. CMJ loaded power output, bar displacement, peak, and mean power (watts) are recorded by using a distance encoder attached to one end of the bar. The distance encoder records the position and direction of the bar to an accuracy of 0.0003 m. A dynamic measurement system automatically calculates the relevant kinematic and kinetic parameters of every repetition of CMJ loaded performed throughout the whole range of motion, providing real-time information on screen and stores data on a disk for subsequent analysis. The RFD max is assessed in the concentric phase – the portion of the jump before take-off in which the change in displacement is positive. Adequate recovery is allowed between all trials (2–3 minutes). Strong verbal encouragement is given to all subjects to motivate them to perform each test action as maximally and rapidly as possible [39].

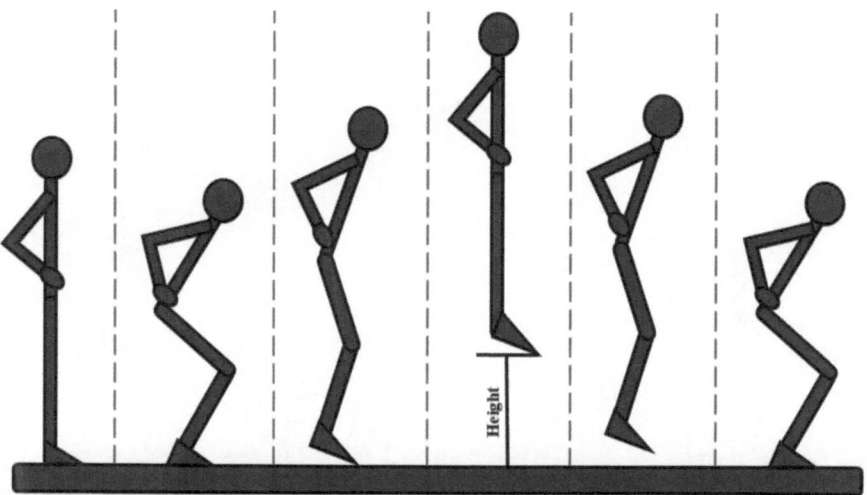

FIGURE 5.3   Countermovement jump test.

Abalakov Jump (ABK) Test. In this test, arm swinging is allowed to assist in generating maximum height. The player stands upright in socks or bare feet, as still as possible on the mat with weight evenly distributed over both feet. When all is ready, the player squats down until the knees are bent at 90 degrees, while swinging the arms back behind the body. Without pausing, the arms are swung forward and the athlete jumps as high as possible, landing back on the mat on both feet at the same time. The take-off must be from both feet, with no initial steps or shuffling, and the player must also not pause at the base of the squat. Record the best result of at least three attempts. One minute of rest is allocated between each trial (Figure 5.4) [40].

Drop Jump (DJ) Test. This test is performed from five standardized drop heights: 20 cm, 40 cm, 60 cm, 80 cm, and 100 cm. In this test, no arm swinging is allowed. The player stands on the box, adjacent to the timing mat. Hands are placed on the hips and stay there throughout the test. The athlete then drops down off the box onto the mat, bending the knees on landing, and then immediately going into a maximal vertical jump. The technique is as per the CMJ. The player jumps vertically as high as possible and back on the mat with both feet landing at the same time. This jump requires players with a good degree of leg strength as the forces through the body are much higher than for a standard vertical jump test. The standard size boxes are not readily available and may even need to be custom-made. Record the best result of at least three attempts. One minute of rest is allocated between each trial (Figure 5.5) [38].

Standing Long Jump Test (Broad Jump). The Broad Jump is a common and easy-to-administer test of explosive leg power. The player stands behind a line marked on the ground with feet slightly apart. A two-foot take-off and landing

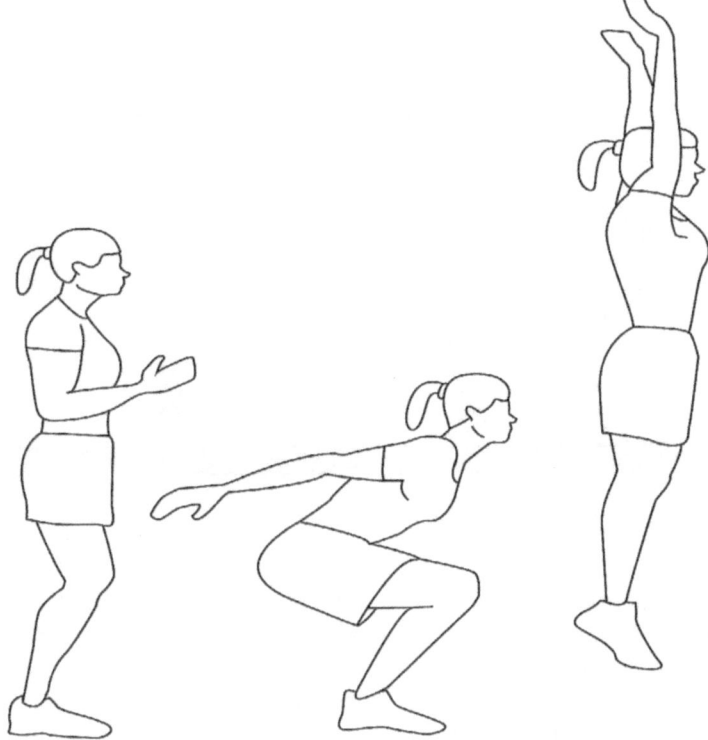

FIGURE 5.4 Abalakov jump test.

is used, with swinging of the arms and bending of the knees to provide forward drive. The subject attempts to jump as far as possible, landing on both feet without falling backward. The measurement is taken from the take-off line to the nearest point of contact on the landing (back of the heels). Record the longest distance jumped, the best of three attempts. One minute of rest is allocated between each trial (Figure 5.6) [41].

5.5.3 Strength tests

Maximal strength test using 1RM or % of 1RM.

Exercise intensity during resistance training has been commonly identified with relative load (percentage of one-repetition maximum, 1RM) or with performing a given maximal number of repetitions in each set (XRM: 5RM, 10RM, 15RM, etc.). However, for several reasons, none of these methods is entirely appropriate for precisely monitoring the real effort the athlete is performing in each training session. Direct assessment of 1RM, however, has some potential disadvantages worth noting. It may be associated with injury when performed incorrectly or by novice subjects, and it is time-consuming and impractical for large groups. Furthermore,

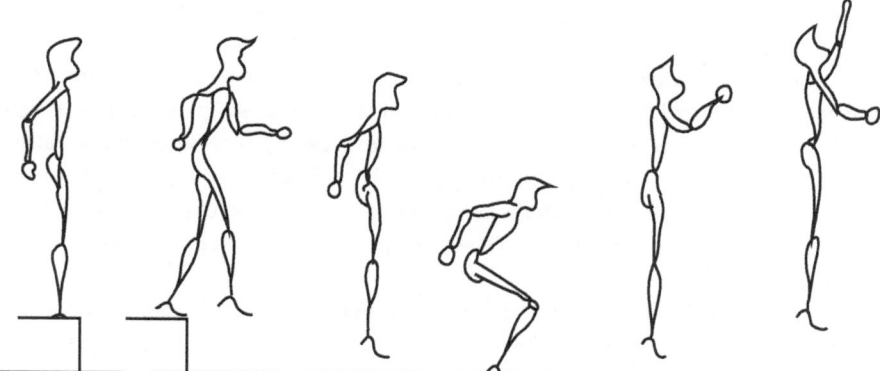

FIGURE 5.5 Drop jump test.

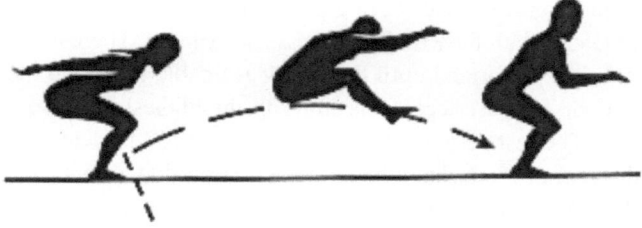

FIGURE 5.6 Standing long jump test.

experience tells us that the actual RM can change quite rapidly after only a few training sessions, and often the obtained value is not the subject's true maximum.

An alternative way to prescribe loading intensity is to determine, through trial and error, the maximum number of repetitions that can be performed with a given submaximal weight. The benefits of a multiple RM test compared to a maximal 1RM test are

- most athletes are not accustomed to using 1RM in training; therefore, multiple repetitions provide greater familiarity to training sets.
- multiple repetitions allow for assessment of the technique during performance of test and allow for the early detection of technique deterioration.
- multiple repetitions can provide for greater reliability in the assessment of strength and power.

Maximal Strength Test using 1 repetition maximum (1RM).

Full Squat. For the maximal dynamic strength (1RM) of the lower limb, full squat (FS) is selected to provide data on maximum strength through the full range of motion of the muscles involved. Players perform an FS assuming an extended position starting from the knee angle (about 180°), with shoulders in contact with a bar. On command, the players perform a controlled eccentric leg flexion until 60°. Then, a concentric leg extension (as fast as possible) starting from the flexed position (60°) to reach full extension of 180° against the resistance determined by the weight plates added to both ends of the bar. The trunk is kept as straight as possible. A safety belt is used by all players. The tests can be performed in a squatting apparatus or with free weight. Warm-ups consist of a set of ten repetitions at loads of 40–60% of the perceived maximum. The last acceptable extension with highest possible load is determined as 1RM. The rest period between actions is always 3 minutes.

Bench Press. For the upper body, the 1RM bench press (BP) is chosen because it involves some arm muscles that are specific to overhand throwing. The test can also be performed in a Smith machine or free weight with an Olympic bar (20 kg) as for the FS. The players lower the bar from a fully extended arm position until the bar is at chest height but not touching and then immediately extend the arms as fast as possible to return to the starting position. Warm-up consists of a set of ten repetitions at loads of 40–60% of the perceived maximum. Thereafter, 4–6 separate single attempts are performed until the player is unable to extend the arms to the required position. The last acceptable lift with the highest possible load is determined as 1RM. The rest period between trials is always 3 minutes.

Maximal Strength Test using a linear velocity transducer (m/s).

Full Squat. A Smith machine or free weight with an Olympic bar (20 kg) can be used to perform the progressive loading test. The full squat (FS) is performed with players starting from the upright position with the knees and hips fully extended, parallel feet stance approximately shoulder width apart, and the barbell resting across the back at the level of the acromion. Each player descends in a continuous motion until the top of the thighs is below the horizontal plane, the posterior thighs and shanks making contact with each other (~35–40° knee flexion), and immediately reversed motion and raise back to the upright position. Unlike the eccentric phase that is performed at a controlled mean velocity (~0.50–0.65 m/s), players are required to always execute the concentric phase at maximal intended velocity. One set of eight repetitions with 20 kg is performed before testing as a warm-up protocol. The initial load is 30 kg and is progressively increased in 10-kg increments until the attained repetition velocity is lower than 0.68 m/s. This results in total increasing loads performed by each player. One set of three repetitions is performed for light loads (1.14 m/s), and only two repetitions are performed for moderate loads (< 1.14 m/s). Strong verbal encouragement is provided to motivate participants to give a maximal effort. Inter-set recoveries range from 3 min (light) to 5 min (heavy loads). The velocity used to calculate the 1RM is the mean propulsive velocity (MPV), which is defined as that fraction of the concentric phase during which barbell acceleration is greater than the acceleration because of gravity [42]. With this progressive loading test are analyzed four variables: (a) estimated 1RM value, which is calculated from the MPV attained against the heaviest load of the test; (b) the average MPV attained against all absolute loads common to pretest and posttest; (c) the average MPV attained for absolute loads moved at velocities equal to or faster than 1 m/s; and (d) average MPV attained for absolute loads moved slower than 1 m/s [42].

Bench Press. A Smith machine or free weight with an Olympic bar (20 kg) can be used to perform the progressive loading test. Players lay supine on a flat bench, with their feet resting flat on the floor and hands placed on the bar slightly wider (2–3 cm) than shoulder width. The position on the bench is carefully adjusted so that the vertical projection of the bar corresponded with each player's intermammary line. The individual position on the bench as well as grip widths are measured so that they can be reproduced on every lift. Players are not allowed to bounce the bar off their chests or raise the shoulders or trunk off the bench. The bar holders are positioned so that the bar stops ~1 cm above each player's chest. After lowering the bar at a controlled mean eccentric velocity (~0.30–0.50 m/s), players stop for ~1.5 sec at the bar holders (momentarily releasing the weight but keeping contact with the bar), and thereafter they perform a purely concentric push at maximal intended velocity. This momentary pause between phases is imposed in order to minimize the contribution of the rebound effect and allow for more reliable, consistent measures [43]. Each player is carefully instructed to always perform the concentric phase of each repetition in an explosive manner, exploding the bar off the chest as fast as possible. Warm-up consists of 5 min of joint mobilization exercises, followed by two sets of eight and six repetitions (3-min rest) with loads of 20 and 30 kg. The initial load is set at 20 kg for all players and is gradually increased in 10-kg increments. The test ends for each player when the attained concentric MPV is lower than 0.35 m/s, which corresponds to ~88% 1RM [44, 45]. During the test, three repetitions are executed for light (MPV > 0.95 m/s), two for medium (0.95 m/s > MPV > 0.55 m/s), and only one for the heaviest (MPV < 0.55 m/s) loads. Inter-set rests range from 2 (light loads) to 4 min (heavy loads). The estimation of 1RM is done for each player from the MPV attained against the heaviest load (kg) lifted in the progressive loading test, as follows: $(100 \cdot \text{load}) / (8.4326 \cdot \text{MPV}^2) - (73.501 \cdot \text{MPV}) + 112.33$ [44].

5.5.4 Field testing

5.5.4.1 Power test

5 Jump Test (5JT). This test is performed on the grass with the players equipped with appropriate football boots. The 5JT consists of five consecutive strides with joined feet position at the start and end of the jumps. From the starting joined feet position, the player is not allowed to perform any back step with any foot; rather, he has to directly jump to the front with a leg of his choice. After the first four strides, i.e., alternating left and right feet for two times each, he has to perform the last stride and end the test again with joined feet. If the player fell back on completion of the last stride, the test is performed again. 5JT performance is measured with a

tape measure from the front edge of the player's feet at the starting position to the rear edge of the feet at the final position. The person assessing the landing has to focus on the last stride of the player in order to exactly determine the last footprint on the grass as the players cannot always stay on their feet on landing. The starting position is set on a fixed point [21].

Throwing-in. This test evaluated the power of the upper body [46]. The standing players are asked to throw the football with both hands as far as possible in the fashion of throwing-in in a real game. The distance is measured to the nearest 0.2 m (Figure 5.7).

Standing Kick. This test assesses both the power of the lower body and the kicking skill [47, 48]. Players are instructed to kick the ball without a run-up (i.e., while the player is stationary) for maximal distance. They are standing with the nondominant leg positioned beside the stationary ball and, while using a preparatory countermovement swing of the kicking leg, kick the ball as fast as possible. The kicking distance is measured to the nearest 0.2 m.

5.5.4.2 Sprint test

10-m Sprint. The ability to rapidly accelerate from a standing position is measured over a 10-m dash initiated from a standing position. The stopwatch starting pedal is positioned behind the starting line. The player must start from a standing position placing his forward foot just behind the starting line and his rear foot on the pedal after having positioned the pedal according to his natural starting position. The timing starts as soon as the foot of the player leaves the pedal. Before testing, each player performs a submaximal sprint to familiarize himself with the test procedure.

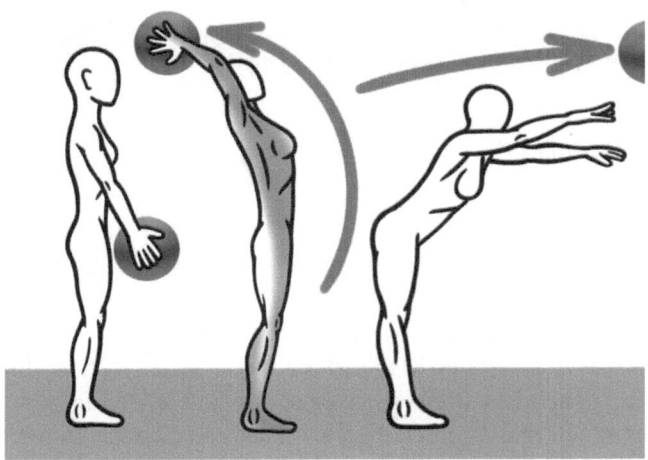

FIGURE 5.7　Throwing-in test.

Flying 20-m Sprint. This test assesses the sprinting ability over a short distance, which should be of particular importance for football [6, 49]. The running time along 20 m following the 10-m maximal acceleration is measured. As a consequence, the players are instructed to run with maximal speed over 30 m, and both the 10-m (i.e., acceleration) and 20-m (i.e., maximal speed over a short distance) tests are obtained from the same trial.

5.5.4.3   Agility and change of direction tests

10 × 5 m Shuttle Test. This test assesses running agility from required rapid changes in directions [5]. Marker cones and/or lines are placed 5 meters apart. Start with a foot at one marker. When instructed by the timer, the player runs to the opposite marker, turns, and returns to the starting line. This is repeated five times without stopping (covering 50 meters in total). At each marker, both feet must fully cross the line. Record the total time taken to complete the 50-m course (Figure 5.8).

Zigzag Test. This test assesses running agility from changes in direction. A zigzag course consists of 4–5-m sections set out at 100° angles. The selection of this test is based on rapid acceleration, deceleration, and balance control required for short running time, which represents the result of the test [6] (Figure 5.9).

Pro Agility Shuttle or 5-10-5 Shuttle Test. Three marker cones are placed along a line 5 meters apart. The player straddles the middle line and puts one hand down in a three-point stance. The player can start by going either to the right or left direction. For example, on the signal "Go," the player turns and runs 5 meters to the right side and touches the line with his right hand. He then runs 10 meters to his left and touches the other line with his left hand and then finally turns and finishes by running back through the start/finish line. The player is required to touch the line at each turn. The time to complete the test in seconds to the nearest two decimals is recorded. The score is the best time of three trials [50].

Illinois Test. The length of the course is 10 meters, and the width is 5 meters. Four cones are used to mark the start, finish, and the two turning points. Another four cones are placed down the center an equal distance apart. Each cone in the center is spaced 3.3 meters apart. Subjects should lie on their front (head to the start line) and hands by their shoulders. On the "Go" command, the stopwatch is

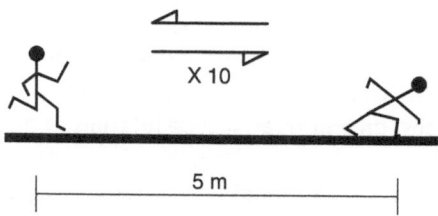

FIGURE 5.8   10 × 5 m Shuttle Test.

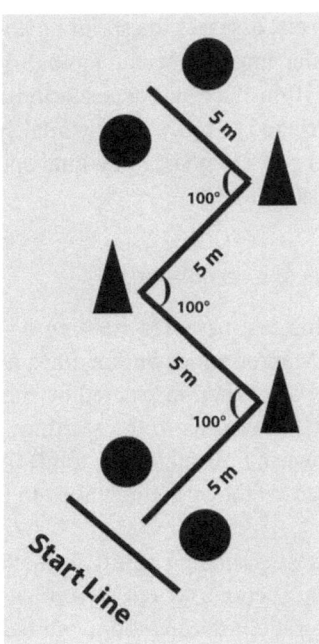

FIGURE 5.9   Diagram of the course used in the zigzag test. Each straight sprint is 5 m and each turn at a flag is 100°.

started, and the athlete gets up as quickly as possible and runs forward 10 meters to run around a cone, then back 10 meters, and then runs up and back through a slalom course of four cones. Finally, the player runs another 10 meters up and back past the finishing cone, at which the timing is stopped. Several trials should be completed, with the best score recorded (Figure 5.10).

T-Test. It should be emphasized that the T-test is clearly a preplanned change of direction speed test rather than a reactive agility test. Set out four cones (5 m and 10 m). The subject starts at cone A. On the command of the timer, the subject sprints to cone B and touches the base of the cone with their right hand. They then turn left and shuffle sideways to cone C and also touches its base, this time with their left hand and then shuffling sideways to the right to cone D and touching the base with the right hand. They then shuffle back to cone B touching with the left hand and run backward to cone A. The stopwatch is stopped as they pass cone A. The trial will not be counted if the subject crosses one foot in front of the other, while shuffling fails to touch the base of the cones or fails to face forward throughout the test. Take the best time of three successful trials to the nearest 0.1 seconds (Figure 5.11) [51, 52].

5-0-5 Agility Test. For the 5-0-5 agility test, two timing gates are placed 5 m from a designated turning point. Athletes assume a starting position 10 m from the timing gates (and therefore 15 m from the turning point). Athletes are instructed to

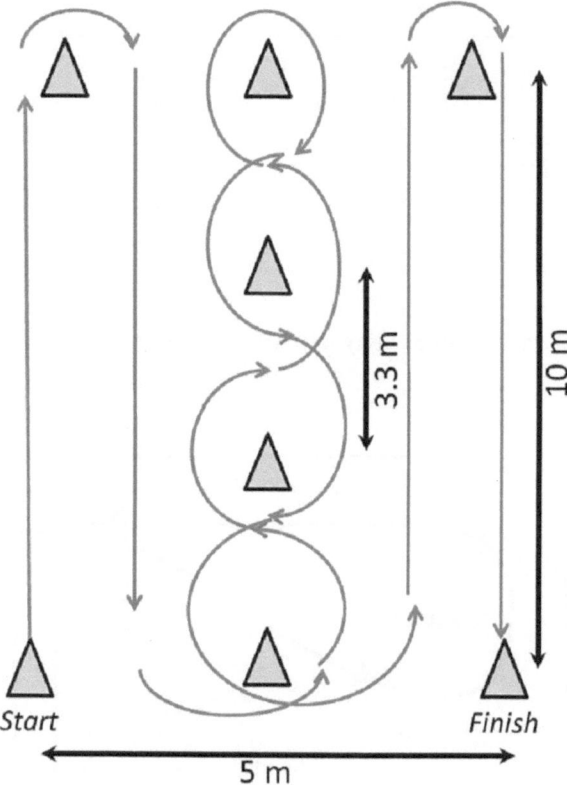

FIGURE 5.10   Diagram of the course used in the Illinois test.

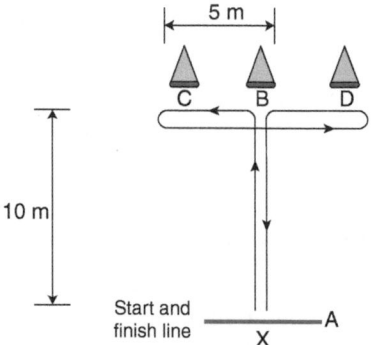

FIGURE 5.11   Diagram of T-test. Adapted from Semeick [52].

accelerate as quickly as possible through the timing gates, pivot on the 15-m line, and return as quickly as possible through the timing gates. The best of two trials is recorded. The turning ability on each leg should be tested. The subject should be encouraged to not overstep the line too much as this will increase their time.

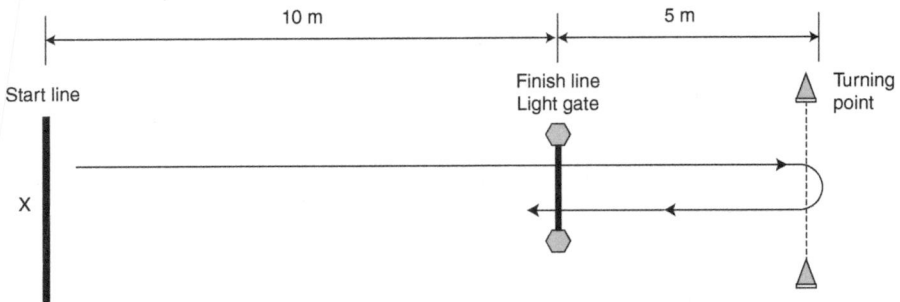

FIGURE 5.12   Diagram of 5-0-5 agility test. Adapted from Gabbett et al. [54].

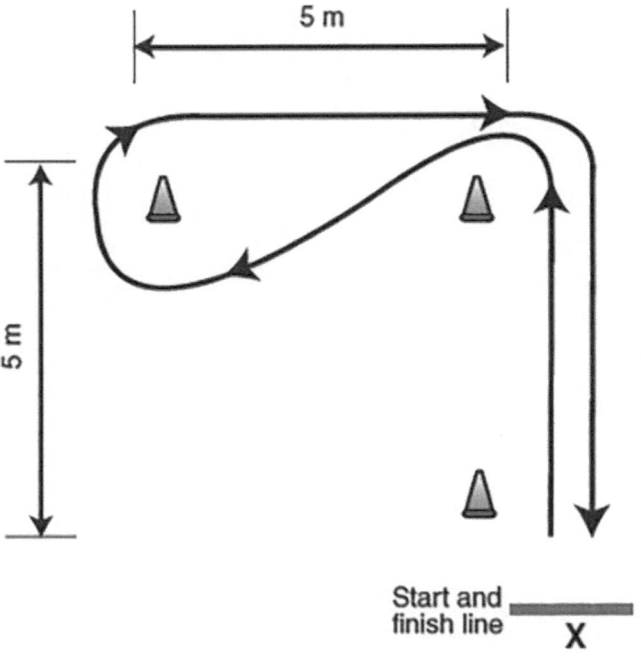

FIGURE 5.13   Diagram of L-run test. Adapted from Gabbett et al. [54].

Record the best time for turning on each side and also the average of both. The change of direction deficit can also be calculated by dividing the 5-0-5 time by the straight line 10-m sprint time (Figure 5.12) [53].

L-Run Test. In this preplanned running test, the player runs 5 m, turns 90° to the left, runs 5 m, makes a full 180° turn around a cone, returns to the original cone, makes another 90° turn, and returns to the start position (Figure 5.13) [54].

Hexagonal Agility Test. Using an athletic tape, mark a hexagon (six-sided shape) on the floor. The length of each side should be 60.5 cm, and each angle

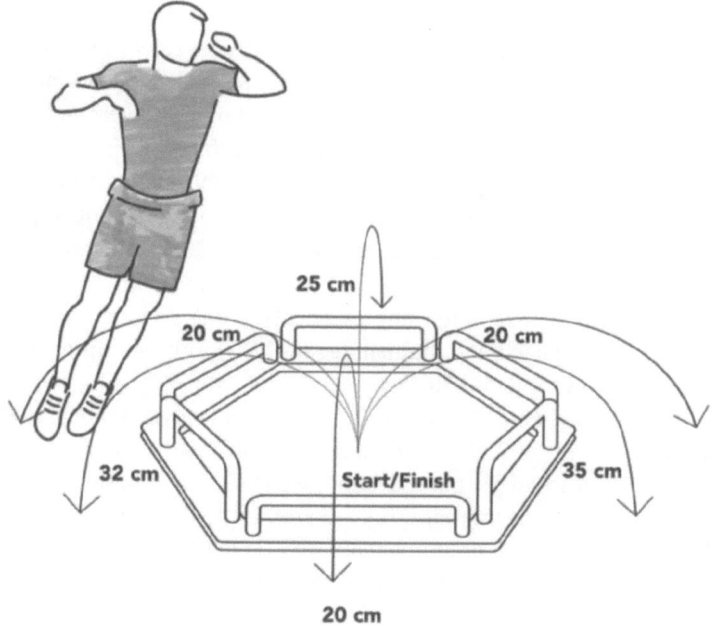

25 cm

20 cm   20 cm

32 cm   Start/Finish   35 cm

20 cm

FIGURE 5.14   Hexagonal agility test.

should work out to be 120 degrees. The player begins with both feet together in the middle of the hexagon facing the front line. On the command "Go," they jump ahead across the line and then back over the same line into the middle of the hexagon. Then, continuing to face forward with the feet together, they jump over the next side and back into the hexagon. Continue this pattern for three full revolutions, continuing to face forward throughout the test. Perform the test both clockwise and anti-clockwise. The player score is the time taken to complete three full revolutions. The best score from two trials is recorded. Comparison of the anti-clockwise and clockwise directions will show if any imbalances exist between left and right movement skills (Figure 5.14).

5.6   Adaptations associated to strength and muscle power in football players after explosive training

5.6.1   Power adaptations specific to football

Although a considerable number of studies reported football-specific adaptations after explosive training (EXT) programs, most of these focused on the kicking ability of youth male football players [55–65]. Although not all studies reported significant changes [66], among those that reported significant improvements, the age of the participants ranges from 10.3 to 15.5 years, and the training programs lasted between 6 and 12 weeks, with improvements in kicking velocity between 7 and 16% and in kicking distance between 11 and 37%. Greater improvements were observed after EXT programs that incorporated a progressive load increase (e.g., volume) [67], a combination of vertical–horizontal and unilateral–bilateral drills [68], loaded jumps [59, 65], and different types of surfaces [64].

Similar findings were noted among youth female [69], young adult female [62, 70], and young adult male football players [71], with significant improvements in kicking velocity (8–13%) and kicking distance (~23%) after 8–12 weeks of training.

For those studies that reported improvements in the kicking performance for the dominant (7–12%) and non-dominant leg (8–13%), similar improvements were observed between legs [40, 56, 70, 71].

Aside from kicking velocity/distance, two studies analyzed the effects of EXT on the dribbling ability [72, 73], with somewhat different findings. In one study, youth (age 12–17 years) male players improved (6–33%) in 20-m sprint with ball dribbling after 6 weeks of training [72]. In contrast, male youth players (age ~11 years) showed no significant improvement (~3%) in the Illinois test while dribbling a football [73] after 8 weeks of training. If differences between the testing conditions or between the training programs might explain the different findings between studies, future studies should clarify this.

Overall, evidence suggests that improvements in some relevant football-specific outcomes may be induced with EXT programs. Such adaptations may offer to the football player some advantage over its opponent during matches. The mechanisms underlying football-specific improvements are not clear, with further research needed to clarify these.

5.6.2 Balance

The effects of EXT on balance performance have been analyzed among male youth football players between ~11 and ~16 years of age, after interventions between 4 and 8 weeks [74–82]. Balance was measured using field-based tests (i.e., stork balance test; Y balance test) and laboratory-based tests (e.g., balance-force plates), under different conditions (i.e., stable surface, unstable surface, one-leg stance, two-leg stance, eyes open, and eyes closed) and different directions (i.e., mediolateral/anterior, anterior–posterior, and medial–lateral), with improvements between 3% and 211% (Effect Size [ES] = 0.2 up to 5.3).

Greater improvement in balance was noted when EXT included an unstable surface [79], although such finding was not replicated in another study [75]. However, the combination of stable and unstable surfaces seems to offer some advantage over a stable surface only [80]. Similarly, the combination of unilateral–bilateral and vertical–horizontal drills seems to offer greater balance improvements [61]. When jump drills are combined with balance drills, it seems that the application of balance drills before jumping exercises seems particularly effective [74, 76].

Overall, improvements in balance may be expected after 4–8 weeks of training. The combination of stable and unstable surfaces, unilateral–bilateral and vertical–horizontal jump drills, in addition to balance drills (particularly when these are applied before jumping exercises), might offer greater chances of meaningful balance improvements after EXT interventions. However, most evidence currently comes from youth male football players. Further studies may be needed in other specific groups of football players before robust conclusions can be derived.

5.6.3 Maximal strength

Only one study reported maximal strength among youth female football players (age ~17 years) [83]. After 10 weeks of training (resistance training [RT] and high-intensity anaerobic sprints, mixed with jumps), within-group increases were noted for 1RM squat, leg extension, and calves (~5–30 kg). However, strength measurements were conducted only in the experimental group, precluding a comparison with the control group.

Similarly, only two studies reported strength-related outcomes in adult female football players. One study recruited young adult players (age ~19 years) [84]. After 10 weeks of training (jumps mixed with RT, sprint, and agility drills), no significant within-group changes (−1.6–6.3%) were noted for maximal isometric strength of knee flexors or extensors in the dominant or non-dominant leg. Similarly, among young adult female football players (age ~19 years) [85], after 10 weeks of training (jumps mixed with RT, sprint, and agility drills), no significant within-group changes were observed. The lack of changes included the normalized peak isometric strength of the hip internal and external rotators, knee flexors or extensors, and hip abductors, for both legs. A lack of changes was noted also for the hip extensors (right leg) and hip adductors (left leg). Only the hip extensors (left leg), hip flexors (both legs), and adductors (right leg) increased normalized peak isometric strength.

One study [86] reported a mixed sample of adult female and male football players. After 11 weeks of either traditional RT combined with weightlifting drills, or RT combined with jumps, a meaningful improvement (~300%) was noted in 4RM squat, although the improvement was similar between the groups.

Among youth male football players, one study recruited players (mean age 17.3–17.6 years) during 8 weeks of training (jumps combined with RT), using either unilateral or bilateral drills [62]. The bilateral group showed significant within-group improvements in 1RM knee extension (13%, ES, ~0.8) and flexion (7%, ES, ~0.5). The unilateral group showed a marginal significant improvement only in knee extension 1RM (2%; ES, ~0.3). Another study with youth male football players (age ~16 years) included 8 weeks of EXT or jump plus RT [87]. Compared to a control group, only the group that combined jumps plus RT achieved a significant improvement in 1RM half squat (~46%). In another study with youth male football players (mean age 14.7 years) [88], after 6 weeks of training (jumps, combined with RT, sprints, and COD drills), a significant increase in 1RM squat (28.5%) was noted compared to a control group. Similarly, in another study [89] with youth male football players (mean age 12.7 years), after 6 weeks of training (jumps, combined with RT, sprints, and COD drills), a significant increase in 1RM squat (52.0%) was noted compared to a control group. In another study [58] with youth male football players (mean age 10.7 years), after 12 weeks of EXT, a significant increase in back squat strength (28.0%) was noted compared to a control group. In another study [74] with male youth football players (age 13–14 years), after 8 weeks of training (jumps, combined with balance drills), a significant within-group increase in knee extensor maximal voluntary isometric strength was noted. Of note, after training involving balance and jumps in the same set (78%) or after training involving balance sets completed before jump sets (59%), the improvements were similar. In another study [90] with youth male football players (mean age 12.6 years), after 8 weeks of EXT, an increase in isometric peak torque (15.4%) but not dynamic peak torque (6.4%) was noted compared to a control group. In another study [73], compared to a control group, youth male football players (age 11 years) showed no significant improvements in the strength performance of the back extensor (15.9%; 12.6%) or knee extensor muscles (39.0%; 41.2%) after 8 weeks of jump training combined with either balance or COD drills, respectively. In another study [91], youth male football players (age 17.8 years), after 5 weeks of training (jumps, combined with RT, sprints, and COD drills), showed no improvement in a series of strength measures (0.5–8.7%; dominant and non-dominant leg peak torque of knee flexor and extensor muscles) compared to a group that used RT only. In another study [92], in youth male football players (age 12.7 years), after 12 weeks of EXT, an increase in half-squat maximal strength (4.2%) was noted compared to a control group. In another study [62] with youth male football players (mean age 13–14 years), compared to a control group, after 7 weeks of EXT, a significant improvement was noted in 5RM squat after training with a fixed drop jump height (10.6%) or an optimal drop jump height (18.1%). In another study [63], among youth male football players (age 13.2 years), after 7 weeks of EXT, a significant improvement in 5RM squat (11.9%) was noted compared to the control group.

Among adult male football players (median age 21 years; range 18–24.5), 11 studies provided outcome measures related to maximal strength. In one study [93], after 8 weeks of training (jumps combined with RT and sprints), no significant improvement in 1RM squat (21.7%) was noted compared with a control group that completed an RT program. In another study [94], after 6 weeks of training (jumps, combined with RT and sprints), a within-group increase was noted in 1RM squat (7.4%) after a complex training approach, but not after a block training approach (7.3%). In another study [95], after 8 weeks of either loaded EXT or unloaded jumps (i.e., body-mass only), relatively greater improvements were noted after loaded training, including 1RM squat (13% and 7%, respectively), quadriceps concentric (16% and 10%, respectively), and eccentric peak torque

(24% and 15%, respectively), as well as hamstring eccentric peak torque (15% and 17%, respectively). In another study [96], after 8 weeks of EXT combined with RT (i.e., either as complex training, traditional training, or contrast training), within-group improvements were noted in half-squat 1RM (46–53%). In another study [97], 7 weeks of training (jumps, mixed with RT and sprint drills) induced meaningful improvements (4–15%) in several measures of maximal strength (i.e., peak toque in concentric and eccentric quadriceps and hamstring muscle actions, dominant and non-dominant limbs) when compared to a control group. In another study [98], after 9 weeks of EXT, significant improvements were noted in several measures of maximal strength (i.e., 1RM squat, 1RM plantar flexors dominant and non-dominant limbs, 1RM knee extensor dominant and non-dominant limbs, quadriceps concentric peak torque dominant limb, and hamstrings concentric and eccentric peak torque dominant and non-dominant limbs) when compared to a control group. However, slightly greater improvements were noted after EXT combined with RT (i.e., complex training) (mean 17%, range 4–39%) compared to EXT alone (mean 10%, range 0–31%). In another study [99], after 7 weeks of training (jumps, combined with RT, sprints, and COD drills), significant improvements (17–29%) were noted in several measures of maximal strength (i.e., 1RM half squat, isometric peak force bilateral, dominant, and non-dominant limbs) when compared to a control group. In another study [100], after 6 weeks of EXT, a significant improvement (7.5%) was noted for knee extensors' maximal voluntary isometric strength when compared to a control group. In another study [101], after 6 weeks of training EXT, 3RM squat showed a within-group improvement of ES 0.27 (absolute, kg) and 0.35 (relative, kg.kg-1). In another study [102], after 8 weeks of training (jumps combined with RT), although a significant within-group improvement was noted for 1RM half squat (22.9%), when compared to a control group (i.e., RT only; improvement 25.9%), no significant difference was noted between the groups. In another study [103], after 6 weeks of training (jumps, combined with RT, sprints, and COD drills), 1RM squat increased 13.4% compared to a control group.

Overall, contrasting finding was noted on the effects of EXT on maximal strength, with significant improvements in some, but not all studies and/or groups of football players. Significant improvements were more consistent after EXT combined with RT. It seems that EXT drills with greater/optimal intensity, including overloads (e.g., jump squat) and more specific to the strength measure (e.g., bilateral jumps for bilateral squat), may increase the effectiveness of EXT interventions for the improvement of maximal strength performance.

References

1. Impellizzeri, FM, Marcora, SM, Castagna, C, Reilly, T, Sassi, A, Iaia, FM, and Rampinini, E. Physiological and performance effects of generic versus specific aerobic training in soccer players. *Int J Sports Med* 27, 483–492, 2006.

2. Bangsbo, J, Norregaard, L, and Thorso, F. Activity profile of competition soccer. *Can J Sport Sci* 16, 110–116, 1991.

3. Reilly, T, and Thomas, V. A motion analysis of work-rate in different positional roles in professional football match-play. *J Hum Mov Stud* 2, 87–97, 1976.

4. Castagna, C, D'Ottavio, S, and Abt, G. Activity profile of young soccer players during actual match play. *J Strength Cond Res* 17, 775–780, 2003.

5. Reilly, T, Bangsbo, J, and Franks, A. Anthropometric and physiological predispositions for elite soccer. *J Sports Sci* 18, 669–683, 2000.

6. Little, T and Williams, AG. Specificity of acceleration, maximum speed, and agility in professional soccer players. *J Strength Cond Res* 19, 76–78, 2005.

7. Delecluse, CH, Van Coppenolle, H, Willems, E, Diels, R, Goris, M, and Van Leemputte, M. Analysis of 100m sprint performance as a multi-dimensional skill. *J Hum Mov Stud* 28, 87–101, 1995.

8. Moir, G, Sanders, R, Button, C, and Glaister, M. The effect of periodised resistance training on accelerative sprint performance. *Sports Biomech* 6, 285–300, 2007.

9. Bradley, PS, Sheldon, W, Wooster, B, Olsen, P, Boanas, P, and Krustrup, P. High intensity running in English FA Premier League soccer matches. *J Sports Sci* 27, 159–168, 2009.

10. Stolen, T, Chamari, K, Castagna, C, and Wisloff, U. Physiology of soccer: An update. *Sports Med* 35, 501–536, 2005.

11. Chelly, MS, Cherif, N, BenAmar, M, Hermassi, S, Fathloun, M, Bouhlel, E, Tabka, Z, and Shephard, R. Relationships of peak leg power, 1-RM half back squat and leg muscle volume to 5-m sprint performance of junior soccer players. *J Strength Cond Res* 24, 266–271, 2010.

12. Chelly, MS, Fathloun, M, Cherif, N, Ben Amar, M, Tabka, Z, and Van Praagh, E. Effects of a back squat training program on leg power, jump- and sprint performances in junior soccer players. *J Strength Cond Res* 23, 2241–2249, 2009.

13. Mirkov, D, Nedeljkovic, A, Kukolj, M, Ugarkovic, D, and Jaric, S. Evaluation of the reliability of soccer-specific field tests. *J Strength Cond Res* 22, 1046–1050, 2008.

14. Young, WB, McDowell, MH, and Scarlett, BJ. Specificity of sprint and agility training methods. *J Strength Cond Res* 15, 315–319, 2001.

15. Wisløff, U, Helgerud, J, and Hoff, J. Strength and endurance of elite soccer players. *Med Sci Sports Exerc* 30, 462–467, 1998.

16. Verheijen, R. Handbuch fur Fussballkondition. In: Sporis, G, Jukic, I, Milanovic, L, and Vucetic, V. Reliability and factorial validity of agility tests for soccer players. *J Strength Cond Res* 24(3), 679–686, 2010.

17. Bangsbo, J. Time and motion characteristics of competition soccer. In: Reilly, T and Korkusuz, F, eds. *Science football* (vol 6). London: Routledge, 1992, pp. 34–40.

18. Hoff, J, and Helgerud, J. Endurance and strength training for soccer players: Physiological considerations. *Sports Med* 34, 165–180, 2004.

19. Sáez de Villarreal, E, Suarez-Arrones, L, Requena, B, Haff, GG, and Ferrete, C. Effects of plyometric and sprint training on physical and technical skill performance in adolescent soccer players. *J Strength Cond Res* 29(7), 1894–1903, 2015.

20. Ferrete, C, Requena, B, Suarez-Arrones, L, and Saez de Villarreal, E. Effect of strength and high-intensity training on jumping, sprinting, and intermittent endurance performance in prepubertal soccer players. *J Strength Cond Res* 28(2), 413–422, 2014.

21. Chamari, K, Chaouachi, A, Hambli, M, Kaouech, F, Wisloff, U, and Castagna, C. The five-jump test for distance as a field test to assess lower limb explosive power in soccer players. *J Strength Cond Res* 22(3), 944–950, 2008.

22. Ronnestad, BR, Kvamme, NH, Sunde, A, and Raastad, T. Short-term effects of strength and plyometric training on sprint and jump performance in professional soccer players. *J Strength Cond Res* 22, 773–780, 2008.
23. Nuzzo, JL, McBride, JM, Cormi, P, and McCaulley, GO. Relationship between countermovement jump performance and multijoint isometric and dynamic tests of strength. *J Strength Cond Res* 23, 699–707, 2008.
24. Tanner, RK and Gore, CJ. *Physiological tests for elite athletes.* Champaigne, IL: Human Kinetics, 2000.
25. Abernethy, P, Wilson, G, and Logan, P. Strength and power assessment: Issues, controversies and challenges. *Sports Med* 19(6), 401–417, 1995.
26. Nosaka, K, Sakamoto, K, Newton, M, and Sacco, P. The repeated bout effect of reduced-load eccentric exercise on elbow flexor muscle damage. *Eur J Appl Physiol* 85, 34–40, 2001.
27. Vukovich, M and Michaelis, J. Effect of two different creatine supplementation products on muscular strength and power. *Sports Med Training and Rehab* 8(4), 369–383, 1999.
28. Volek, JF, Duncan, ND, Mazzetti, SA, Staron, RS, Putukian, M, Gomez, AL, Pearson, DR, Fink, WJ, and Kraemer, WJ. Performance and muscle fibre adaptations to creatine supplementation and heavy resistance training. *Med Sci Sports Exercise* 31(8), 1147–1156, 1999.
29. Stout, J, Eckerson, J, Ebersole, K, Moore, G, Perry, S, Housh, T, Bull, A, Cramer, J, and Batheja, A. Effect of creatine loading on neuromuscular fatigue threshold. *J Appl Physiol* 88, 109–112, 2000.
30. Izquierdo, M, Ibanez, J, Gonzalez-Badillo, JJ, and Gorostiaga, EM. Effects of creatine supplementation on muscle power, endurance, and sprint performance. *Med. Sci. Sports Exercise* 34(2), 332–343, 2002.
31. Atkinson, G, and Reilly, T. Circadian variation in sports performance. *Sports Med* 21(4), 292–312, 1996.
32. Winget, CM, DeRoshia, CW, and Holley, DC. Circadian rhythms and athletic performance. *Med Sci Sports Exerc* 17(5), 498–516, 1985.
33. Harris, J, and Elbourn, J. *Warming up and cooling down.* 2nd edition, Champaigne, IL: Human Kinetics, 2002.
34. Murphy, AJ, and Wilson, GJ. The assessment of human dynamic muscular function: A comparison of isoinertial and isokinetic tests. *J Sports Med Phys Fit* 36, 169–177, 1996.
35. MacDougall, JD, and Wenger, HA. The purpose of physiological testing. In: MacDougall JD, Wenger HA, Green HJ, eds. *Physiological testing of high-performance athlete.* Champaign, IL: Human Kinetics, 1991, pp. 1–5.
36. Svensson, M, and Drust, B. Testing soccer players. *J Sports Sci* 23, 601–618, 2005.
37. Kotzamanidis, C, Chatzopoulos, D, Michailidis, C, Papaiakovou, G, and Patikas, D. The effect of a combined high intensity strength and speed training program on the running and jumping ability of soccer players. *J Strength Cond Res* 19(2), 369–375, 2005.
38. Saez de Villarreal, E, Gonzalez-Badillo, JJ, and Izquierdo, M. Low and moderate plyometric training frequency produce greater jumping and sprinting gains compared with high frequency. *J Strength Cond Res* 22, 715–725, 2008.
39. Sáez de Villarreal, E, Izquierdo, M, and Gonzalez-Badillo, JJ. Enhancing jump performance after combined vs. Maximal power, heavy-resistance, and plyometric training alone. *J Strength Cond Res* 25(12), 3274–3281, 2011.
40. Sáez de Villarreal, E, Suarez-Arrones, L, Requena, B, Haff, GG, and Ferrete, C. Effects of plyometric and sprint training on physical and technical skill performance in adolescent soccer players. *J Strength Cond Res* 29(7), 1894–1903, 2015.

41. Domınguez-Dıez, M, Castillo, D, Raya-Gonzalez, J, Sanchez-Dıaz, S, Soto-Celix, M, Rendo Urteaga, T, and Lago-Rodríguez, Á. Comparison of multidirectional jump performance and lower limb passive range of motion profile between soccer and basketball young players. *PLoS ONE* 16(1), e0245277, 2021.

42. Sanchez-Medina, L, Perez, CE, and Gonzalez-Badillo, JJ. Importance of the propulsive phase in strength assessment. *Int J Sports Med* 31, 123–129, 2010.

43. Pallarés, JG, Sánchez-Medina, L, Pérez, CE, de la Cruz-Sánchez, E, and Mora-Rodríguez, R. Imposing a pause between the eccentric and concentric phases increases the reliability of isoinertial strength assessments. *J Sports Sci* 32, 1165–1175, 2014.

44. González-Badillo, JJ, and Sánchez-Medina, L. Movement velocity as a measure of loading intensity in resistance training. *Int J Sports Med* 31, 347–352, 2010.

45. Sánchez-Medina, L, González-Badillo, JJ, Pérez, CE, and Pallarés, JG. Velocity- and power-load relationships of the bench pull vs. bench press exercises. *Int J Sports Med* 35, 209–216, 2014.

46. Kukolj, M, Ugarkovic, D, and Jaric, S. Profiling anthropometric characteristics and functional performance of 12 to 18 years-old elite junior soccer players. *J Hum Mov Stud* 45, 403–418, 2003.

47. Markovic, G, Dizdar, D, and Jaric, S. Evaluation of tests of maximum kicking performance. *J Sports Phys Fitness* 46, 215–220, 2006.

48. McCrudden, M, and Reilly, TA. A Comparison of the punt and the drop-kick. In: Reilly T, Clarrys J, and Stibbe A, eds. *Science and football* II. London: E & FN Spon, 1993, pp. 362–368.

49. Cometti G, Maffiuletti NA, Pousson M, Chatard, JC, and Maffulli, N. Isokinetic strength and anaerobic power of elite, subelite and amateur French soccer players. *Int J Sports Med* 22, 45–51, 2001.

50. Holmberg, P. Preseason preparatory training for a division III women's college basketball team. *Strength Cond J* 32(6), 42–54, 2010.

51. Pauole, K, Madole, K, Garhammer, J, Lacourse, M, and Rozenek, R. Reliability and validity of the t-test as a measure of agility, leg power, and leg speed in collegeaged men and women. *J Strength Cond Res* 14(4), 443–450, 2000.

52. Semenick, D. Tests and measurements: the T test. *Nat Strength Cond Assoc J* 12(1), 36–37, 1990.

53. Draper, JA, and Lancaster, MG. The 505 test: A test for agility in the horizontal plane. *Aus J Sci Med Sport* 17(1), 15–18, 1985.

54. Gabbett, TJ, Kelly, JN, and Sheppard, JM. Speed, change of direction speed, and reactive agility of rugby league players. *J Strength Cond Res* 22(1), 174–181, 2008.

55. Bouguezzi, R, Chaabene, H, Negra, Y, Ramirez-Campillo, R, Jlalia, Z, Mkaouer, B, and Hachana, Y. Effects of different plyometric training frequency on measures of athletic performance in prepuberal male soccer players. *J Strength Cond Res* 34(6), 1609–1617, 2020.

56. García-Pinillos, F, Martínez-Amat, A, Hita-Contreras, F, Martínez-López, EJ, and Latorre-Román, PA. Effects of a contrast training program without external load on vertical jump, kicking speed, sprint, and agility of young soccer players. *J Strength Cond Res* 28(9), 2452–2460, 2014.

57. Marques, MC, Pereira, A, Reis, IG, and van den Tillaar, R. Does an in-season 6-week combined sprint and jump training program improve strength-speed abilities and kicking performance in young soccer players? *J Hum Kinet* 39, 157–166, 2013.

58. Michailidis, Y, Fatouros, IG, Primpa, E, Michailidis, C, Avloniti, A, Chatzinikolaou, A, and Kambas, A. Plyometrics trainability in preadolescent soccer athletes. *J Strength Cond Res* 27(1), 38–49, 2013.

59. Negra, Y, Chaabene, H, Sammoud, S, Prieske, O, Moran, J, Ramirez-Campillo, R, and Granacher, U. The increased effectiveness of loaded versus unloaded plyometric jump training in improving muscle power, speed, change of direction, and kicking-distance performance in prepubertal male soccer players. *Int J Sports Physiol Perform* 15(2), 189–195, 2020.

60. Ramirez-Campillo, R, Meylan, C, Alvarez, C, Henriquez-Olguin, C, Martinez, C, Canas-Jamett, R, and Izquierdo, M. Effects of in-season low-volume high-intensity plyometric training on explosive actions and endurance of young soccer players. *J Strength Cond Res* 28(5), 1335–1342, 2014.

61. Ramirez-Campillo, R, Henriquez-Olguin, C, Burgos, C, Andrade, DC, Zapata, D, Martinez, C, and Izquierdo, M. Effect of progressive volume-based overload during plyometric training on explosive and endurance performance in young soccer players. *J Strength Cond Res* 29(7), 1884–1893, 2015.

62. Ramirez-Campillo, R, Sanchez-Sanchez, J, Gonzalo-Skok, O, Rodriguez-Fernandez, A, Carretero, M, and Nakamura, FY. Specific changes in young soccer player's fitness after traditional bilateral vs. unilateral combined strength and plyometric training. *Front Physiol* 9, 265, 2018.

63. Ramirez-Campillo, R, Alvarez, C, Garcia-Pinillos, F, Gentil, P, Moran, J, Pereira, LA, and Loturco, I. Effects of plyometric training on physical performance of young male soccer players: potential effects of different drop jump heights. *Pediatr Exerc Sci* 31(3), 306–313, 2019.

64. Ramirez-Campillo, R, Alvarez, C, Garcia-Pinillos, F, Garcia-Ramos, A, Loturco, I, Chaabene, H, and Granacher, U. Effects of combined surfaces vs. single-surface plyometric training on soccer players' physical fitness. *J Strength Cond Res* 34(9), 2644–2653, 2020.

65. Rosas, F, Ramirez-Campillo, R, Diaz, D, Abad-Colil, F, Martinez-Salazar, C, Caniuqueo, A, and Izquierdo, M. Jump training in youth soccer players: effects of haltere type handheld loading. *Int J Sports Med* 37(13), 1060–1065, 2016.

66. Ramirez-Campillo, R, Alvarez, C, García-Pinillos, F, Sanchez-Sanchez, J, Yanci, J, Castillo, D, and Izquierdo, M. Optimal reactive strength index: is it an accurate variable to optimize plyometric training effects on measures of physical fitness in young soccer players? *J Strength Cond Res* 32(4), 885–893, 2018.

67. Ramirez-Campillo, R, Burgos, CH, Henriquez-Olguin, C, Andrade, DC, Martinez, C, Alvarez, C, and Izquierdo, M. Effect of unilateral, bilateral, and combined plyometric training on explosive and endurance performance of young soccer players. *J Strength Cond Res* 29(5), 1317–1328, 2015.

68. Ramirez-Campillo, R, Gallardo, F, Henriquez-Olguin, C, Meylan, CM, Martinez, C, Alvarez, C, and Izquierdo, M. Effect of vertical, horizontal, and combined plyometric training on explosive, balance, and endurance performance of young soccer players. *J Strength Cond Res* 29(7), 1784–1795, 2015.

69. Rubley, MD, Haase, AC, Holcomb, WR, Girouard, TJ, and Tandy, RD. The effect of plyometric training on power and kicking distance in female adolescent soccer players. *J Strength Cond Res* 25(1), 129–134, 2011.

70. Sedano Campo, S, Vaeyens, R, Philippaerts, RM, Redondo, JC, de Benito, AM, and Cuadrado, G. Effects of lower-limb plyometric training on body composition,

explosive strength, and kicking speed in female soccer players. *J Strength Cond Res* 23(6), 1714–1722, 2009.

71. Sedano, S, Matheu, A, Redondo, JC, and Cuadrado, G. Effects of plyometric training on explosive strength, acceleration capacity and kicking speed in young elite soccer players. *J Sports Med Phys Fitness* 51(1), 50–58, 2011.

72. Asadi, A, Ramirez-Campillo, R, Arazi, H, and Saez de Villarreal, E. The effects of maturation on jumping ability and sprint adaptations to plyometric training in youth soccer players. *J Sports Sci* 36(21), 2405–2411, 2018.

73. Makhlouf, I, Chaouachi, A, Chaouachi, M, Ben Othman, A, Granacher, U, and Behm, DG. Combination of agility and plyometric training provides similar training benefits as combined balance and plyometric training in young soccer players. *Front Physiol* 9, 1611, 2018.

74. Chaouachi, M, Granacher, U, Makhlouf, I, Hammami, R, Behm, DG, and Chaouachi, A. Within session sequence of balance and plyometric exercises does not affect training adaptations with youth soccer athletes. *J Sports Sci Med* 16(1), 125–136, 2017.

75. Granacher, U, Prieske, O, Majewski, M, Büsch, D, and Muehlbauer, T. The role of instability with plyometric training in sub-elite adolescent soccer players. *Int J Sports Med* 36(5), 386–394, 2015.

76. Hammami, R, Granacher, U, Makhlouf, I, Behm, DG, and Chaouachi, A. Sequencing effects of balance and plyometric training on physical performance in youth soccer athletes. *J Strength Cond Res* 30(12), 3278–3289, 2016.

77. Huang, PY, Chen, WL, Lin, CF, and Lee, HJ. Lower extremity biomechanics in athletes with ankle instability after a 6-week integrated training program. *J Athl Train* 49(2), 163–172, 2014.

78. Myer, GD, Ford, KR, Brent, JL, and Hewett, TE. The effects of plyometric vs. dynamic stabilization and balance training on power, balance, and landing force in female athletes. *J Strength Cond Res* 20(2), 345–353, 2006.

79. Negra, Y, Chaabene, H, Sammoud, S, Bouguezzi, R, Abbes, MA, Hachana, Y, and Granacher, U. Effects of plyometric training on physical fitness in prepuberal soccer athletes. *Int J Sports Med* 38(5), 370–377, 2017.

80. Negra, Y, Chaabene, H, Sammoud, S, Bouguezzi, R, Mkaouer, B, Hachana, Y, and Granacher, U. Effects of plyometric training on components of physical fitness in prepuberal male soccer athletes: the role of surface instability. *J Strength Cond Res* 31(12), 3295–3304, 2017.

81. Sporri, D, Ditroilo, M, Rodriguez, ECP, Johnston, RJ, Sheehan, WB, and Watsford, ML. The effect of water-based plyometric training on vertical stiffness and athletic performance. *PLoS One* 13(12), 11, 2018.

82. Trecroci, A, Cavaggioni, L, Caccia, R, and Alberti, G. Jump rope training: balance and motor coordination in preadolescent soccer players. *J Sports Sci Med* 14(4), 792–798, 2015.

83. Siegler, J, Gaskill, S, and Ruby, B. Changes evaluated in soccer-specific power endurance either with or without a 10-week, in-season, intermittent, high-intensity training protocol. *J Strength Cond Res* 17(2), 379–387, 2003.

84. Grieco, CR, Cortes, N, Greska, EK, Lucci, S, and Onate, JA. Effects of a combined resistance-plyometric training program on muscular strength, running economy, and Vo2peak in division I female soccer players. *J Strength Cond Res* 26(9), 2570–2576, 2012.

85. Greska, EK, Cortes, N, Van Lunen, BL, and Oñate, JA. A feedback inclusive neuro-muscular training program alters frontal plane kinematics. *J Strength Cond Res* 26(6), 1609–1619, 2012.

86. Moore, EWG, Hickey, MS, and Reiser Ii, RF. Comparison of two twelve-week off-season combined training programs on entry level collegiate soccer players' performance. *J Strength Cond Res* 19(4), 791–798, 2005.

87. Hammami, M, Gaamouri, N, Shephard, RJ, and Chelly, MS. Effects of contrast strength vs. plyometric training on lower-limb explosive performance, ability to change direction and neuromuscular adaptation in soccer players. *J Strength Cond Res* 33(8), 2094–2103, 2019.

88. Franco-Márquez, F, Rodríguez-Rosell, D, González-Suárez, JM, Pareja-Blanco, F, Mora-Custodio, R, Yañez-García, JM, and González-Badillo, JJ. Effects of combined resistance training and plyometrics on physical performance in young soccer players. *Int J Sports Med* 36(11), 906–914, 2015.

89. Rodríguez-Rosell, D, Franco-Márquez, F, Pareja-Blanco, F, Mora-Custodio, R, Yáñez-García, JM, González-Suárez, JM, and González-Badillo, JJ. Effects of 6 weeks resistance training combined with plyometric and speed exercises on physical performance of pre-peak-height-velocity soccer players. *Int J Sports Physiol Perform* 11(2), 240–246, 2016.

90. McKinlay, BJ, Wallace, P, Dotan, R, Long, D, Tokuno, C, Gabriel, DA, and Falk, B. Effects of plyometric and resistance training on muscle strength, explosiveness, and neuromuscular function in young adolescent soccer players. *J Strength Cond Res* 32(11), 3039–3050, 2018.

91. Lehnert, M, Psotta, R, and Botek, Z. The effects of high-resistance and plyometric training on adolescent soccer players: A comparative study. *Gazzetta Medica Italiana Archivio Per Le Scienze Mediche* 171(5), 567–576, 2012.

92. Negra, Y, Chaabene, H, Stöggl, T, Hammami, M, Chelly, MS, and Hachana, Y. Effectiveness and time-course adaptation of resistance training vs. plyometric training in prepubertal soccer players. *J Sport Health Sci* 2016.

93. Spineti, J, Figueiredo, T, Bastos De Oliveira, V, Assis, M, Fernandes De Oliveira, L, Miranda, H, and Simao, R. Comparison between traditional strength training and complex contrast training on repeated sprint ability and muscle architecture in elite soccer players. *J Sports Med Phys Fit* 56(11), 1269–1278, 2016.

94. Wallenta, C, Granacher, U, Lesinski, M, Schünemann, C, and Mühlbauer, T. Effects of complex versus block strength training on the athletic performance of elite youth soccer players. *Sportverletzung-Sportschaden* 30(1), 31–37, 2016.

95. Coratella, G, Beato, M, Milanese, C, Longo, S, Limonta, E, Rampichini, S, and Esposito, F. Specific adaptations in performance and muscle architecture after weighted jump squat vs. body mass squat jump training in recreational soccer players. *J Strength Cond Res* 32(4), 921–929, 2018.

96. Kobal, R, Loturco, I, Barroso, R, Gil, S, Cuniyochi, RR, Ugrinowitsch, C, and Tricoli, V. Effects of different combinations of strength, power, and plyometric training on the physical performance of elite young soccer players. *J Strength Cond Res* 31(6), 1468–1476, 2017.

97. Mendiguchia, J, Martinez-Ruiz, E, Morin, JB, Samozino, P, Edouard, P, Alcaraz, PE, and Mendez-Villanueva, A. Effects of hamstring-emphasized neuromuscular training on strength and sprinting mechanics in football players. *Scand J Med Sci Sports* 25(6), e621–629, 2015.

98. Brito, J, Vasconcellos, F, Oliveira, J, Krustrup, P, and Rebelo, A. Short-term performance effects of three different low-volume strength-training programs in college male soccer players. *J Hum Kinet* 40, 121–128, 2014.

99. Faude, O, Roth, R, Giovine, DD, Zahner, L, and Donath, L. Combined strength and power training in high-level amateur football during the competitive season: A randomised-controlled trial. *J Sports Sci* 31(13), 1460–1467, 2013.

100. Váczi, M, Tollár, J, Meszler, B, Juhász, I, and Karsai, I. Short-term high intensity plyometric training program improves strength, power and agility in male soccer players. *J Human Kin* 36(1), 17–26, 2013.

101. Lockie, RG, Murphy, AJ, Schultz, AB, Knight, TJ, and de Jonge, X. The effects of different speed training protocols on sprint acceleration kinematics and muscle strength and power in field sport athletes. *J Strength Cond Res* 26(6), 1539–1550, 2012.

102. Ronnestad, BR, Kvamme, NH, Sunde, A, and Raastad, T. Short-term effects of strength and plyometric training on sprint and jump performance in professional soccer players. *J Strength Cond Res* 22(3), 773–780, 2008.

103. Rodríguez-Rosell, D, Torres-Torrelo, J, Franco-Márquez, F, González-Suárez, JM, and González-Badillo, JJ. Effects of light-load maximal lifting velocity weight training vs. combined weight training and plyometrics on sprint, vertical jump and strength performance in adult soccer players. *J Sci Med Sport* 20(7), 695–699, 2017.

6

ASSESSMENT OF FOOTBALL-SPECIFIC ENDURANCE

Alejandro Rodríguez-Fernández
and Javier Sánchez-Sánchez

6.1 Introduction

Football match play is characterized by intermittent high-intensity activity, underpinned by high levels of aerobic and anaerobic fitness [1]. During a football match, players perform accelerations, sprinting, changes of direction, jumping, side stepping, tackling, and game-specific technical skills at high intensity during the match, but most of the distance is covered walking or at low intensity [2]. Therefore, aerobic capacity is a key factor to fuel the extensive running and movement required during a match and to aid recovery from these high-intensity actions [3]. In this highly demanding scenario, aerobic training is traditionally an important component of physical training in football, and assessment of aerobic endurance is essential for trainers and practitioners [4].

Aerobic fitness assessment tests are important for performance monitoring since they provide objective data on player physical status and team performance during the season [5]. These data can be used by the coach to select training programs and references on when to return to play [6]. Additionally, these tests provide feedback and motivation for players. Sports scientists can use information from physiological tests to create individual profiles in the sport and include strengths and weaknesses of the players and the team [5].

6.2 Main variables used to determine football-specific endurance performance

Aerobic endurance performance has been assessed by determining maximal oxygen uptake (VO_2max), anaerobic threshold, and running economy [7]. The VO_2max is the highest amount of oxygen that the body can utilize during exhaustive exercise

DOI: 10.4324/9781032637006-6

while breathing air at sea level [8]. Previous studies indicated that the VO_2max of male international football players was between 50 and 75 ml/kg/min [2]. These VO_2max values are sufficient for football players and can delay the emptying of muscle glycogen stores [9] and have a better recovery from high-intensity efforts [10] to improve participation in decisive actions [11].

6.3 Importance of endurance assessment

In football, endurance capacity was assessed by laboratory tests, which require a controlled environment to gain measurement precision [12]. Although the results were more reliable, the lack of specificity of a laboratory test prevented transference of the results to specific training and to explain match performance. In addition, laboratory tests had other limitations [1], (i) the time needed for application and preparation, which is not always possible within the football training process; (ii) require highly qualified material and personnel only available to professional clubs; (iii) do not replicate the football player's activity, which makes the player uncomfortable, causing them to lose motivation to express their full potential. For these reasons, laboratory tests lost importance in favor of field tests that were commonly used in modalities other than football [13]. These tests were performed with protocols of a continuous nature, with running stages performed at progressively increasing speed, (e.g., Multistage shuttle) or linear runs at constant intensity to try to reach the maximum distance in the allowed time (e.g., 12-minute run test), both aimed at reaching a maximum rate that could be used in an equation for the indirect estimation of VO_2max. Although these tests reported the football player's aerobic fitness, their ecological value was low since the protocols did not reproduce the football activity profile [14]. For this reason, performance specialists in team sports began to devise protocols that simulated game activity through activities that combined efforts of progressive intensity and recovery, as well as runs with change of direction [15]. In this way, aerobic fitness could be determined by performance in these actions, with high transfer capacity to individualize and quantify resistance training loads [16].

6.4 Field tests to assess endurance in football

6.4.1 Yo-Yo intermittent recovery test

The Yo-Yo intermittent recovery test (YYIR) assesses the capacity to carry out intermittent exercise, leading to maximal activation of the aerobic system [15]. Additionally, there is a variant of the YYIR defined as level 2 (YYIR2), which determines an individual's ability to recover from repeated exercise, with a high contribution from the anaerobic system [17]. Both tests present reasonably high reproducibility and existing low coefficients of variation when analyzing performance in the YYIR and YYIR2 carried out in different sessions (i.e., tests separated by one week) in professional [14] and amateur [18] football players.

The YYRI consists of repeated exercise bouts performed at progressively increasing speeds, interspersed with 10-second active rest periods and performed until exhaustion [14]. Football players perform repeated 2 × 20 meter runs back and forth between the starting, turning, and finishing lines at a progressively increased speed controlled by audio bleeps from specific software. After the finishing line, there is a 5-meter zone that marks the running distance during the active recovery period. The test consists of four running bouts at 10–13 km/h and seven runs at 13.5–14 km/h, followed by 0.5 km/h speed increments after every eight running bouts. The test ends when the football player twice fails to reach the finishing line in time. The test result is taken as the total distance covered. The VO_2max (ml/kg/min) can be estimated according to the equation: YYIR: distance (m) × 0.0084 + 36.4; YYIR2: distance (m) × 0.0136 + 45.3.

The physiological response to the YYIR and YYIR2 has been described in previous studies [14, 17]. Progressive increases in the heart rate have been observed in both tests, but with a greater increase in the YYIR2 than YYIR. The incremental response of the heart rate is maximum at the end of the test. This allows these tests to be used to determine the individual maximum heart rate and to quantify internal load in training activities [19]. In relation to the metabolic response, both tests provoke maximum activity of the aerobic system, with a greater degree of activation of the anaerobic pathway in the YYIR2 [15]. For this, the creatine phosphate level at the end of the test was lower in the YYIR2 than in the YYIR [14]. This response may explain the higher lactate concentration observed at the end of the YYIR2 compared to YYIR due to the greater use of glucolysis to cope with repeated high-intensity efforts [17]. Activation of this energy pathway will cause the emptying of glycogen in fast fibers, which can contribute to the development of a specific fatigue in the player during the performance of repeated high-intensity exercises [20].

Both versions of the test (YYIR or YYIR2) have been used to assess the physical fitness of different groups of athletes. Top-elite male football players had a higher performance level in the YYIR than elite players at a lower level or sub-elite and moderately trained players (2420 meters versus 2190 meters, 2030 meters, and 1810 meters, respectively) [11, 14, 21–23]. In addition, both the YYIR and YYIR2 showed differences in performance according to demarcations (i.e., central defenders and attackers covering less distance than midfield players and fullbacks). Differences in test performance according to competitive level and demarcation can indicate to coaches the ability of football players to perform high-speed actions during the game [11]. These results may suggest that there is a basic level of fitness necessary to perform at a high level and in a certain position.

In female football players, despite significant correlation coefficients between the VO_2max in the laboratory test and distance covered in the YYIR in amateur

($r = 0.83$) [24] or elite ($r = 0.55$) female football players [25], the YYIR1 did not provide an accurate prediction of VO$_2$max since YYIR1 significantly underestimated VO$_2$max by 9.4% [24]. It is possible that the different nature of the field tests and laboratory test (i.e., intermittent efforts, changes of direction, and duration), female physiological factors, and the equation used, which is usually designed specifically for male players, gave rise to these differences. For this reason, a gender-specific equation to estimate VO$_2$max has been proposed [24]. However, although the relevance of VO$_2$max has been questioned in football performance [21], a strong correlation ($r = 0.81$) with high-intensity running during a match has been obtained [36]. For these reasons, VO$_2$max cannot be considered the single best indicator of female football-specific physical performance [35], but coaches can use this measure to discriminate elite and sub-elite players and detect large changes in the fitness status as a result of specific training regimens [26].

6.4.2 The 30–15 intermittent fitness test

The 30–15 intermittent fitness test (30–15 IFT) consists of repeated exercise of 30-second shuttle runs interspersed with 15 seconds of passive recovery periods [13]. The velocity starts at 8 km/h for the first 30-second run and is increased by 0.5 km/h every 45-second stage thereafter, with a speed controlled by audio beeps. The football players perform runs, back and forth between two lines set 40 meters apart, with an intermediate line at 20 meters. During the 15-second recovery period, the football player walks in a forward direction to reach the closest line, from where they begin the next run stage. The test ends when a football player can no longer maintain the imposed running speed and is unable to reach a zone by the audio signal three times consecutively. The velocity attained during the final completed stage is determined as the players' velocity intermittent fitness test (VIFT), and the VO$_2$max (ml/kg/min) can be estimated from the VIFT according to the equation [16]: $28.3 - 2.15G - 0.741A - 0.0357W + 0.0586A \times VIFT + 1.03VIFT$ [G, gender: female = 2 and male =1; A, age; W, weight].

The classic continuous field tests [27, 28] allowed the end velocity of the test to be obtained (consequently, indirectly, the VO$_2$max of athletes) but not the maximal aerobic velocity (MAV, determined by gas exchange analysis, is the lowest running velocity that elicits VO$_2$max or the minimum velocity that elicits VO$_2$max) [29]. Therefore, neither VO$_2$max nor MAV corresponds to the end velocity of the test, and this cannot be obtained with an indirect test [16]. The end velocity of the test includes an anaerobic component that can be expressed differently in two athletes with the same VO$_2$max speed [16]. The different performance during intensity efforts higher than the VO$_2$max speed means that MAV cannot be used to individualize resistance training with change of direction, intermittent efforts, and, especially, to prescribe high-intensity loads. For this reason, it is necessary to have indicators to ensure that all athletes, when performing high-intensity runs in their endurance training sessions, develop aerobic and anaerobic loads according to their level of conditioning. One way to achieve this could be through the anaerobic velocity reserve (AVR), which can be determined by the difference between the player's maximum velocity (i.e., 40-m sprint test) and the final speed achieved in an incremental test [16]. Another way is from the VIFT (end velocity reached in 30–15 IFT test) because it is obtained simultaneously with maximal aerobic function, anaerobic capacity (or at least the proportion of AVR used), neuromuscular qualities, and change of direction and inter-effort recovery abilities. In addition, VIFT was shown to be more accurate for the individualization of high intermittency aerobic training [29]. This makes the 30–15 IFT a useful test for assessing intermittent aerobic fitness, prescribing endurance training, and monitoring workloads in team sports [30].

6.5 Specific assessment of aerobic fitness

The specific assessment of physical fitness in football has been carried out using different strategies: the inclusion of technical elements in field tests (football-specific "dribbling track") [4], simulating the activity pattern of a football match (Loughborough Intermittent Shuttle Test) [31], or evaluation through game-based situations (small-sided games) [32].

During the competitive season, coaches and practitioners seek information about their players' fitness level in order to reinforce training prescription (training process) and balance the positive and negative training status of the athlete (training monitoring) [30]. Different test protocols are designed to reproduce specific match demand and physical qualities such as intermittent endurance through the Yo-Yo IR test [14], TIVRE football test [12], and 30–15 IFT [33] or maximal repeated effort [34]. However, during the competitive season, maximal tests are not usually employed [35]. In addition, since submaximal parameters of aerobic fitness could be more sensitive to training [26], the use of submaximal tests has been proposed [36, 37]. On the other hand, during the competitive season, time is limited, which on many occasions does not allow the application of these protocols. In addition, no football-specific assessments have been reported, which allow technical, tactical, and physical staff to fully integrate sport-specific involvement within training situations in order to maximize training content. For this, recently, the use of small-sided games (SSGs) has been analyzed as a tool to assess physical fitness in football players [32, 38]. Owen et al. [32] obtained moderate-to-very large associations between an SSG (5 versus 5 within a 25 × 25 m with 3 × 3 min games) and distance covered in the Yo-Yo IR1 test, highlighting the correlation with the total distance ($r = 0.88$) and dynamic stress load ($r = 0.80$) in the SSG, registered by GPS in elite football players. Similarly, Stevens et al. [39] obtained a *moderate* to *large* relationship ($r = 0.45$ to $r = 0.70$) between the SSG (6 versus 6 within a 40 × 34 m with 4 × 7 min including goalkeepers), locomotor performance (time motion analysis), and Yo-Yo IR2 distance. In addition, a significant negative relationship was observed between the ability to recover from SSGs (heart rate recovery after 4 versus 4 within a 40 × 30 m pitch with standard goals, with six bouts of 90 seconds separated by 90 seconds of passive recovery) and the general aerobic endurance performance determined by velocity and heart rate at a fixed blood lactate concentration of 4 mmol L^{-1} ($r = -0.91$ and $r = -0.69$, respectively) in semiprofessional football players [38]. Considering these results, coaches could potentially utilize the SSG protocol as a fitness assessment tool during the season, with the advantage that this protocol is already a frequently used training methodology at all levels, ages, and sexes [40, 41] of football cohorts, in addition to presenting the ecological validity [32]. However, the differences were relatively small in SSG performance compared to the differences among levels (i.e., professional, amateur, or female) in Yo-Yo IR2 performance [39]. In addition, significant negative correlations were found for internal load (heart rate and RPE) with Yo-Yo IR2 distance. Riboli et al. [37] found that SSG demands showed poor overall internal (heart rate) and external (distance and locomotor performance) responsiveness to the training-induced aerobic adaptations, as assessed by Yo-Yo submax (20-m shuttle lasting 4 min). This aspect suggests that SSGs have several limitations to assess physical fitness in football players: (i) a ceiling effect (fitness and technical) for exercise intensity, with lower intensity in fit players; (ii) the influence of motivation in SSG locomotor performance; (iii) the influence of tactical elements; (iv) the variability in external and internal load, which is greater when the intensity is increased; and (v) poor internal and external responsiveness to determine training-induced aerobic adaptations. For these reasons, SSGs cannot be used to assess physical endurance capacities or aerobic adaptations in football players and standardized maximal or submaximal testing seem to be required.

6.6 Relationship between aerobic fitness and match performance

After high-intensity interval training, an increase of 10.8% in VO_2max has been associated with an increase not only in global aspects (lactate threshold or running economy of 16% and 6.7%, respectively) but also with an increase in total distance covered (20%), average number of sprints per player (100%), and number of involvements with the ball (24.1%) in a match [42]. These results will increase the interest in VO_2max training and in the analysis of the relationship between physical fitness tests and locomotor performance in a match. Obviously, better VO_2max and higher locomotor performance during a match do not guarantee success in football, which is a complex sport, but they will increase the chances that the player reaches the ball before their rival in situations, which may affect the final result. Castagna et al. [43] obtained a large to very large association between several physical match activities that have been demonstrated to be a football-specific dependent variable (i.e., high-intensity activity and high-intensity running or sprinting) and the Yo-Yo IR1 and Multistage Shuttle run test, supporting the direct validity for assessment of physical fitness in male youth football players. However, the Hoff test demonstrated a large association only with the distance covered while sprinting ($r = 0.70$). A modified version of the University of Montreal Track Test, a better predictor of VO_2max ($r = 0.96$ with VO_2max), was a consistently better predictor of game running performance than repeated sprint ability, sprint, acceleration, or lower limb explosive strength [44]. However, playing position and its associated tactical roles need to be taken into consideration when examining the relationship between physical capacities and match running performance since results of the University of Montreal Track Test explained more than 25% of total distance, high-intensity distance, sprinting, and even peak running speed reached in second strikers and strikers [44]. Contrary to these results, Rebelo et al. showed that the distance covered in the Yo-Yo IR1 was associated with match locomotor performance (time spent in sprinting), but the Yo-Yo IR2 and VO_2max were not correlated with the activity during the match. The Yo-Yo IR1 version is a more sensitive measure to variations in match physical performance than VO_2max. It is possible that other aerobic-dependent factors than VO_2max (e.g., ability to recover from high-intensity intermittent exercise and peak running speed during incremental tests) can be used to assess specific physiological components of football performance [45]. Previous studies highlight the importance of locomotor factors (i.e., peak incremental test speeds) in comparison with VO_2max and $VO_2kinetics$ for greater repeated-sprint performance [46], a determinant factor in football performance [47].

References

1. Jemni M, Prince MS, Baker JS. Assessing cardiorespiratory fitness of soccer players: Is test specificity the issue? – A review. *Sports Med.* 2018;4(28):1–18.
2. Stølen T, Chamari K, Castagna C, Wisløff U. Physiology of soccer. *Sports Med.* 2005;35(6):501–536.
3. Rodríguez-Fernández A, Sánchez-Sánchez J, Rodríguez-Marroyo JA, Casamichana D, Villa JG. Effect of 5-weeks pre-season training with small-sided game in RSA according to physical fitness. *J Sport Med Phys Fitness.* 2017;57(5):529–536.
4. Hoff J. Training and testing physical capacities for elite soccer players. *J Sports Sciences* [Internet]. 2005 June [cited 2012 July 18];23(6):573–582. Available from: https://www.ncbi.nlm.nih.gov/pubmed/16195006
5. Svensson M, Drust B. Testing soccer players. *J Sports Sci* [Internet]. 2005 June [cited 2013 June 16];23(6):601–618. Available from: https://www.ncbi.nlm.nih.gov/pubmed/16195009
6. Rösch D, Hodgson R, Peterson L, Graf-BAumann T, Junge A, Chomiak J, et al. Assessment and evaluation of football performance. *Am J Sports Med.* 2000;28(5):29–39.
7. Joyner MJ, Coyle EF. Endurance exercise performance: The physiology of champions. *J Physiol* [Internet]. 2008;586(1):35–44. Available from: https://www.pubmedcentral.nih.gov/articlerender.fcgi?artid=2375555&tool=pmcentrez&rendertype=abstract%5Cn https://www.pubmedcentral.nih.gov/articlerender.fcgi?artid=2375555%7B&%7Dtool=pmcentrez%7B&%7Drendertype=abstract

8. Midgley AW, McNaughton LR, Polman R, Marchant D. Criteria for determination of maximal oxygen uptake: A brief critique and recommendations for future research. *Sports Med* (Auckland, NZ) [Internet]. 2007 Jan;37(12):1019–1028. Available from: https://www.ncbi.nlm.nih.gov/pubmed/18027991

9. Thomas V, Reilly T. Fitness assessment of English league soccer players through the competitive season. *Br J Sports Med.* 1979 Sep;13(3):103–109.

10. Glaister M. Multiple sprint work: Physiological responses, mechanisms of fatigue and the influence of aerobic fitness. *Sports Med.* 2005;35(9):757–777.

11. Mohr M, Krustrup P, Bangsbo J. Match performance of high-standard soccer players with special reference to development of fatigue. *J Sports Sci.* 2003 July;21(7):519.

12. Drust B, Gregson W. Fitness testing. In: Williams AM, Ford P, Drust B (eds), *Science and soccer.* Routledge;2013. p. 55–76.

13. Buchheit M. The 30–15 intermittent fitness test: Accuracy for individualizing interval training of young intermittent sport players. *J Strength Cond Res.* 2008;22(2):365–374.

14. Krustrup P, Mohr M, Amstrup T, Rysgaard T, Johansen J, Steensberg A, et al. The yo-yo intermittent recovery test: Physiological response, reliability, and validity. *Med Sci Sports Exerc.* 2003;35(4):697–705.

15. Bangsbo J, Iaia FM, Krustrup P. The yo-yo intermittent recovery test. A useful tool for evaluation of physical performance in intermittent sports. *Sports Med.* 2008;38(1):37–51.

16. Buchheit M. The 30–15 intermittent fitness test: 10 year review. *Myorobie J.* 2010;1:1–9.

17. Krustrup P, Mohr M, Nybo L, Jensen JM, Nielsen JJ, Bangsbo J. The Yo-Yo IR2 test: Physiological response, reliability, and application to elite soccer. *Med Sci Sports Exerc.* 2006;38(9):1666–1673.

18. Thomas A, Dawson B, Goodman C. The yo-yo test: Reliability and association with a 20-m shuttle run and VO(2max). *Int J Sports Physiol Perform.* 2006;1(2):137–149.

19. Sanchez-Sanchez J, Hernandez D, Casamichana D, Martinez C, Ramírez-Campillo R, Sampaio J. Heart rate, technical performance and session-RPE in elite youth soccer small-sided games played with wildcard player. *J Strength Cond Res.* 2017;31(10):2678–2685.

20. Rodríguez-Fernández A, Sanchez-Sanchez J, Ramirez-Campillo R, Nakamura FY, Rodríguez-Marroyo JA, Villa-Vicente JG. Relationship between repeated sprint ability, aerobic capacity, intermittent endurance, and heart rate recovery in youth soccer players. *J Strength Cond Res.* 2019 Dec;33(12):3406–3413.

21. Castagna C, Impellizzeri FM, Chamari K, Carlomagno D, Rampinini E. Aerobic fitness and yo-yo continuous and intermittent tests performances in soccer players: A correlation study. *J Strength Cond Res* [Internet]. 2006 May;20(2):320–325. Available from: https://www.ncbi.nlm.nih.gov/pubmed/16689621

22. Ferrari Bravo D, Impellizzeri FM, Rampinini E, Castagna C, Bishop D, Wisloff U. Sprint vs. interval training in football. *Int J Sports Med* [Internet]. 2008 Aug [cited 2012 Mar 27];29(8):668–674. Available from: https://www.ncbi.nlm.nih.gov/pubmed/18080951

23. Rampinini E, Impellizzeri FM, Castagna C, Abt G, Chamari K, Sassi A, et al. Factors influencing physiological responses to small-sided soccer games. *J Sports Sci* [Internet]. 2007 Apr [cited 2013 Mar 7];25(6):659–666. Available from: https://www.ncbi.nlm.nih. gov/pubmed/17454533

24. Martínez-Lagunas V, Hartmann U. Validity of the Yo-Yo intermittent recovery test level 1 for direct measurement or indirect estimation of maximal oxygen uptake in female soccer players. *Int J Sports Physiol Perform* [Internet]. 2014 Sep [cited 2017 Oct 4];9(5):825–831. Available from: https://journals.humankinetics.com/doi/10.1123/ ijspp.2013-0313

25. Krustrup P, Mohr M, Ellingsgaard H, Bangsbo J. Physical demands during an elite female soccer game: Importance of training status. *Med Sci Sports Exerc.* 2005;37(7):1242–1248.
26. Impellizzeri FM, Rampinini E, Marcora SM. Physiological assessment of aerobic training in soccer. *J Sports Sci.* 2005;23(June):583–592.
27. Léger LA, Mercier D, Gadoury C, Lambert J. The multistage 20 metre shuttle run test for aerobic fitness. *J Sports Sci* [Internet]. 1988;6(2):93–101. Available from: https://www.tandfonline.com/doi/abs/10.1080/02640418808729800
28. Leger L, Boucher R. An indirect continuous running multistage field test: The Universite de Montreal track test. *Can J Appl Sport Sci.* 1980;5(2):77–84.
29. Buchheit M. The 30–15 intermittent fitness test: Accuracy for individualizing interval training of young intermittent sport players. *J Strength Cond Res.* 2008;22(2):365–374.
30. Scott TJ. Testing, prescribing and monitoring training in team sports: The efficiency and versatility of the 30–15 Intermittent Fitness Test. *Sports Perform.* 2018;10:1–5.
31. Nicholas CW, Nuttall FE, Williams C. The Loughborough Intermittent Shuttle Test: A field test that simulates the activity pattern of soccer. *J Sports Sci* [Internet]. 2000;18(2):97–104. Available from: https://www.ncbi.nlm.nih.gov/pubmed/10718565
32. Owen AL, Newton M, Shovlin A, Malone S. The use of small-sided games as an aerobic fitness assessment supplement within elite level professional soccer. *J Human Kinet.* 2020;71(1):243–253.
33. Thomas C, Dos'Santos T, Jones PA, Comfort P. Reliability of the 30-15 intermittent fitness test in semiprofessional soccer players. *Int J Sports Physiol Perform.* 2016 Mar;11(2):172–175.
34. Di Mascio M, Ade J, Musham C, Girard O, Bradley PS. Soccer-specific reactive repeated-sprint ability in elite youth soccer players: Maturation trends and association with various physical performance tests. *J Strength Cond Res.* 2020;34(12):3538–3545.
35. Halson SL. Monitoring training load to understand fatigue in athletes. *Sports Med.* 2014;44:139–1347.
36. Impellizzeri FM, Mognoni P, Sassi A, Rampinini E. Validity of a submaximal running test to evaluate aerobic fitness changes in soccer players. *J Sports Sci.* 2004;22:547.
37. Riboli A, Dellal A, Esposito F, Coratella G. Can small-sided games assess the training-induced aerobic adaptations in elite football players? *J Sports Med Phys Fitness.* 2022;62(10):1313–1322..
38. Reinhardt L, Schulze S, Kurz E, Schwesig R. An investigation into the relationship between heart rate recovery in small-sided games and endurance performance in male, semi-professional soccer players. *Sports Med.* 2020;6(1):43.
39. Stevens TGA, de Ruiter CJ, Beek PJ, Savelsbergh GJP. Validity and reliability of 6-a-side small-sided game locomotor performance in assessing physical fitness in football players. *J Sports Sci.* 2016;34(6):527–534.
40. Bujalance-Moreno P, Latorre-Román PÁ, García-Pinillos F. A systematic review on small-sided games in football players: Acute and chronic adaptations. *J Sports Sci* [Internet]. 2018;October:1–29. Available from: https://www.ncbi.nlm.nih.gov/pubmed/30373471
41. Clemente FM, Ramirez-Campillo R, Afonso J, Sarmento H. Effects of small-sided games vs. running-based high-intensity interval training on physical performance in soccer players: A meta-analytical comparison. *Front Physiol.* 2021;12:642703.
42. Helgerud J, Engen LC, Wisloff U, Hoff J. Aerobic endurance training improves soccer performance. *Med Sci Sports Exerc* [Internet]. 2001 Nov;33(11):1925–1931. Available from: https://www.ncbi.nlm.nih.gov/pubmed/11689745

43. Castagna C, Manzi V, Impellizzeri F, Weston M, Carlos J. Relationship between endurance field tests and match performance in young soccer players. *J Strength Cond Res.* 2010;24:3227–3233.

44. Buchheit M, Mendez-Villanueva A, Simpson BM, Bourdon PC. Match running performance and fitness in youth soccer. *Int J Sports Med.* 2010;31(11):818–825.

45. Rampinini E, Bishop D, Marcora S, Ferrari Bravo D, Sassi R, Impellizzeri F. Validity of simple field tests as indicators of match-related physical performance in top-level professional soccer players. *Int J Sports Med.* 2007;28(3):228–235.

46. Buchheit M. Repeated-sprint performance in team sport players: Associations with measures of aerobic fitness, metabolic control and locomotor function. *Int J Sports Med.* 2012;33(3):230–239.

47. Girard O, Mendez-Villanueva A, Bishop D. Repeated-sprint ability – Part I. *Sports Med* [Internet]. 2011;41(8):673–694. Available from: https://link.springer.com/10.2165/1159 0550-000000000-00000

7

STATIC AND DYNAMIC NEUROMUSCULAR BALANCE FIELD-BASED ASSESSMENTS

Marc Madruga Parera, Rodrigo Ramírez-Campillo and Víctor Moreno-Pérez

7.1 Lower limb assessment

The assessment of lower limb neuromuscular control will be discussed in this section, including assessment of static and dynamic neuromuscular control, asymmetries, joint control, and change of direction.

7.1.1 Assessment of static neuromuscular control

One of the most popular tests to assess lower limb neuromuscular control is the single-leg standing test. This test is often used as a measure of static postural stability and a threshold test to determine readiness to begin high-level exercise programs such as plyometrics [1]. The ability to single-leg standing can be used to detect differences between lower limbs and assist clinicians to determine if impairment is present [2, 3]. Indeed, a study in female football players found that those with poorer pre-season unilateral balance values were more prone to ankle sprains during the season [4]. Watson [5] assessed football players' postural sway in the 15-seconds single-leg standing test, and athletes unable to perform it without touching down were classified as having an abnormal postural sway.

The single-leg standing test may involve stable and unstable surfaces (similar to the Balance Error Scoring System described by Riemann et al. [6]), qualitative measures, or more objective measures (e.g., center of pressure measurements using a force plate). Additionally, the test can be performed with eyes open or closed.

However, the relevance of static assessment as a predictor of sports injuries has been criticized, mainly because of the dynamic nature of football, suggesting the need for dynamic assessments.

DOI: 10.4324/9781032637006-7

7.1.2 Assessment of dynamic neuromuscular control

The Star Excursion Balance Test and the Y-Balance Test

The Star Excursion Balance Test (SEBT) is commonly used to assess the athlete's dynamic neuromuscular control (Figure 7.1), associated to physical fitness, chronic ankle instability, and injury risk [7, 8]. The SEBT involves maintaining postural stability with one foot in the floor, while the contralateral foot must reach eight different directions in order to assess the dynamic neuromuscular control in such directions. To reduce the time needed to complete the SEBT, Plisky et al. [9] developed a short version of the test, deemed as the Y-Balance test. The Y-Balance test requires to complete three balance directions (anterior, posterolateral, and posteromedial). Both the SEBT and Y-Balance tests are low cost, easily applicable, and with high reliability (e.g., ICC for intrarater reliability ranged from 0.85 to 0.91) [9]. Both the SEBT and the Y-Balance Test allow the assessment of dynamic balance in the sagittal, transversal, and frontal planes, although they may involve different neuromuscular demands [7, 9].

The SEBT and the Y-Balance Test may predict sport injuries. For example, inter-limb differences of ≥4 cm might increase injury risk [10]. Indeed, Samaan et al. [11] applied the SEBT pre- and post-anterior cruciate ligament (ACL) intervention and observed greater differences in the anterior direction (compared to other directions) after ACL intervention, considering that SEBT is a useful tool to assess return-to-play readiness. Additionally, McCann et al. [12] indicated that the SEBT may predict chronic ankle instability. Moreover, the relationship between neuromuscular control and athletic performance can be assessed with the SEBT.

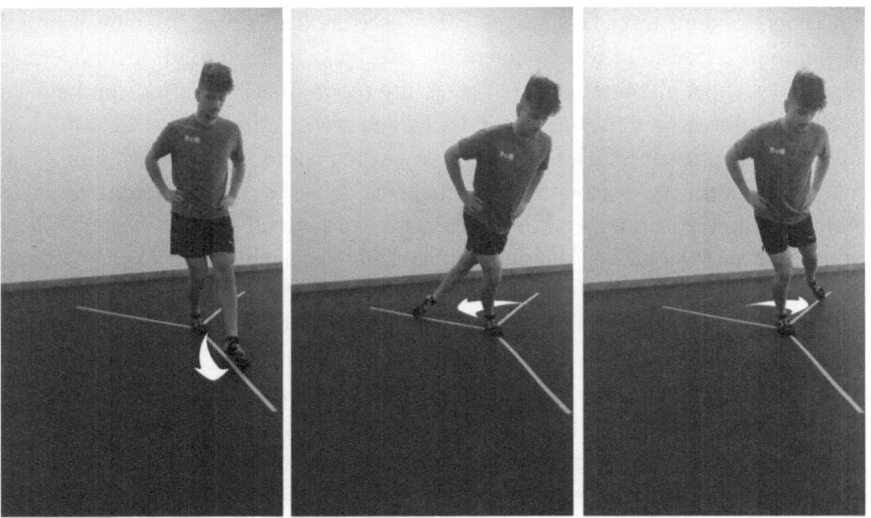

FIGURE 7.1 Y-Balance Test (modified from Plisky et al. [9]. A: anterior; B: posterolateral; C: posteromedial).

For example, Gonzalo-Skok et al. [13] observed a relationship between the SEBT (anterior direction), 5-m sprint ($p = 0.03$; $r = 0.560$) and 180° change of direction speed ($p = 0.01$; $r = 0.630$), as well as between SEBT (medial direction), 5-m sprint ($p = 0.029$; $r = 0.563$), and 180° change of direction speed ($p = 0.04$; $r = 0.552$).

However, the kinematics of these tests are not specific to football and the associated actions commonly encountered during matches such as decelerations and landings. Additionally, football actions commonly require instability due to the variability of the game, the environment, or unexpected situations.

7.1.3 Leg asymmetry assessment

7.1.3.1 Single-leg jumps and hops test

Jump and hop tests (Figure 7.2) may be used to assess neuromuscular control, particularly unilateral jump and hop tests, and include the assessment of both the impulse and landing phases of the jump–hop action [14–17]. Jump tests such as the squat jump, countermovement jump, or drop jump and hop tests such as the single hop for distance, triple hop for distance, cross-over hop for distance, and 6-m timed hop have been used in the assessment of neuromuscular control, in relation to athletic performance, injury prevention, and return to play [16].

Jump tests have high reproducibility, standardization, low variability, and reduced coordination requirements, detecting meaningful small-magnitude changes (i.e., highly sensitive) in inter-limb neuromuscular asymmetries (i.e., dominant versus nondominant limb) [18, 19]. This is a relevant assessment feature, considering that asymmetries might involve a neuromuscular risk factor for injury [20]. However, asymmetries (and its magnitude) are modulated by the type of test being used for assessment, chronological age, maturity, sex, type of sport, period of the season, and modulators that may preclude the establishment of a particular threshold for increased injury risk [15, 21]. However, independent of the magnitude of asymmetry, such assessment may help identify dominant and nondominant limbs in particular actions, helping identify a better profile risk and provide meaningful information to identify relevant follow-up asymmetry variations. In addition, functional asymmetries (up to a certain magnitude for specific actions) should also be considered during assessment.

In addition, the hop tests (e.g., single hop for distance, triple hop for distance, cross-over hop for distance, and 6-m timed hop) can be used to assess the ACL return to play process, considering their characteristics associated to the dynamic stability of the knee joint [16, 22]. Further, single, triple, and cross-over hops for distance have strong reliability [17], with ICC values of 0.92, 0.88, and 0.84, respectively. However, the 6-m timed hop has consistently reported lower ICC values (0.66–0.82), although it is important to consider the qualitative parameters that this test can assess, allowing different dimensions of assessment for knee joint stability (according to the direction of the test). In a review, Davies et al. [16] demonstrated that the single

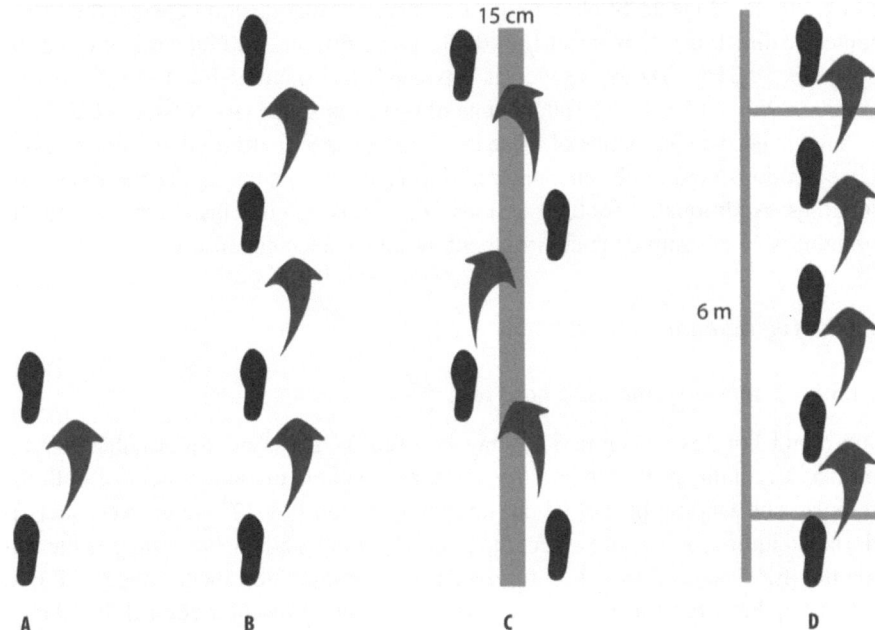

FIGURE 7.2 Four single-leg hop tests. A: single hop for distance; B: triple hop for distance; C: cross-over hop for distance; D: 6-m timed hop [16].

hop and triple jump tests may offer relevant information regarding several variables related to knee joint stability (dynamic and neuromuscular control of the leg). However, it is also important to assess the specific neuromuscular control profile of the athlete according to the specific abilities required in the sport [14, 19].

7.1.4 Knee control assessment and leg asymmetry assessment

The knee sustains one of the highest percentages of injuries of the lower limb joints in soccer players [23]. Biomechanical evidence supports that impaired movement patterns are a modifiable risk factor for ACL tears and other serious lower limb injuries, such as iliotibial band syndrome and patellofemoral joint pain [23]. It is well known that ACL tears may occur due to deficits in neuromuscular control and specific movement tasks, including decreased sagittal plane joint flexion of the knee, hip, and trunk, in combination with increased knee valgus and leg rotation [24].

7.1.4.1 Clinic-based nomogram to predict high knee abduction loads

Biomechanical laboratory assessment showed that the high knee abduction moment landing task has high sensitivity and specificity, although expensive biomechanical laboratory equipment and complex measurement protocols are required to assess individual athletes [25]. However, in the last years, a field-based nomogram was validated [26] and may predict high knee abduction status derived from the landing phase of a drop vertical jump, helping in the identification of athletes at high risk to ACL injury [27]. Knee valgus motion, relative quadriceps recruitment, knee flexion range of motion, tibia length, and body mass are among the key variables included in the nomogram [26].

7.1.4.2 Landing Error Scoring System

The Landing Error Scoring System (LESS) test is used to assess biomechanical patterns during a jump-landing task and to identify athletes at potentially high risk of injury [28, 29]. Moreover, the LESS has been used to quantify changes in neuromuscular and biomechanical performance after prevention programs in youth football players [30] and residual functional impairments in intercollegiate athletes with a previous injury and in patients following ACL reconstruction [31]. The LESS is an inexpensive field-based clinical assessment tool [28] to possessing moderate-to-excellent criterion validity, with good-to-excellent reliability [29].

According to Padua et al. [28], the measurement of a jump-landing task requires the use of two standard video cameras to capture the sagittal and frontal plane of movement (i.e., landing). The jump-landing task incorporated vertical and horizontal movements as participants jumpdown from a 30-cm-high box to a distance of 50% of their height away from the box, down to a firm surface (force platform in case of laboratory assessment), and immediately rebounded for a maximal vertical jump on landing (Figure 7.3).

The LESS test was originally developed using a standardized checklist of 17 technique error items. Athletes with higher scores (i.e., > 6, poor score; < 4, excellent score) would display kinematics indicative of poor landing mechanics [28]. Specifically, a set of items address lower limb and trunk positioning at the time of initial contact with the ground (items 1–6). Another set of items assess errors in positioning of the feet (items 7–11) and are scored at initial ground contact (item 11), at the time the entire foot is in contact with the ground (items 7 and 8), and at the time of initial contact and maximum knee flexion (items 9 and 10), at maximum knee flexion angle (items 12–14), and at maximum knee valgus angle (item 15). Finally, two *global* items address overall sagittal plane movement and the rater's general perception of landing quality (items 16 and 17) [28].

7.1.4.3 Tuck jump test

The Tuck jump test is a clinic field-based tool developed for the identification of the neuromuscular deficits in the lower extremity landing technique during a repetitive plyometric activity [32]. Previous studies suggested that the observation of these neuromuscular deficits could be indicative of quadriceps dominance, ligament

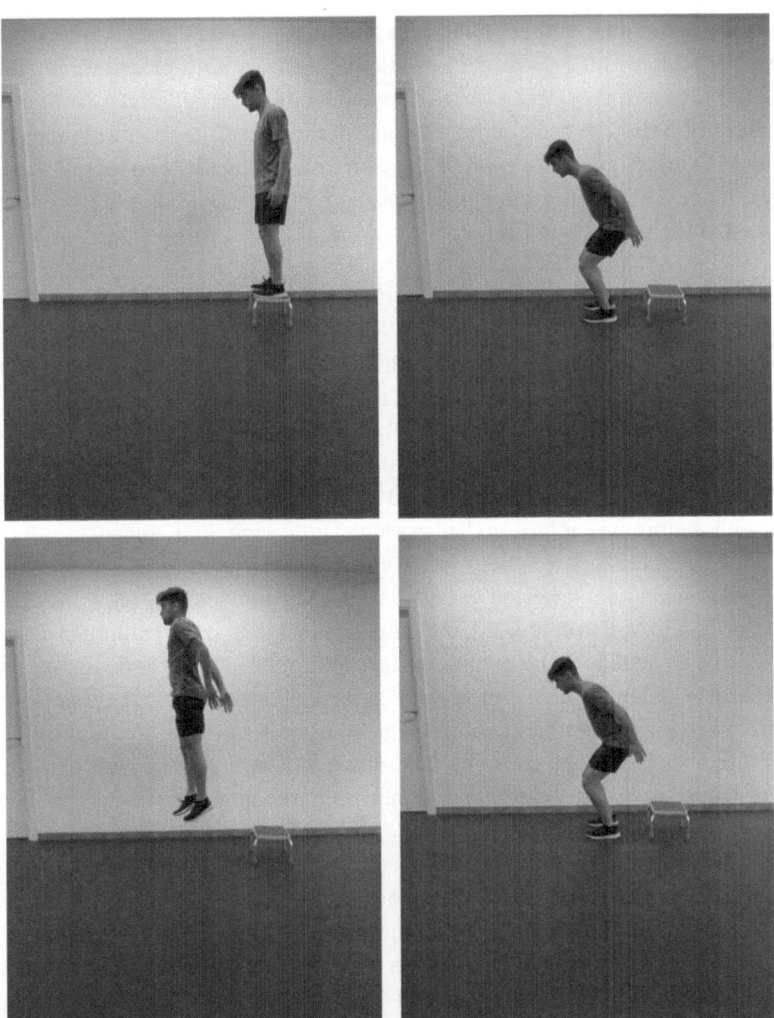

FIGURE 7.3 Landing Error Scoring System.

dominance, leg dominance, and/or trunk dominance, all of which are known risk factors for lower limb injury [33, 34]. The Tuck jump test requires the athlete to jump in place for a period of 10 seconds [33]. During this period, the participant performs a countermovement before a maximal vertical jump, simultaneously pulling their knees up toward their chest, while the ground contact must be minimized, using a toe to mid-foot rocking landing strategy, using the same footprint with each jump (Figure 7.4). Participants are assessed using a 10-point rating scale during

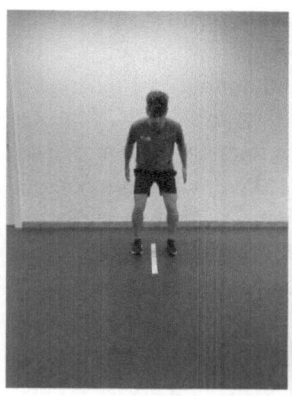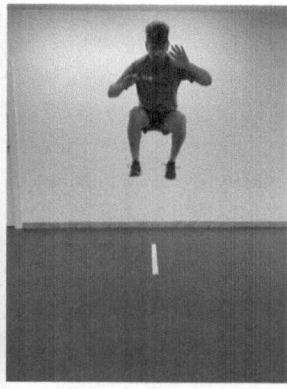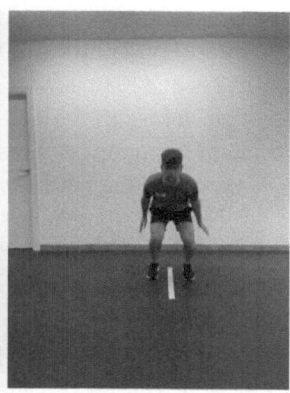

FIGURE 7.4   Tuck jump test.

the procedure, with higher scores associated to increased injury risk (similar to the LESS test) [33]. The Tuck jump has demonstrated a high intrarater reliability of 0.84 (range 0.72–0.97).

7.1.5 Change of direction

Change of direct tests closely resembles the kinematic and coordination needs of the sport [18]. Dynamic neuromuscular control during change of direction is important for athletic performance (e.g., faster change of direction) assessment of neuromuscular injury risk factors and to assess the return to play process [35, 36].

The change of direction tests allow the assessment of neuromuscular and coordination strategies in relation to joint angles (lower limbs; trunk positioning) [37, 38], use of dominant or non-dominant legs, and injured or non-injured leg, where neuromuscular asymmetries may be indicative of injury risk (Rouissi et al.) [37].

There are several tools available for the assessment of change of direction in neuromuscular control [35, 39, 40]. For example, Dos'Santos et al. [41] developed a qualitative assessment tool deemed as "The Cutting Movement Assessment Score (CMAS)" aimed at preventing ACL injuries, showing an excellent intra-rater reliability for CMAS total score (ICC = 0.946) (Dos'Santos et al.) [35]. The CMAS assesses the position of the foot, knee, hip, and trunk during the change of direction action, allowing the assessment of a potential relationship between its different measured items and ACL injury risk.

Additionally, a quantitative assessment, such as inter-limb asymmetries during change of direction actions, may help identify neuromuscular risk factors. For example, Madruga-Parera et al. [18] assessed team sport athletes, observing asymmetries of 3.39% in the double 90° change of direction test (ICC dominant leg, 0.69, range 0.42–0.85; non-dominant leg, 0.99, range 0.97–0.99) and

2.12% in the double 180° change of direction test (ICC dominant leg, 0.96, range 0.92–0.98; non-dominant, 0.98, range 0.96–0.99). Moreover, asymmetry values of 10.52% and 5.48% were noted for the double 90° and double 180° change of direction deficit tests (ICC 0.89, range 0.79–0.94) [18]. Additionally, repeated change of direction tests may also be sensitive to assess inter-limb asymmetries, as demonstrated in with handball players, where a 5.5% asymmetry was noted in an 8-repeated 180° change of direction test [15]. The neuromuscular risk factors have also been assessed using an overloaded change of direction test, potentially a more sensitive test to detect asymmetries. Indeed, Madruga-Parera et al. [18] observed asymmetry values of 10.72–12.67% (mean ICC 0.70–0.81, range 0.46–0.93) in a lateral shuffle step test with an iso-inertial device and asymmetry values of 9.80–11.79% (mean ICC 0.70–0.87, range 0.46–0.94) in a crossover step with an iso-inertial device. In this sense, tests that allow the assessment of change of direction deficit, change of direction repeated ability, as well as overloaded change of direction test may be particularly sensitive to assess asymmetries as potential neuromuscular risk factors.

7.2 Trunk dominance assessment

7.2.1 Core stability biomechanical assessment

7.2.1.1 Unstable sitting paradigms

Trunk stability has been also assessed using the unstable sitting paradigm test. In this test, the athletes use an unstable sitting approach, over a force plate, while fluctuations in the center of pressure are measured [42]. This test allows the assessment of trunk stability deficit (i.e., trunk instability) and lower-back syndrome [43]. Additionally, the test allows to assess the relationship with knee injury in female athletes [44]. Indeed, Zazulak et al. [44] reported that impaired trunk proprioception and deficits in trunk control are predictors of knee injury in female athletes. Specifically, these authors found a higher trunk displacement in collegiate athletes with knee injuries compared to uninjured athletes.

However, these measures were derived during artificial conditions and postures in which the pelvis is immobilized, thus reducing ecological validity. In addition, the test requires expensive laboratory equipment and laborious measurement protocols.

7.2.2 Field-based core stability tests

The different available field-based core stability tests can be broadly grouped into (i) muscular-based tests, (ii) lower back and pelvis control-based tests, and (iii) balance-based tests [42].

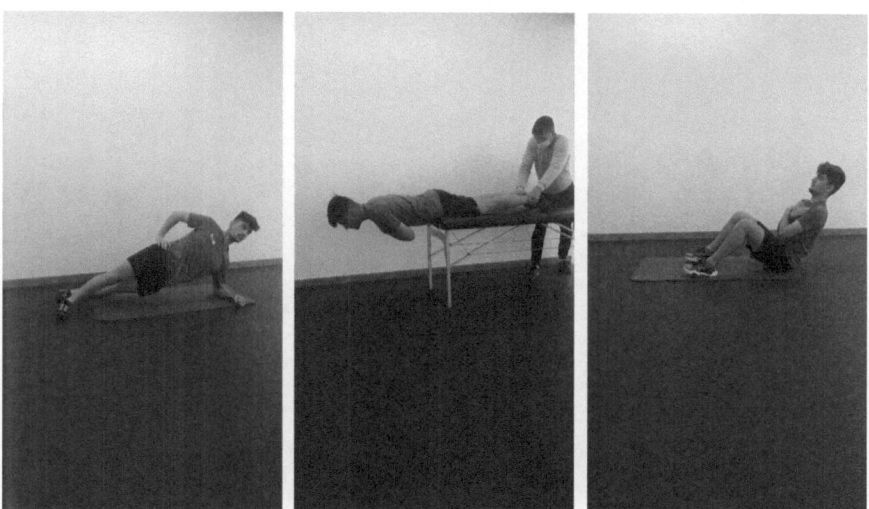

FIGURE 7.5   Muscular-based core stability tests.

7.2.3   Muscular-based tests

Previous studies proposed the use of static muscle endurance tests (e.g., Biering–Sorensen test, side bridge test, and plank-to-fatigue test) or strength power tests (e.g., front abdominal *power* test and side abdominal *power* test) to assess core stability based on the assumption that core strength equals core stability [45, 46].

Among the muscle endurance core tests, the protocol of McGill [47] is one of the most commonly reported in the literature to assess core stability in athletes and physically active participants. McGill [48] developed a battery of four isometric muscle endurance tests to assess core stability (Figure 7.5). The test battery requires no special equipment and displayed a strong reliability (ICC range 0.97–0.99) [47].

However, field-based muscle endurance core tests usually involve the use of the participant's own body for the assessment, with anthropometric characteristics greatly affecting the test results [49]. In addition, the ecological validity of such measures may be questioned based on their prolonged isometric actions and non-functionality [50]. In this sense, movement abnormalities (indicating a loss of core control) may be detectable using more dynamic approaches, such as during the Tuck jump assessment [33] or the LESS test [28].

7.2.4   Core tests based on lower back and pelvis control

Tests such as the double leg lowering test [45, 51] (Figure 7.6) and the Sahrmann core stability test [52, 53] may be included in this category of field-based core stability assessment tests. The aforementioned tests mainly require the control of

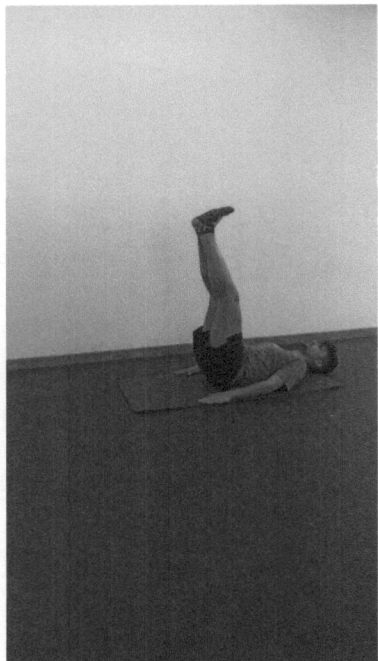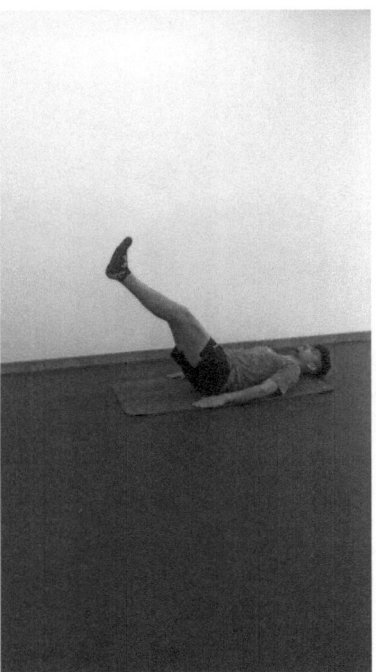

FIGURE 7.6   Double leg lowering test.

the lower back and pelvis to face the forces initiated by the movement of the lower limbs [42].

The Sahrmann core stability test involves five levels of increasing difficulty, progressing from static position efforts toward active movements requiring multi-joint actions [53]. The use of different difficulty levels may help classify the stabilizing muscles functional state. The Sahrmann test is commonly used in research reports to assess the effects of lumbar pelvic stability training interventions on athlete's performance measures, and also in more clinical contexts [52].

Although the double leg lowering test and the Sahrmann core stability test demonstrated good reliability, studies related to their validity are lacking [51, 53]. However, both tests have proved to be of practical relevance to help the soccer player gain a more comprehensive assessment of their progress during core stability training.

7.2.4.1   Balance-based tests to assess core stability.

Some popular tests in this category are the three-plane core test (Figure 7.7), the one leg standing balance test, and the one leg squat test [54, 55]. However, although used in practical settings, their validity through research is yet to be established [42].

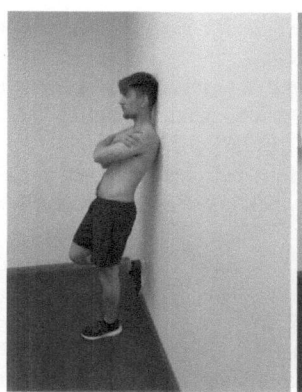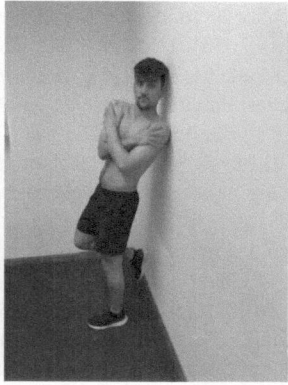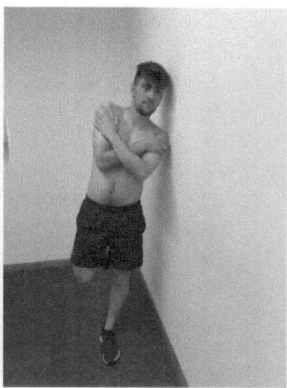

FIGURE 7.7 Three-plane core test, A: sagittal plane; B: transverse plane; C: frontal plane.

References

1. Feigenbaum LA, Kim KJ, Gaunaurd IA, Kaplan LD, Scavo VA, Bennett C, Gailey RS. Post-concussive changes in balance and postural stability measured with canesense and the balance error scoring system (BESS) in división I collegiate football players: a case series. *Int J Sports Phys Ther*. 2019; 14(2): 296–307.
2. Chmielewski TL, Myer GD, Kauffman D, Tillman SM. Plyometric exercise in the rehabilitation of athletes: physiological responses and clinical application. *J Orthop Sports Phys Ther*. 2006; 36(5):308–319.
3. Kim KJ, Agrawal V, Bennett C, Gaunaurd I, Feigenbaum L, Gailey R. Measurement of lower limb segmental excursion using inertial sensors during single-limb stance. *J Biomech*. 2018; 71:151–158.
4. Söderman K, Alfredson H, Pietilä T, Werner S. Risk factors for leg injuries in female soccer players: a prospective investigation during one out-door season. *Knee Surg Sports Traumatol Arthrosc*. 2001; 9(5):313–321.
5. Watson AW. Ankle sprains in players of the field-games Gaelic football and hurling. *J Sports Med Phys Fitness*.1999; 39(1):66–70.
6. Riemann BL, Guskiewicz KM, Shields EW. Relationship between clinical and force-plate measures of postural stability. *J Sport Rehabil*. 1999; 8:71–82.
7. Gribble PA, Hertel J, Plisky P. Using the Star Excursion Balance Test to assess dynamic postural-control deficits and outcomes in lower extremity injury: a literature and systematic review. *J Athl Train*. 2012; 47(3):339–357. doi: 10.4085/1062-6050-47.3.08.
8. Ko J, Rosen AB, Brown CN. Functional performance tests identify lateral ankle sprain risk: a prospective pilot study in adolescent soccer players. *Scand J Med Sci Sports*. 2018; 28(12):2611–2616. doi: 10.1111/sms.13279.
9. Plisky PJ, Gorman PP, Butler RJ, Kiesel KB, Underwood FB, Elkins B. The reliability of an instrumented device for measuring components of the star excursion balance test. *N Am J Sports Phys Ther*. 2009; 4(2):92–99.
10. Plisky PJ, Rauh MJ, Kaminski TW, Underwood FB. Star Excursion Balance Test as a predictor of lower extremity injury in high school basketball players. *J Orthop Sports Phys Ther*. 2006; 36(12):911–919. https://doi.org/10.2519/jospt.2006.2244
11. Samaan, M, Ringleb, S, Bawab, S, Greska, E, and Weinhandl, J. Altered lower extremity joint mechanics occur during the star excursion balance test and single leg hop after

ACL-reconstruction in a collegiate athlete. *Comput Methods Biomech Biomed Engin.* 2018; 21(4):344–358. doi: 10.1080/10255842.2018.1452203

12. McCann RS, Crossett ID, Terada M, Kosik KB, Bolding BA, Gribble PA. Hip strength and star excursion balance test deficits of patients with chronic ankle instability. *J Sci Med Sport.* 2017; 20(11):992–996. doi: 10.1016/j.jsams.2017.05.005.

13. Gonzalo-Skok O, Serna J, Rhea MR, Marín PJ. Relationships between functional movement test and performance test in young elite male basketball players. *Int J Sports Phys Ther.* 2015; 10(5):628–638.

14. Bishop C, Lake J, Loturco I, Papadopoulos K, Turner A, Read P. Interlimb asymmetries: the need for an individual approach to data analysis. *J Strength Cond Res.* 2021; 35(3):695–701. doi: 10.1519/JSC.0000000000002729.

15. Madruga-Parera M, Bishop C, Read P, Lake J, Brazier J, Romero-Rodriguez D. Jumping-based asymmetries are negatively associated with jump, change of direction, and repeated sprint performance, but not linear speed, in adolescent handball athletes. *J Hum Kinet.* 2020; 31(71):47–58. doi: 10.2478/hukin-2019-0095.

16. Davies WT, Myer GD, Read PJ. Is it time we better understood the tests we are using for return to sport decision making following ACL reconstruction? A critical review of the hop tests. *Sports Med.* 2020; 50(3):485–495. doi: 10.1007/s40279-019-01221-7.

17. Reid A, Birmingham TB, Stratford PW, Alcock GK, Giffin JR. Hop testing provides a reliable and valid outcome measure during rehabilitation after anterior cruciate ligament reconstruction. *Phys Ther.* 2007; 87(3):337–349. doi: 10.2522/ptj.20060143.

18. Madruga-Parera M, Bishop C, Beato M, Fort-Vanmeerhaeghe A, Gonzalo-Skok O, Romero-Rodríguez D. Relationship between interlimb asymmetries and speed and change of direction speed in youth handball players. *J Strength Cond Res.* 2021; 35(12):3482–3490. doi: 10.1519/JSC.0000000000003328.

19. Madruga-Parera, M. *Inter-limb asymmetries and sports performance. From assessment to the application of sport-specific iso-inertial resistance training in young athletes.* Doctoral Thesis. University of Girona, Spain. 2020.

20. Fort-Vanmeerhaeghe A, Romero-Rodriguez D, Montalvo A, Kiefer A, Lloyd R, Myer G. Integrative neuromuscular training and injury prevention in youth athletes. Part I. *J Strength Cond Res.* 2016; 38(3):36–48.

21. Bishop C, Read P, Chavda S, Jarvis P, Brazier J, Bromley T, Turner A. Magnitude or direction? Seasonal variation of interlimb asymmetry in elite academy soccer players. *J Strength Cond Res.* 2022;36(4):1031–1037. doi: 10.1519/JSC.0000000000003565

22. Gustavsson A, Neeter C, Thomeé P, Silbernagel, KG, Augustsson J, Thomeé R, Karlsson J. A test battery for evaluating hop performance in patients with an ACL injury and patients who have undergone ACL reconstruction. *Knee Surg Sports Traumatol Arthrosc.* 2006; 14(8):778–788. doi: 10.1007/s00167-006-0045-6

23. Powers CM. The influence of abnormal hip mechanics on knee injury: a biomechanical perspective. *J Orthop Sports Phys Ther.* 2010; 40(2):42–51. doi: 10.2519/jospt.2010.3337.

24. Read PJ, Oliver JL, de Ste Croix MB, Myer GD, Lloyd RS. Reliability of the tuck jump injury risk screening assessment in elite male youth soccer players. *J Strength Cond Res.* 2016; 30(6):1510–1516. doi: 10.1519/JSC.0000000000001260.

25. Myer GD, Ford KR, Khoury J, Succop P, Hewett TE. Clinical correlates to laboratory measures for use in non-contact anterior cruciate ligament injury risk prediction algorithm. *Clin Biomech.* 2010; 25(7):693–9. doi: 10.1016/j.clinbiomech.2010.04.016.

26. Myer GD, Ford KR, Khoury JK, Hewett TE. Three-dimensional motion analysis validation of a clinic based nomogram designed to identify high ACL injury risk in females. *Phys Sports Med.* 2011; 39(1):19–28. doi: 10.3810/psm.2011.02.1858.
27. Myer GD, Ford KR, Khoury J, Succop P, Hewett TE. Development and validation of a clinic based prediction tool to identify female athletes at high risk of ACL injury. *Am J Sports Med.* 2010b; 38:2025–2033.
28. Padua DA, Marshall SW, Boling MC, Thigpen CA, Garrett WE Jr, Beutler AI. The Landing Error Scoring System (LESS) is a valid and reliable clinical assessment tool of jump-landing biomechanics: the JUMP-ACL study. *Am J Sports Med.* 2009; 37(10):1996–2002. doi: 10.1177/0363546509343200.
29. Hanzlíková I, Hébert-Losier K. Is the landing error scoring system reliable and valid? A systematic review. *Sports Health.* 2020; 12(2):181–188. doi: 10.1177/1941738119886593.
30. DiStefano LJ, Padua DA, DiStefano MJ, Marshall SW. Influence of age, sex, 200 technique, and exercise program on movement patterns after an anterior cruciate 201 ligament injury prevention program in youth soccer players. *Am J Sports Med.* 2009 Mar; 37(3):495–505. doi: 10.1177/0363546508327542.
31. Gokeler A, Eppinga P, Dijkstra PU, Welling W, Padua DA, Otten E, Benjaminse A. Effect of fatigue on landing performance assessed with the landing error scoring system (LESS) in patients after ACL reconstruction. A pilot study. *Int J Sports Phys Ther.* 2014; 9(3):302–311.
32. Myer GD, Ford KR, Hewett TE. Rationale and clinical techniques for anterior cruciate ligament injury prevention among female athletes. *J Athl Train.* 2004; 39(4):352–364.
33. Myer GD, Ford KR, Hewett TE. Tuck jump assessment for reducing anterior cruciate ligament injury risk. *Athl Ther Today.* 2008; 13(5):39–44.
34. Myer GD, Brent JL, Ford KR, Hewett TE. Real-time assessment and neuromuscular training feedback techniques to prevent ACL injury in female athletes. *Strength Cond J.* 2011;33(3):21–35. doi: 10.1519/SSC.0b013e318213afa8.
35. Dos'Santos, T, Bishop, C, Thomas, C, Comfort, P, and Jones, PA. The effect of limb dominance on change of direction biomechanics: a systematic review of its importance for injury risk. *Phys Ther Sport.* 2019; 37:179–189.
36. Dos'Santos, T, Mcburnie, A, Donelon, T, Thomas, C, Comfort, and Jones, PA. A qualitative screening tool to identify atheletes with "high-risk" movement mechanics during cutting: the cutting movement assessment score (CMAS). *Phys Ther Sport.* 2019; 38:152–161. doi: 10.1016/j.ptsp.2019.05.004.
37. Rouissi M, Haddad M, Bragazzi NL, Owen AL, Moalla W, Chtara M, Chamari K. Implication of dynamic balance in change of direction performance in young elite soccer players is angle dependent. *J Sports Med Phys Fitness.* 2018; 58(4):442–449. doi: 10.23736/S0022-4707.17.06752-4.
38. Dos'Santos, T, McBurnie, A, Thomas, C, Comfort, P, and Jones, PA. Biomechanical determinants of the modified and traditional 505 change of direction speed test. *J Strength Cond.* 2020; 34:1285–1296.
39. Hewit, JK, Cronin, JB, and Hume, PA. Understanding change of direction performance: a technical analysis of a 180° ground-based turn and sprint task. *Int J Sports Sci Coach.* 2012; 7:493–501.
40. Nimphius, S, Callaghan, SJ, Spiteri, T, and Lockie, RG. Change of direction deficit: a more isolated measure of change of direction performance than total 505 time. *J Strength Cond Res.* 2016;30(11):3024–3032. doi: 10.1519/JSC.0000000000001421.

41. Dos'Santos, T, Thomas, C, McBurnie, A, Comfort, P, and Jones, P. Biomechanical determinants of performance and injury risk during cutting: a performance-injury conflict? *Sports Med.* 2021;51(9):1983–1998. doi: 10.1007/s40279-021-01448-3.

42. Vera-García FJ, Barbado D, Moreno-Pérez V, Hernández-Sánchez S, Juan-Recio C, Elvira JLL. Core stability: evaluación y criterios para su entrenamiento. *Rev Andal Med Deporte.* 2015; 8(3):130–137.

43. Van Dieen JH, Koppes LL, Twisk JW. Low back pain history and postural sway in unstable sitting. *Spine.* 2010; 35(7):812–817.

44. Zazulak BT, Hewett TE, Reeves NP, Goldberg B, Cholewicki J. Deficits in neuromuscular control of the trunk predict knee injury risk: a prospective biomechanical-epidemiologic study. *Am J Sports Med.* 2007; 35:1123–1130. doi. org/10.1177/0363546507301585.

45. Leetun DT, Ireland ML, Willson JD, Ballantyne BT, Davis IM. Core stability measures as risk factors for lower extremity injury in athletes. *Med Sci Sports Exerc.* 2004; 36(6):926–934.

46. Nesser TW, Huxel KC, Tincher JL, Okada T. The relationship between core stability and performance in division I football players. *J Strength Cond Res.* 2008; 22(6):1750–1754.

47. McGill SM, Childs A, Liebenson C. Endurance time for low back stabilization exercises: clinical targets for testing and training from a normal database. *Arch Phys Med Rehabil.* 1999; 80:941–944.

48. McGill SM. *Low Back Disorders. Evidence-Based Prevention and Rehabilitation.* Champaign: Human Kinetics, 2002.

49. Juan-Recio C, López-Plaza D, Barbado Murillo D, García-Vaquero MP, Vera-García FJ. Reliability assessment and correlation analysis of 3 protocols to measure trunk muscle strength and endurance. *J Sports Sci.* 2018; 36(4):357–364. doi: 10.1080/02640414.2017.1307439.

50. Read PJ, Oliver JL, De Ste Croix MBA, Myer GD, Lloyd RS. A review of field-based assessments of neuromuscular control and their utility in male youth soccer players. *J Strength Cond Res.* 2019; 33(1):283–299. doi: 10.1519/JSC.0000000000002069.

51. Krause DA, Youdas JW, Hollman JH, Smith J. Abdominal muscle performance as measured by the double leg-lowering test. *Arch Phys Med Rehabil.* 2005; 86(7):1345–1348.

52. Stanton R, Reaburn PR, Humphries B. The effect of short-term Swiss ball training on core stability and running economy. *J Strength Cond Res.* 2004; 18(3):522–528.

53. Faries MD, Greenwood M. Core training: stabilizing the confusion. *Natl Strength Condition Assoc.* 2007; 29(2):10–25.

54. Kibler WB, Press J, Sciascia A. The role of core stability in athletic function. *Sports Med.* 2006; 36(3):189–198.

55. Weir A, Darby J, Inklaar H, Koes B, Bakker E, Tol JL. Core stability: Inter- and intraobserver reliability of 6 clinical tests. *Clin J Sport Med.* 2010; 20(1):34–38.

8

KINEMATIC AND KINETIC ASSESSMENT IN PROFESSIONAL FOOTBALL PLAYERS

Javier Courel-Ibáñez and Raúl Domínguez Herrera

8.1 Linear sprinting assessment

Linear sprints are an essential component of soccer performance [1, 2] and involved in most of goal situations [3]. Current trends in soccer strength and conditioning (S&C) are speeding up the game [1], making the sprinting ability of utmost importance. Descriptive studies examining players behaviors during competition revealed that professional soccer players normally perform sprint no longer than 30 m [4] and lasting 2–4 s [5], accounting for 1–11% of the total distance covered during a match [6]. Table 8.1 summarizes the common sprint outcomes in soccer. Of note, different studies have reported that the time to cover 10 m is strongly related with soccer performance [7–9], while longer runs > 30 m may better reflect the maximum speed [5].

8.1.1 Testing procedures for sprinting assessment

Warm-up: dynamic warm-up including jogging, joint mobility, and progressive accelerations (e.g., 2 × 15 m at self-controlled 30–50% and 50–70% of maximum speed) with 1 min of rest in between and one practice trial for familiarization. To avoid injuries, players should avoid sudden breaks to finish the test and smoothly decrease velocity, while crossing the finish line.

Set-up and execution: the test starts with the player in a natural standing position (i.e., ready to start a sprint), with one foot behind the start line. The executer must initiate the test with a maximum acceleration and try to cover the distance on the shortest time possible. Besides a traditional stopwatch, photoelectric cells (i.e., photocells) and radars are widely used to increase the accuracy of the outcomes. If using photocells, players should start 0.5 m behind the first gate to avoid starting the chronometer before crossing the cell. The starting position may account for the results, so it must be standardized.

DOI: 10.4324/9781032637006-8

TABLE 8.1 Examples for sprinting outcomes in soccer players

Sample	0–5 m	0–10 m	0–20 m	0–30 m	0–40 m
Men					
Spanish first division	1.38 ± 0.06		3.38 ± 0.12		
Spanish second division	1.40 ± 0.03		3.42 ± 0.08		
Spanish third division	1.43 ± 0.06		3.46 ± 0.11		
Spanish fifth division	1.44 ± 0.06		3.54 ± 0.13		
Grecian youth National Team		1.95 ± 0.34			
Grecian youth National division		2.14 ± 0.41			
French first division		1.80 ± 0.06		4.22 ± 0.19	
French second division		1.82 ± 0.08		4.25 ± 0.14	
Danish National team		1.67	3.05	4.35	5.64
Danish First division		1.70	3.11	4.43	5.75
Danish junior elite		1.70	3.12	4.44	5.77
British junior elite				4.31 ± 0.04	
British junior sub-elite				4.46 ± 0.21	
Younger Tunisian elite		1.87 ± 0.10		4.38 ± 0.18	
British first and second division		1.83 ± 0.08			
Turkish different league				4.26 ± 0.13	
Females					
Spanish first division	1.50 ± 0.05		3.72 ± 0.12		
Spanish second division	1.50 ± 0.05		3.78 ± 0.11		
Spanish first division				4.9 ± 0.2	
Spanish second division				5.0 ± 0.2	

Data are seconds [5, 7–13].

8.2 Agility and change-of-direction (COD)

The ability to quickly accelerate and decelerate and effectively change direction (COD) plays a key role in soccer both to enhance scoring actions and avoid conceding a goal [4]. Enhancing agility (i.e., the ability to perform COD rapidly) is one of the most important objectives of the S&C programs on soccer players, especially during the off-season period [14]. Besides physical conditioning, agility is related to perceptual and decision-making skills, particularly during very rapid actions [15]. Indeed, agility development is also essential during formative stages to facilitate skill transfer, enabling the learning of new skills, reducing incidence of injury, and facilitating re-learning of old skills during rehabilitation and return-to-play processes [16].

Critical evaluations of COD assessment with best-practice guidelines examining over 40 tests have been recently published [17–19]. Because there is not a single comprehensively valid test of COD or agility, practitioners should design or select their own tests by considering the number of COD, time to complete the test, total distance, and angles of COD [17]. The typical measure of agility and COD is done by recording the total time to complete the test. Despite highly reliable, total time has been criticized to be biased to linear sprint ability and thus masking actual COD ability [17, 20]. Recent approaches suggest using the COD deficit measure (i.e., subtracting athletes' equidistant linear sprint time from the COD test) [20, 21] as a more isolated measure of COD, both as an absolute score or z-score. The COD deficit can be easily calculated and often requires minimal effort because 10-m sprint times are typically measured along with 505 performances in testing batteries.

COD deficit = COD test − Equidistant linear sprint test

Future perspectives for COD are focused in enhancing the ecological value to determine the perceptual and decision-making skills as a reaction to a given stimulus (e.g., anticipating to an attacker cutting manoeuvre) [19]. Alternative tests emerged a few years ago to measure the reactive agility using lights [4, 22, 23]. Human stimuli are also advisable for a more ecologically valid stimulus without compromising the test reliability [18]. Indeed, latest reviews highlighted that most agility tests occur in simple contexts, whereby only two possible responses are possible, concluding the need of creating more specific and complex environments that challenge the cognitive process of high-level athletes [19].

8.2.1 Testing procedures for agility and COD assessment

Here, we briefly explain four common COD tests (Figures 8.1 and 8.2); for a detailed description of COD and agility tests, see [17–19]. The starting position may account for the results, so it must be standardized. If using photocells, players should start 0.5 m behind the first gate to avoid starting the chronometer before crossing the cell. The turning ability on each leg should be tested. Some tests may also be adapted for sport-specific testing by dribbling a ball through the course.

505 test [24]: Players assumed a starting position 10 m from the start line, ran as quickly as possible through the start/finish line, pivoted 180° at the 15-m line and returned as fast as possible. The time taken to cover the 5 m up and back distance – 10 m total is recorded. The subject should be encouraged to not overstep the line by too much as this will increase their time.

Zigzag COD [25,26]: This test requires the player to run a course around cones in the shortest possible time. A common configuration is to complete four splits of 5 m with 100° angle.

T-Test (modified) [27]: This test involves forward, lateral, and backward movements. Players complete five sprints as follows: 5 m forward, side-shuffle 2.5 m to the left, side shuffle 5 m to the right, side-shuffle 2.5 m to the left, and 5 m backwards until crossing the starting line.

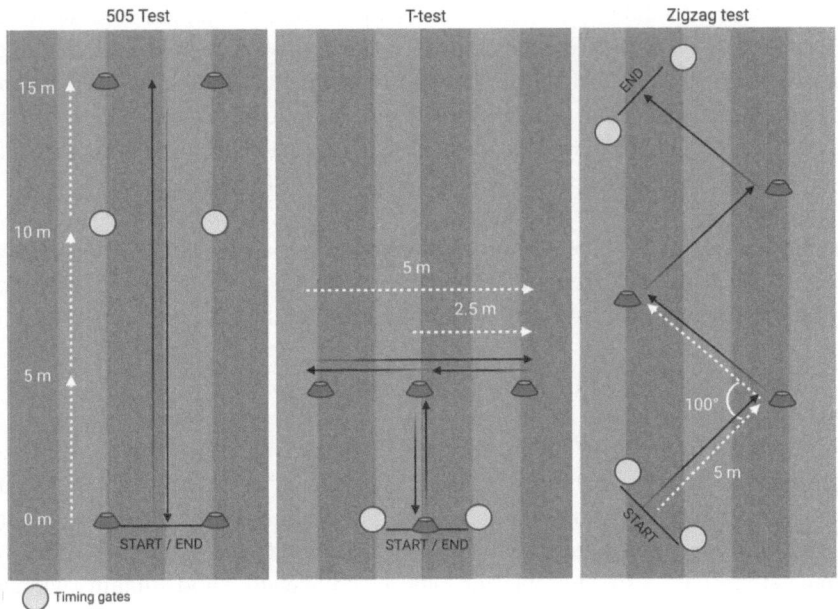

FIGURE 8.1 Three common agility and Change of Direction (COD) tests in soccer.

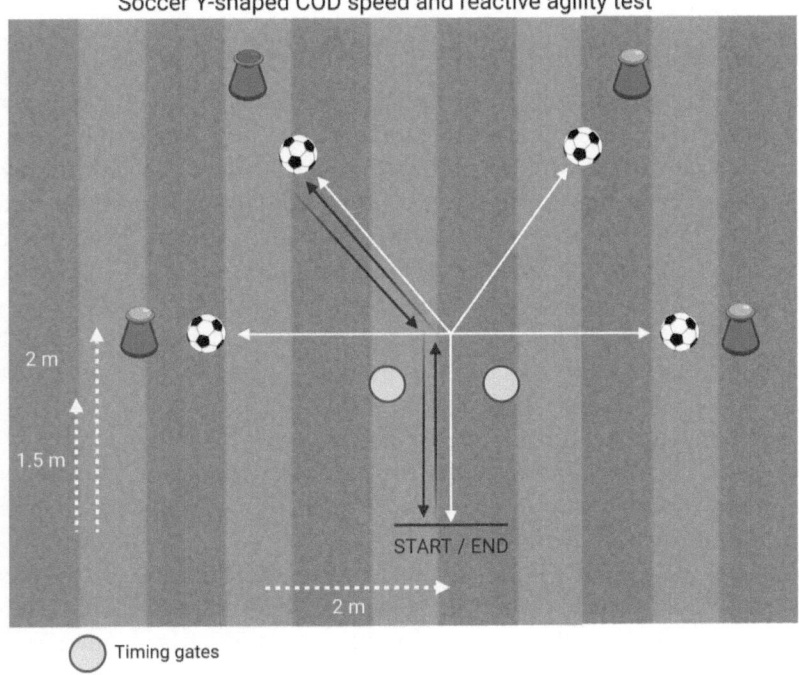

FIGURE 8.2 The soccer-specific, Y-shaped COD speed and reactive agility test.

Soccer-specific Y-shaped COD speed and reactive agility test [23]: Players start from the start line and run toward the timing gate (1.5 m forward). When the player crosses, a hardware module light in one of the four LEDs is placed inside the 30-cm-high cones. Players had to assess which cone was lit, run to the particular cone, kick (rebound) the ball in front of the cone placed at the specially constructed stand positioned 3 cm above the ground, and return to the start line as quickly as possible.

8.3 Jumping assessment

Vertical jumps are universally used to determine players' lower body strength and power by examining how much force players are able to produce in a very short time period [28, 29]. As other sports, common vertical jumping tests in soccer are the countermovement jump (CMJ, Figure 8.4), squat jump (SJ, Figure 8.5), and the Abalakov test (Figure 8.6) [7–10, 12, 30–32]. Besides, drop jumps (DJ, Figure 8.7) from 10-cm to 40-cm boxes are frequently used to examine the ability to quickly switch from an eccentric to a concentric contraction [33].

In essence, vertical jump involves three phases (Figure 8.3): an initial contact phase lowering the body against the ground that ends with a take-off (TO) from the ground, leading to a flight phase or time in the air (TIA) and a landing final phase. The contact phase is also divided into a downward or eccentric phase and an upward or concentric phase.

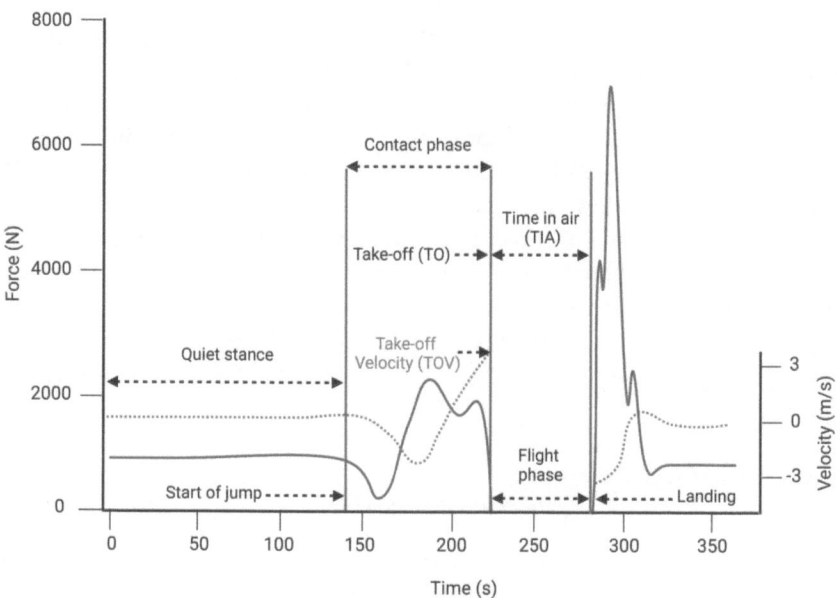

FIGURE 8.3 An example of jumping phases and force–time–velocity curves from a Countermovement Jump (CMJ). TOV: Take-off velocity.

Recording time, force, and/or displacement during a jump provides a number of useful metrics (Tables 8.2 and 8.3). Jump height is probably the most popular metric. The gold standard method to determine the vertical jump height requires a force platform to obtain the take-off velocity (TOV) and applying the equation [29]:

$$\text{TOV jump height} = \frac{TOV^2}{2g}$$

*g = 9.81 m·s^{-2} (gravitational acceleration); TOV = take-off velocity

However, the costs of the force platform and its low ecological value on the majority of sports including soccer (i.e., don't allow jumping on the field or using the soccer boots) have given rise to more practical and accessible technologies that estimate jump height from the time in the air (TIA), such as contact platforms, photocells mats [34], or smartphone apps [35]. TIA jump height estimation relies on the biomechanical inherent relationship between velocity, displacement, and time; hence, the jump height can be indirectly estimated from the total flight time using the equation:

$$\text{TIA jump height} = 1/2g \left(\frac{TIA}{2} \right)^2$$

*g = 9.81 m·s^{-2} (gravitational acceleration); TIA = time in the air

Despite its popularity, there is growing evidence suggesting that height may not be a good indicator of lower limb power or maximal power output capability [41]. Some authors proposed the external maximal power output capacity (P_{max}) and the jump condition power output (P_{jump}) as better variables to account for performance in soccer. Furthermore, the S&C community is recently falling out to see the process (i.e., the jump strategy) as a far better performance indicator than the output (i.e., jump height) [42]. These approaches will be later explained in the sections "Force-velocity-power (FVP) profiling" and "Rate of Force Development (RFD)."

Additionally, DJ allows the calculation of the Reactive Strength Index (RSI), a common variable used in soccer to examine the rapid force development ability and to optimize the plyometric training [43, 44]. A higher value of the RSI reflects a more efficient performance of the movement in the stretch-shortening cycle. Therefore, a great ground contact time (e.g., > 0.25 s) may suggest that the intensity of that particular exercise is too difficult for the athlete and needs to be adapted or replaced [43, 44].

$$\text{RSI} = jump\ height(cm) \Big/ ground\ contact\ time(s)$$

Latest studies suggest that jumping metrics are also useful indicators of neuromuscular fatigue-overload in soccer and may facilitate individualized load monitoring [45]. Jump height loss in a CMJ has been shown as an effective measure used to quantify the fatigue induced during the training session [46, 47]. DJ performance

TABLE 8.2 Performance, kinetic, and temporal jumping metrics. Modified from Cohen et al. [32]

Metric	Definition
Jump height (cm)	Determined using the TOV or TIA methods
Reactive strength index, RSI	Jump height/contraction time (time from initiation of movement to take-off)
Downward (eccentric) phase	
Deceleration impulse (Ns)	Net impulse (force x time) during the eccentric deceleration phase (from maximum negative velocity to zero velocity)
Yielding RFD (N/s)	Average rate of force development (Δ force/Δ time) calculated between the start of the yielding phase (i.e., minimum force) and the start of jump-deceleration phase (when velocity crosses zero)
Deceleration RFD (N/s)	Average rate of force development (Δ force/Δ time) between the start of the jump-deceleration phase and the jump-concentric phase
Force at 0 velocity (N)	Force at timepoint of zero velocity (end of eccentric/ beginning of jump-concentric phase)
Peak velocity (m/s)	Maximal negative velocity during the jump-eccentric phase
Peak power (W)	Maximal negative power during the jump-eccentric phase
Unloading phase duration (s)	Time between the point of minimum force and point of maximum negative velocity in the jump-eccentric phase
Yielding phase duration (s)	Time between the point of minimum force and point of maximum negative velocity in the jump-eccentric phase
Deceleration duration (s)	Time between minimum velocity and end of jump-eccentric phase (zero velocity/countermovement depth)
Countermovement depth (cm)	maximal center of mass displacement during jump-eccentric phase
Upward (concentric) phase	
Peak force (N)	Maximal force value during the jump-concentric phase
Force at peak power (N)	Force value at the timepoint of peak power during jump-concentric phase
Impulse (Ns)	Maximal velocity value during the jump-concentric phase
Peak velocity (m/s)	
Peak power (W)	Maximal power value during the concentric phase
Duration (s)	Time between the start of the concentric phase to take-off
Landing phase	
Peak force (N)	Maximal force during the landing phase
Landing RFD (N/s)	Average rate of force development (Δ force/Δ time) calculated between the landing timepoint and timepoint of peak landing force
Com depth at peak force (cm)	Center of mass displacement between the landing timepoint and the timepoint of peak landing force
Max landing cm depth (cm)	Maximum center of mass displacement during landing phase
Time to max landing depth (s)	Time from landing to timepoint of the maximum center of mass displacement

TOV = take-off velocity. TIA = time in the air. RFD: Rate of force development [36–40].

TABLE 8.3 Examples for jumping outcomes in soccer players

Sample	Squat Jump (SJ)	Countermovement Jump (CMJ)	Abalakov jumping test
Men			
Spanish first division		43.7 ± 2.2	50.1 ± 4.2
Spanish second division			
Spanish junior fourth division		43.9 ± 4.8	51.8 ± 4.8
Spanish different league	37.2	46.5	57.17
French first division	38.5 ± 3.8	41.6 ± 4.2	
French second division	33.8 ± 7.5	39.7 ± 5.2	
Turkish different league	51.3 ± 6.7		
British junior elite			55.8 ± 5.8
British junior sub-elite			50.2 ± 7.6
Females			
Spanish first division	26.1 ± 0.4	26.7 ± 0.3	
Spanish first division		32.6 ± 3.7	38.0 ± 4.8
Spanish second division	24.2 ± 0.3	24.3 ± 0.3	
Spanish junior second division		28.4 ± 2.0	33.1 ± 2.7
Danish National team		30.7 ± 4.1	
Danish First division		28.1 ± 4.1	
Danish junior elite		28.5 ± 4.1	
American youth first division		40.9 ± 5.5	

Data are cm. [7, 9, 10, 12, 30–32].

is used as a readiness-to-train monitoring tool [48] and for injury-risk screening purposes [49]. Furthermore, the analysis of jump landing and eccentric phases seems a promising tool for injury risk and motor control screening in soccer [50, 51].

8.3.1 Testing procedures for jumping assessment

Warm-up: include squatting and dynamic stretching previous to a set of 3–5 jumps at the specific test and increased intensity interspersed by 45 s. The test should start after a 3-min period of rest for ensuring a complete recovery.

Countermovement jump (CMJ): players start the test with the arms on the hip and the legs extended and jump bending the knees ~90° for initiating quickly a synchronously knee extension (concentric action) in an explosive action to attain the maximum height possible. During the flight phase, the knees continue extending and the hand keeping on the hips, avoiding any sideways or backward/forward movements, while the contact with the ground is first made with the toes.

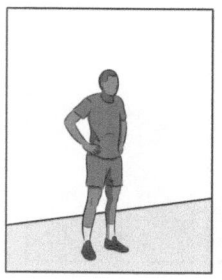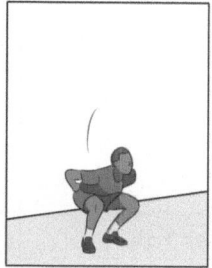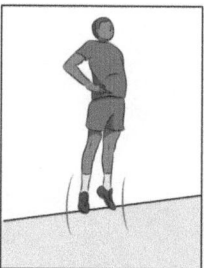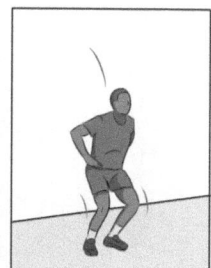

FIGURE 8.4   Countermovement Jump (CMJ).

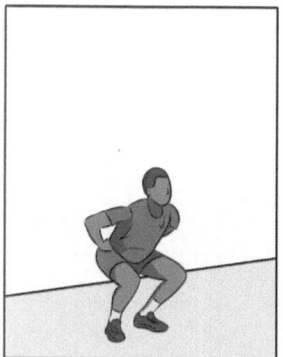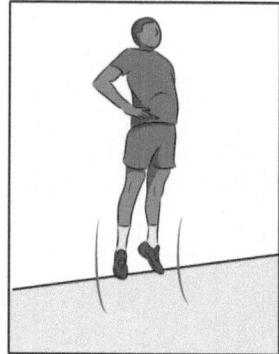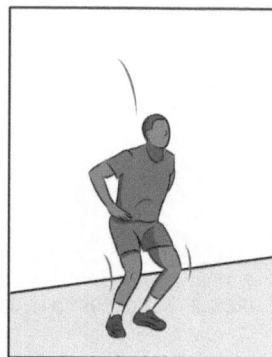

FIGURE 8.5   Squat Jump (SJ).

Squat jump (SJ): players squat until an angle of ~90° (range: 80–100°) and stop during 4 s to avoid any countermovement and, consequently, the elastic component contribution to the jump during the concentric phase [45]. From this position, play-ers perform an explosive extension of the lower limb while they keep the hands on the hips and jump as high as possible. Previous to each jump, players should be instructed to remain inside the jumping area. A manual goniometer or an elastic cord must be located for ensuring the absence of movement during the 2–4 s previ-ous to the beginning of the jumps [45, 52].

Abalakov test: players start with the leg extended and the arm ready for per-forming an impulse when the jump starts. The jump is similar to a CMJ but allow-ing the use of the arms and shoulders to give impulse during the eccentric phase.

Drop jump (DJ): players are asked to drop from a box at a given height (nor-mally from 10 to 40 cm) and perform a maximal vertical jump with the shortest ground-contact time. Players start standing up with their hands placed on the hips and initiated the step-off phase with stepping out of the box with a single leg (not jumping) [33].

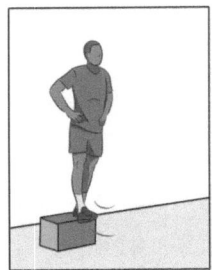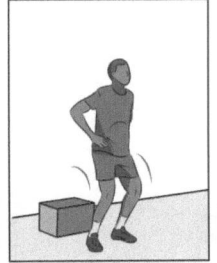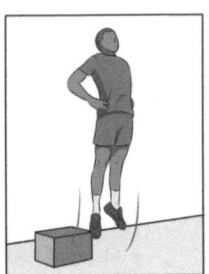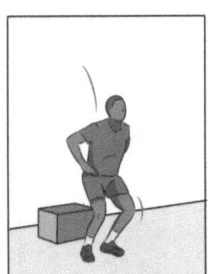

FIGURE 8.6 Abalakov jumping test.

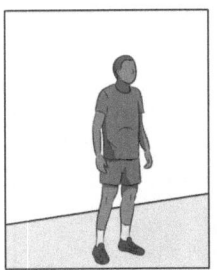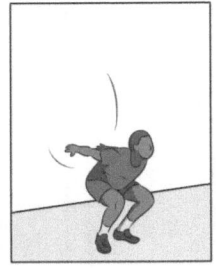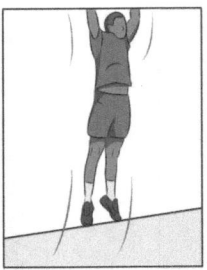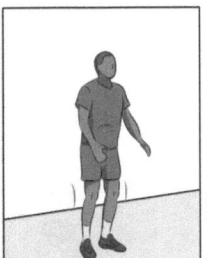

FIGURE 8.7 Drop Jump (DJ).

8.4 Force–Velocity–Power (FVP) profiling

In the last decade, some authors have proposed computing calculations from the jumping and sprinting test to determine the force–velocity–power (FVP) profile to obtain a more detailed information about the physiological and mechanical individual underpinnings of jump performance [53, 54]. Combining the horizontal (sprint-acceleration) and vertical (loaded jumps) force metrics, the FVP profile provides an integrative mechanical representation of the maximal capability of the players [55]. From this profile, one can detect imbalances or deficits in force or velocity and regulate training contents accordingly [56]. Recently, it has been suggested that training based on the FVP profile optimizes sport performance with respect to a traditional training program [52]. So, the FVP profile seems useful in soccer to inform about the muscular capability of the players and to set benchmarks to individualize physical training programs.

Testing procedures for FVP assessment: jumping profile

Jumping FVP profile assessment requires the assessment of two SJ without load (Figure 8.5) with a recovery of 2 minutes and 4–6 sets of loaded SJ (Figure 8.8) in a range of 10–90 kg that are applied in a randomized order (not progressive increasing or decreasing load protocol) [52, 53]. In practice, after familiarization, the full test can be replaced by a quicker 2-load test [57] (0% and 75% of body mass) using an available online Excel® sheet.

Nevertheless, the maximum load used must be considered the external load that impairs a jump height more than 10 cm [54]. The recovery period between sets should be ~2 minutes, and the best jump (highest) is selected for further analysis.

From each trial, practitioners should select the jump height, system mass (body mass of the athlete plus extra load used), and push-off distance. The push-off distance corresponds to the vertical distance covered by the center of mass of the athlete during the take-off. Therefore, the push-off assessment requires measuring the difference between extended lower limb distance (iliac crest to toes with plantar flexed ankle) and the length on the SJ starting position. Thus, the mean power produced during a jump (P_{jump}) is calculated using the following equations [58]:

$$P_{jump} = mg\left(\frac{h}{h_{PO}} + 1\right) \times \sqrt{\frac{gh}{2}}$$

with m the mass of the athlete plus external load, g the gravitational acceleration (9.81 m/s), h the height jump (expressed as m), and h_{PO} the vertical push-off distance. Thus, jump height was defined as the aerial distance covered by the center of mass between the take-off and vertical apex instants.

These procedures are summarized on a YouTube video, and calculations can be computed using a freely available online Excel sheet. For example, Figure 8.9 shows the FVP for a soccer player of 78 kg weight who jumped 27.8 cm in and unloaded SJ and then 11.2 cm with 55 kg (i.e., 75% of body mass).

8.4.1 Testing procedures for FVP assessment: sprinting profile

Sprinting FVP profile assessment requires performing seven maximal sprints: $2 \times 10\,m - 2 \times 15\,m - 20\,m - 30\,m - 40\,m$, which led to establish the force–velocity relationship [59]. Thus, using the best time (i.e., lowest) obtained in each sprint, it is

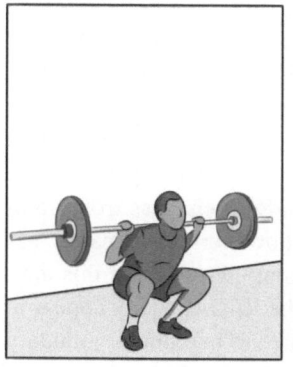
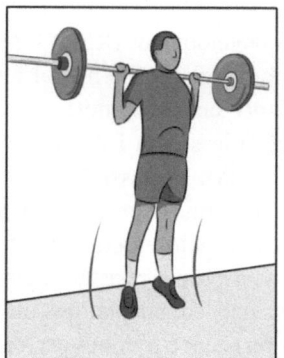
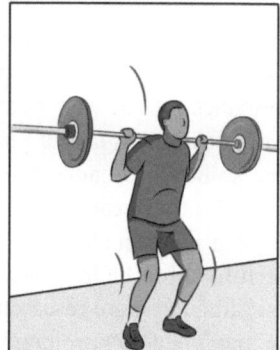

FIGURE 8.8 Loaded Squat Jump.

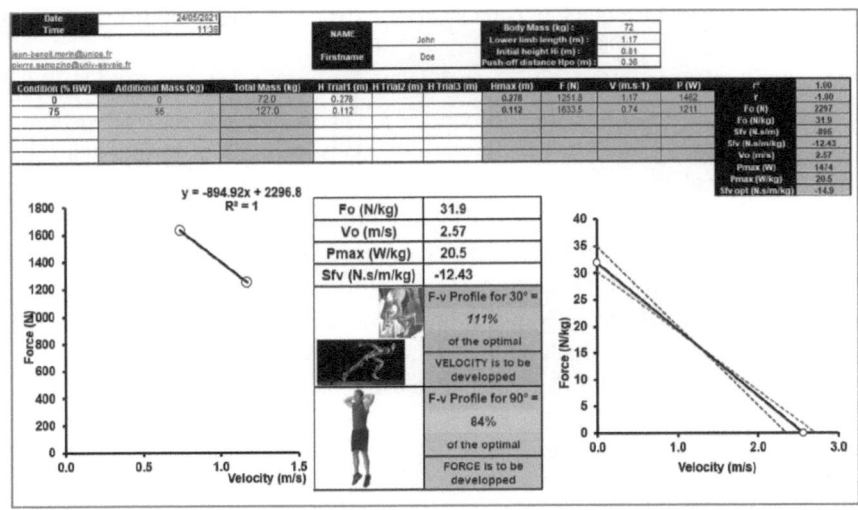

FIGURE 8.9 Example of an FVP profile in jumping using the 2-load method and the available online Excel sheet.

possible to calculate the velocity–time curve and acceleration that, summed to the net horizontal external force, led to calculating the FVP profile. Nevertheless, these authors simplified this method including a simple 30-m sprint test (split times at 5, 10, 15, 20, 25, and 30 m) and data about height (expressed as m), mass (expressed as kg), air temperature (expressed as °C), and air pressure (expressed as hPa).

These procedures are summarized on a YouTube video, and calculations can be computed using a freely available online Excel sheet [59]. For example, Figure 8.10 shows the FVP for a soccer player of 1.77 m height and 72 kg weight who completes a 30-m sprint test in 4.99 s with split times of 5 m: 1.4 s, 10 m: 2.23 s, 15 m: 2.98 s, 20m: 3.64 s, and 25 m: 4.29 s.

8.5 Rate of Force Development (RFD)

In essence, the rate of force development (RFD) refers to the ability to produce force rapidly, and thus it informs about the neural efficiency of motor skill performance [60, 61]. In soccer, players have limited time in which to produce force, with movements taking place in less than 100–200 ms. Thus, increments in players' ability to produce force as fast as possible will result in better performance [60, 62–66]. Because of this neuromuscular component, RFD changes from training can be difficult to detect in a field-based context; however, this capacity has been found to be improved with proper resistance training [61–63]. On this matter, although more research is needed, adaptations on the RFD capacity appear to be maximized by prolonged resistance training performed at maximum voluntary velocity (i.e., ballistic contractions) [67]. Common metrics for the assessment of players' force–time profiling are described in Table 8.4.

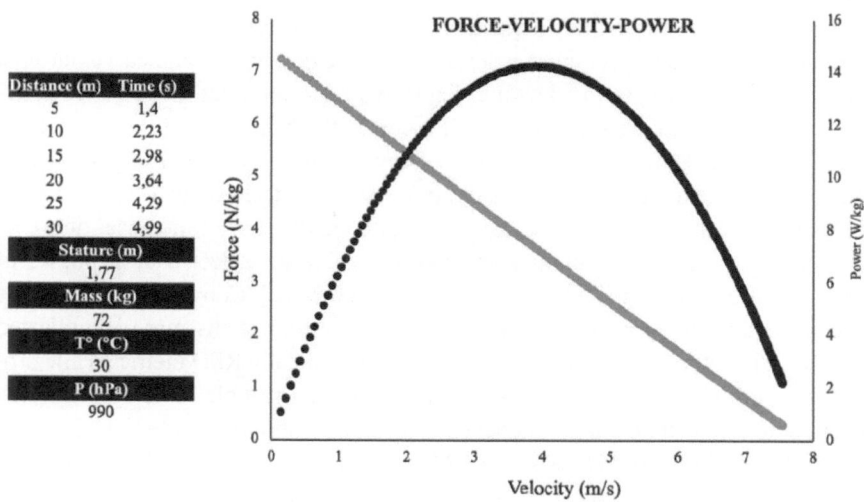

Distance (m)	Time (s)
5	1,4
10	2,23
15	2,98
20	3,64
25	4,29
30	4,99
Stature (m)	
1,77	
Mass (kg)	
72	
T° (°C)	
30	
P (hPa)	
990	

FORCE-VELOCITY-POWER

FIGURE 8.10   A graphical representation of the FVP profile in sprinting. Taken from a free Excel sheet.

TABLE 8.4 Common metrics for RFD assessment

Metric	Definition
Average RFD (N/s)	The slope of the force–time curve (ΔForce/Δtime) calculated by dividing the change in force at the end of the time interval (i.e., initial phase – end phase) by the duration of the time interval (in seconds). Time-interval RFD are calculated for sequential (e.g., 0–50, 50–100, 100–150, and 150–200 ms) or overlapping periods (e.g., 0–50, 0–100, 0–150, and 0–200 ms) to collect measures in different phases of the contraction.
Instantaneous RFD (N/s)	The maximal tangential slope between two adjacent data points (i.e., the change in force is divided by the change in time at every 1-ms time interval).
Peak RFD (N/s)	Peak slope of the force–time curve (i.e., the largest RFD value during a given effort).
Impulse (Ns)	Integration of force over time (i.e., cumulated area under the force–time curve). Like RFD, average impulse can be computed for different RFD periods (e.g., Impulse 0–50, Impulse 0–150, and Impulse 0–250).
Time to peak RFD (ms)	Time to reach the peak RFD.

* *Note*: isokinetic dynamometers report data of rate of torque development (RTD) in $N \cdot m \cdot s^{-1}$, based on the torque signals.

The RFD is a force-time dependent variable; therefore, we need to plot a force–time curve to collect the metrics. An example of a force–time curve during a ballistic, the isometric test is shown in Figure 8.11. Because our interest is to determine the rapid force production, we will focus on the beginning of the contraction onset (<100–150 ms). An optimal time window should be set according to the athlete's experience in the test and the sampling rate of the technology (i.e., the longer the experience and the higher the frequency of data, the shorter the onset time).

Overall, available technologies are highly reliable to collect data at phases of contractions comprising 0–150 ms and 0–250 ms [68–72]. Conversely, an accurate testing for the earliest phases of contractions (<100 ms) seems more complicated [70, 71, 73]. Nowadays, one can easily collect automatically RFD metrics while providing real-time visual feedback using force plates or portable force sensors (e.g., dynamometers or strain gauges) attached to a bench, a post, or a table [70, 73–75].

In addition to isometric tests, the CMJ (Figure 8.4) is commonly used to collect RFD data. In particular, the RFD during the eccentric phase (ECC-RFD) has been suggested as the most determinant force–time determinant for jumping performance [76, 77]. In turn, the peak RFD during the concentric phase is shown unreliable [78]. More recently, the assessment of the ECC-RFD during the yielding phase and the landing phase (see Table 8.2) is done to identify changes in coordination/motor control strategies [31, 32].

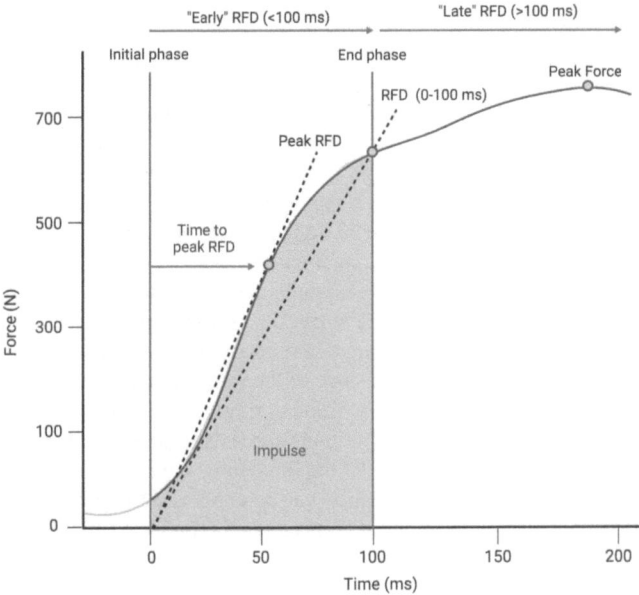

FIGURE 8.11   Rate of Force Development (RFD) measures from the force–time curve during an isometric ballistic test.

RFD is considered a key variable in soccer to optimize the performance by enhancing the muscle strength in rapid movements with fast stretch shortening cycle demands (< 100 ms from the onset of contraction) such as accelerating/decelerating and jumping/landing [60, 79–82]. Increments in the force production at very rapid events (< 50 ms) are critical in minimizing risk of suffering injuries such as anterior cruciate ligament (ACL) [83]. Furthermore, evidence suggests RFD as an early sensitive marker for muscle stiffness, muscle damage, and match-induced fatigue; thus, it is gaining interest as a screening tool for injury rehabilitation management [63, 84–87]. In particular, the RFD hamstring-to-quadriceps ratio (RFD H:Q) [82, 85, 86, 88, 89] and the yielding/landing ECC-RFD during a CMJ [31, 32] seem to be relevant metrics for monitoring soccer players.

8.5.1 Testing procedures for RFD assessment

A number of RFD protocols have been described depending on the purposes. In a field-based context, accessible alternatives such as portable force sensors with strain gauge load cells or hand dynamometers secured with a belt are emerging [71, 72, 74, 90–93], which give coaches and S&C trainers the opportunity to design soccer task-specific testing procedures. Nonetheless, coaches must be careful to create robust methods to collected reliable RFD metrics considering the testing procedures [68, 69], the instructions and focus of attention [94], the athletes' familiarization [71], the signal filtering [70], and the warm-up [95]. Furthermore, because RFD is known to be affected by the muscle group and joint angle at which it is measured, a task-specific assessment approach seems advisable [68, 69].

Warm-up: RFD assessment requires ballistic executions; thus, prior to test, players should perform a specific warm-up including rapid response neuromuscular activation exercises [95]. Familiarization with the test is advisable to increase reliability, especially if measuring very early phases [71].

Execution: Players must perform rapid contractions, as fast and hard as possible, with the emphasis on the explosive/ballistic phase of contraction for 3 s. A countdown of "3, 2, 1, go!" may help in bringing the players to their maximum effort. External cues like "try to break the chain" may also increase performance [94]. Strong verbal encouragement is advisable. Visual inspection of the force–time curve is important to note that all participants reached their maximum capability within 3-s and a 1-s plateau was observed before the contraction ending. Players should complete at least two good trials with 30–45 s rest in between to confirm the results.

Ballistic isometric knee flexion/extension (Figure 8.12): A specific warm-up including two sets of 6 s of three base rotations, side to side over line and 2-inch runs, is advisable [95]. A standardized 3-min warm-up including 12 sub-maximal countermovement jumps and soccer drills (i.e., skipping and short displacements) has also been proposed [86]. If using a dynamometer, follow the manufacturer instructions. If using alternatives such as portable force sensors (e.g., strain gauge), the player sits on a chair, bench, or stretcher with an 80–85° hip flexion and arms crossed. Strapping players to the seat and fixing the free leg could help increase reliability and bring them to their maximum effort. The sensor is secured at one end of the bench at 20–40 cm from the floor and attached at the other to a chain connected to a resistant padded anklet. The anklet must be resistant enough to support the maximal stress, to guarantee the mechanical rigidity, and minimize joint movement. The chain length can be adapted to each players' anthropometric characteristics to achieve mechanical rigidity. Anatomical comfortable knee joint angles may help in reproducibility. Angles can be adapted to the specific task. Common ranges for the knee extension test (quadriceps) are 70–110° of knee flexion [71, 86, 88]. For the knee flexion test (hamstring), common ranges are 60–70° [82, 85, 86, 88, 89]. For greater specificity, tests may be performed at 30° of knee flexion (0° represents full extension) because hamstring and knee ligament injuries are most susceptible to occur at a more extended knee angle [82, 85, 86, 88, 89]. Baseline conditions should be standardized using real-time visual feedback to avoid alterations in the measure due to initial pre-tension and countermovement. If possible, coaches should test both the knee flexion and extension tests sequentially to determine the hamstring-to-quadriceps (H:Q) RFD ratio [82, 85, 86, 88, 89].

Ballistic isometric midthigh clean pull (IMTP): Specific warm-up should include clean derivatives such as the dynamic midthigh pull (Figure 8.12) or sub-maximal IMTP bar for 3–5 s at a self-directed 50%, 75%, and 90% of maximal effort with 60-s recovery. Another proposal is 3 min of cycling, 10 bodyweight squats,

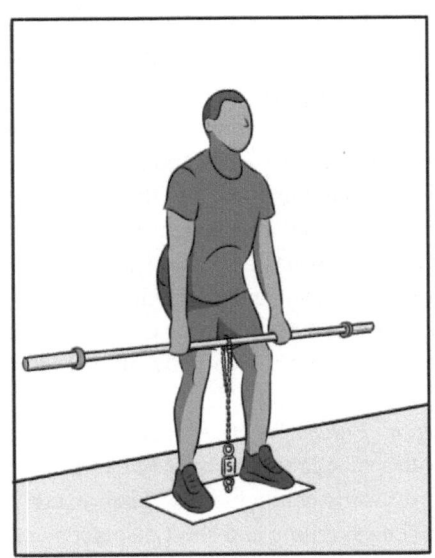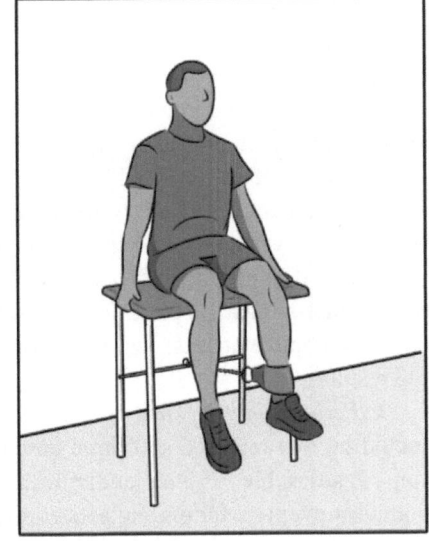

FIGURE 8.12   Isometric midthigh clean pull test (left) and isometric knee flexion test (right).

10 bodyweight walking lunges, and 10 glute bridges [75, 96–99]. The player stands on a force plate, holding an immovable bar. The bar height should be adjusted up or down to allow the player to obtain the optimal knee (125–145°) and hip (140–150°) angles. The body position should be upright torso, slight flexion in the knee resulting in some dorsiflexion, shoulder girdle retracted and depressed, shoulders above or slightly behind the vertical plane of the bar, feet roughly centered under the bar approximately hip width apart, knees underneath and in front of the bar, and thighs in contact with the bar (close to the inguinal crease dependent on limb lengths) [97]. Bar height and individual's angles, grip width, and foot position should be measured and standardized for individuals across sessions [75, 96–99]. The use of lifting straps may help in standardizing the measure and ensure that grip strength is not a limiting factor [97].

8.6 Practical applications and future perspectives

Most of soccer players' actions during a game involve very rapid contraction; thus, the time to produce force is very limited. Hence, the ability to produce force quickly is a critical part of optimizing physical performance.

Maximum speed on test of 30–40 m is very useful, but the acceleration capacity could be more related to soccer success than maximum speed; thus, it is advisable to use splits at 10 m for giving information related to the acceleration capability. Jumping metrics are an effective tool to monitor players' fatigue across a session and assist to individualize the training load.

The FVP could provide relevant information about soccer 'players conditioning from an integrative approach, identifying players' weaknesses, and setting training targets to improve performance in rapid force production actions. The free access to Excel sheets and the increase in accessible technologies make the FVP easy to be determined from sprinting and jumping tests.

Among the number of agility and COD tests, practitioners should adapt them according to the targeted performance requirements to be tested. Recording the COD deficit seems advisable for isolating the performance quality, as well as including complex, decision-making tasks along with the running and cutting abilities.

RFD is a valuable asset for muscle contractility, stiffness, fatigue, and neuromuscular deconditioning. Accordingly, S&C trainers should be focused to shift the force–time curve up (i.e., increasing the magnitude of force) and to the left (i.e., increasing the RFD). Current portable technologies allow the design of practical field-based, task-specific protocols to obtain RFD and impulse measures at different phases of the contraction. However, a proper RFD requires robust assessment methods, a regular monitoring, and a proper data interpretation.

Considering the practical implications of kinetic and kinematic metrics, further understanding of best-practice and testing procedures that can aid the development of practical and useful assessment continues to be of importance.

References

1. Wallace JL, Norton KI. Evolution of world cup soccer final games 1966–2010: Game structure, speed and play patterns. *J Sci Med Sport*. 2014;17(2):223–228. doi:10.1016/j.jsams.2013.03.016
2. Altmann S, Ringhof S, Neumann R, Woll A, Rumpf MC. Validity and reliability of speed tests used in soccer: A systematic review. *PLoS One*. 2019;14(8). doi:10.1371/journal.pone.0220982
3. Faude O, Koch T, Meyer T. Straight sprinting is the most frequent action in goal situations in professional football. *J Sports Sci*. Published online 2012. doi:10.1080/02640414.2012.665940
4. Turner A, Walker S, Stembridge M, et al. A testing battery for the assessment of fitness in soccer players. *Strength Cond J*. 2011;33(5):29–39. doi:10.1519/SSC.0b013e31822fc80a
5. Taşkin H. Evaluating sprinting ability, density of acceleration, and speed dribbling ability of professional soccer players with respect to their positions. *J Strength Cond Res*. 2008;22(5):1481–1486. doi:10.1519/JSC.0b013e318181fd90
6. Wisløff U, Castagna C, Helgerud J, Jones R, Hoff J. Strong correlation of maximal squat strength with sprint performance and vertical jump height in elite soccer players. *Br J Sports Med*. 2004;38(3):285–288.
7. Cometti G, Maffiuletti NA, Pousson M, Chatard JC, Maffulli N. Isokinetic strength and anaerobic power of elite, subelite and amateur French soccer players. *Int J Sports Med*. 2001;22(1):45–51. doi:10.1055/s-2001-11331
8. Gissis I, Papadopoulos C, Kalapotharakos V, Sotiropoulos A, Komsis G, Manolopoulos E. Strength and speed characteristics of elite, subelite, and recreational young soccer players. *Res Sport Med*. 2006;14(3):205–214. doi:10.1080/15438620600854769
9. Reilly T, Williams AM, Nevill A, Franks A. A multidisciplinary approach to talent identification in soccer. *J Sports Sci*. 2000;18(9):695–702. doi:10.1080/02640410050120078
10. Ramos-Campo DJ, Rubio-Arias JA, Carrasco-Poyatos M, Alcaraz PE. Physical performance of elite and subelite Spanish female futsal players. *Biol Sport*. 2016;33(3):297–304. doi:10.5604/20831862.1212633
11. Jiménez-Reyes P, García-Ramos A, Cuadrado-Peñafiel V, et al. Differences in sprint mechanical force–velocity profile between trained soccer and futsal players. *Int J Sports Physiol Perform*. 2019;14(4):478–485. doi:10.1123/ijspp.2018-0402 10.1123/ijspp.2018-0402 10.1123/ijspp.2018-0402 10.1123/ijspp.2018-0402
12. Haugen TA, Tønnessen E, Seiler S. Speed and countermovement-jump characteristics of elite female soccer players, 1995–2010. *Int J Sports Physiol Perform*. 2012;7(4):340–349. doi:10.1123/ijspp.7.4.340
13. Little T, Williams AG. Specificity of acceleration, maximum speed, and agility in professional soccer players. *J Strength Cond Res Cond Res / Natl Strength Cond Assoc*. 2005;19(1):76–78. doi:10.1519/14253.1
14. Sporis G, Jukic I, Milanovic L, Vucetic V. Reliability and factorial validity of agility tests for soccer players. *J Strength Cond Res*. 2010;24(3):679–686. doi:10.1519/JSC.0b013e3181c4d324
15. Sheppard JM, Young W. Agility literature review: Classifications, training and testing. *J Sports Sci*. 2006;24(9):919–932. doi:10.1080/02640410500457109
16. Liefeith A, Kiely J, Collins D, Richards J. Back to the future–in support of a renewed emphasis on generic agility training within sports-specific developmental pathways. *J Sports Sci*. 2018;36(19):2250–2255. doi:10.1080/02640414.2018.1449088

17. Nimphius S, Callaghan SJ, Bezodis NE, Lockie RG. Change of direction and agility tests: Challenging our current measures of performance. *Strength Cond J.* 2018;40(1):26–38. doi:10.1519/SSC.0000000000000309

18. Paul DJ, Gabbett TJ, Nassis GP. Agility in team sports: Testing, training and factors affecting performance. *Sport Med.* 2016;46(3):421–442. doi:10.1007/s40279-015-0428-2

19. Morral-Yepes M, Moras G, Bishop C, Gonzalo-Skok O. Assessing the reliability and validity of agility testing in team sports. *J Strength Cond Res.* 2022;36(7):2035–2049. doi:10.1519/jsc.0000000000003753

20. Thomas TDC, Comfort P, Jones PA. Comparison of change of direction speed performance and asymmetries between team-sport athletes: Application of change of direction deficit. *Sports.* 2018;6(4):174. doi:10.3390/sports6040174

21. Nimphius S, Callaghan SJ, Spiteri T, Lockie RG. Change of direction deficit: A more isolated measure of change of direction performance than total 505 time. *J Strength Cond Res.* 2016;30(11):3024–3032. doi:10.1519/JSC.0000000000001421

22. Fiorilli G, Iuliano E, Mitrotasios M, et al. Are change of direction speed and reactive agility useful for determining the optimal field position for young soccer players? *J Sport Sci Med.* 2017;16(2):247–253.

23. Pojskic H, Åslin E, Krolo A, et al. Importance of reactive agility and change of direction speed in differentiating performance levels in junior soccer players: Reliability and validity of newly developed soccer-specific tests. *Front Physiol.* 2018;9:506. doi:10.3389/fphys.2018.00506

24. Sammoud S, Bouguezzi R, Negra Y, Chaabene H. The reliability and sensitivity of change of direction deficit and its association with linear sprint speed in prepubertal male soccer players. *J Funct Morphol Kinesiol.* 2021;6(2):41. doi:10.3390/jfmk6020041

25. Meylan C, Trewin J, McKean K. Quantifying explosive actions in international women's soccer. *Int J Sports Physiol Perform.* 2017;12(3):310–315. doi:10.1123/ijspp.2015-0520

26. Loturco I, Nimphius S, Kobal R, et al. Change-of direction deficit in elite young soccer players: The limited relationship between conventional speed and power measures and change-of-direction performance. *Ger J Exerc Sport Res.* 2018;48(2):228–234. doi:10.1007/s12662-018-0502-7

27. Sassi RH, Dardouri W, Yahmed MH, Gmada N, Mahfoudhi ME, Gharbi Z. Relative and absolute reliability of a modified agility T-test and its relationship with vertical jump and straight sprint. *J Strength Cond Res.* 2009;23(6):1644–1651. doi:10.1519/JSC.0b013e3181b425d2

28. Barker LA, Harry JR, Mercer JA. Relationships between countermovement jump ground reaction forces and jump height, reactive strength index, and jump time. *J Strength Cond Res.* 2018;32(1):248. doi:10.1519/JSC.0000000000002160

29. Moir GL. Three different methods of calculating vertical jump height from force platform data in men and women. *Meas Phys Educ Exerc Sci.* 2008;12(4):207–218. doi:10.1080/10913670802349766

30. Centeno-Prada RA, López C, Naranjo-Orellana J. Jump percentile: A proposal for evaluation of high level sportsmen. *J Sports Med Phys Fitness.* 2015;55(5):464–470. Accessed May 24, 2021. https://pubmed.ncbi.nlm.nih.gov/26068326/

31. Mujika I, Santisteban J, Impellizzeri FM, Castagna C. Fitness determinants of success in men's and women's football. *J Sports Sci.* 2009;27(2):107–114. doi:10.1080/02640410802428071

32. Vescovi JD, McGuigan MR. Relationships between sprinting, agility, and jump ability in female athletes. *J Sports Sci.* 2008;26(1):97–107. doi:10.1080/02640410701348644

33. Pedley JS, Lloyd RS, Read P, Moore IS, Oliver JL. Drop jump: A technical model for scientific application. *Strength Cond J.* 2017;39(5):36–44. doi:10.1519/SSC.0000000000000331

34. García-López J, Morante JC, Ogueta-Alday A, Rodríguez-Marroyo JA. The type of mat (contact vs. photocell) affects vertical jump height estimated from flight time. *J Strength Cond Res.* 2013;27(4):1162–1167. doi:10.1519/JSC.0b013e31826520d7

35. Balsalobre-Fernández C, Glaister M, Lockey RA. The validity and reliability of an iPhone app for measuring vertical jump performance. *J Sports Sci.* 2015;33(15):1–6. doi:10.1080/02640414.2014.996184

36. Hart LM, Cohen DD, Patterson SD, Springham M, Reynolds J, Read P. Previous injury is associated with heightened countermovement jump force-time asymmetries in professional soccer players. *Transl Sport Med.* 2019;2(5):256–262. doi:10.1002/tsm2.92

37. Harry JR, Paquette MR, Schilling BK, Barker LA, James CR, Dufek JS. Kinetic and electromyographic subphase characteristics with relation to countermovement vertical jump performance. *J Appl Biomech.* 2018;34(4):291–297. doi:10.1123/jab.2017-0305

38. Harry JR, Barker LA, Eggleston JD, Dufek JS. Evaluating performance during maximum effort vertical jump landings. *J Appl Biomech.* 2018;34(5):403–409. doi:10.1123/jab.2017-0172

39. Gathercole RJ, Stellingwerff T, Sporer BC. Effect of acute fatigue and training adaptation on countermovement jump performance in elite snowboard cross athletes. *J Strength Cond Res.* 2015;29(1):37–46. doi:10.1519/JSC.0000000000000622

40. Cormie P, McGuigan MR, Newton RU. Changes in the eccentric phase contribute to improved stretch-shorten cycle performance after training. *Med Sci Sports Exerc.* 2010;42(9):1731–1744. doi:10.1249/MSS.0b013e3181d392e8

41. Morin JB, Jiménez-Reyes P, Brughelli M, Samozino P. When jump height is not a good indicator of lower limb maximal power output: Theoretical demonstration, experimental evidence and practical solutions. *Sport Med.* 2019;49(7):999–1006. doi:10.1007/s40279-019-01073-1

42. Turner AN, Comfort P, McMahon J, et al. Developing powerful athletes, part 1: Mechanical underpinnings. *Strength Cond J.* 2020;42(3):30–39. doi:10.1519/SSC.0000000000000543

43. Ramirez-Campillo R, Alvarez C, García-Pinillos F, et al. Optimal reactive strength index: Is it an accurate variable to optimize plyometric training effects on measures of physical fitness in young soccer players? *J Strength Cond Res.* 2018;32(4):885–893. doi:10.1519/jsc.0000000000002467

44. Flanagan EP, Comyns TM. The use of contact time and the reactive strength index to optimize fast stretch-shortening cycle training. *Strength Cond J.* 2008;30(5):32–38. doi:10.1519/SSC.0b013e318187e25b

45. Armada-Cortés E, Peláez Barrajón J, Benítez-Muñoz JA, Navarro E, San Juan AF. Can we rely on flight time to measure jumping performance or neuromuscular fatigue-overload in professional female soccer players? *Appl Sci.* 2020;10(13):4424. doi:10.3390/app10134424

46. Jimenez-Reyes P, Pareja-Blanco F, Cuadrado-Peñafiel V, Morcillo JA, Párraga JA, González-Badillo JJ. Mechanical, metabolic and perceptual response during sprint training. *Int J Sports Med.* 2016;37(10):807–812. doi:10.1055/s-0042-107251

47. Jiménez-Reyes P, Pareja-Blanco F, Cuadrado-Peñafiel V, Ortega-Becerra M, Párraga J, González-Badillo JJ. Jump height loss as an indicator of fatigue during sprint training. *J Sports Sci.* 2019;37(9):1029–1037. doi:10.1080/02640414.2018.1539445

48. Markwick WJ, Bird SP, Tufano JJ, Seitz LB, Haff GG. The intraday reliability of the reactive strength index calculated from a drop jump in professional men's basketball. *Int J Sports Physiol Perform.* 2015;10(4):482–488. doi:10.1123/ijspp.2014-0265

49. Noyes FR, Barber-Westin SD, Fleckenstein C, Walsh C, West J. The drop-jump screening test: Difference in lower limb control by gender and effect of neuromuscular training in female athletes. *Am J Sports Med.* 2005;33(2):197–207. doi:10.1177/0363546504266484

50. Van Der Does HTD, Brink MS, Benjaminse A, Visscher C, Lemmink KAPM. Jump landing characteristics predict lower extremity injuries in indoor team sports. *Int J Sports Med.* 2016;37(3):251–256. doi:10.1055/s-0035-1559688

51. Cohen DD, Restrepo A, Richter C, et al. Detraining of specific neuromuscular qualities in elite footballers during COVID-19 quarantine. *Sci Med Footb.* 2021;5(supl 1):26–31. doi:10.1080/24733938.2020.1834123

52. Jiménez-Reyes P, Samozino P, Brughelli M, Morin JB. Effectiveness of an individualized training based on force-velocity profiling during jumping. *Front Physiol.* 2017;6:67. doi:10.3389/fphys.2016.00677

53. Jiménez-Reyes P, Samozino P, García-Ramos A, Cuadrado-Peñafiel V, Brughelli M, Morin JB. Relationship between vertical and horizontal force-velocity-power profiles in various sports and levels of practice. *PeerJ.* Published online 2018;13(6):e5937. doi:10.7717/peerj.5937

54. Morin JB, Samozino P. Interpreting power-force-velocity profiles for individualized and specific training. *Int J Sports Physiol Perform.* Published online 2016;11(2):267–272. doi:10.1123/ijspp.2015-0638

55. Samozino P, Rejc E, Di Prampero PE, Belli A, Morin JB. Optimal force-velocity profile in ballistic movements-Altius: Citius or Fortius? *Med Sci Sports Exerc.* Published online 2012;44(2):313–322. doi:10.1249/MSS.0b013e31822d757a

56. Jiménez-Reyes P, Samozino P, Morin J-B. Optimized training for jumping performance using the force-velocity imbalance: Individual adaptation kinetics. Boullosa D, ed. *PLoS One.* 2019;14(5):e0216681. doi:10.1371/journal.pone.0216681

57. García-Ramos A, Pérez-Castilla A, Jaric S. Optimisation of applied loads when using the two-point method for assessing the force-velocity relationship during vertical jumps. *Sport Biomech.* 2021;20(3):274–289. doi:10.1080/14763141.2018.1545044

58. Samozino P, Morin JB, Hintzy F, Belli A. A simple method for measuring force, velocity and power output during squat jump. *J Biomech.* Published online 2008;41(14): 2940–2945. doi:10.1016/j.jbiomech.2008.07.028

59. Samozino P, Rabita G, Dorel S, et al. A simple method for measuring power, force, velocity properties, and mechanical effectiveness in sprint running. *Scand J Med Sci Sport.* Published online 2016;26(6):648–658 doi:10.1111/sms.12490

60. Taber C, Bellon C, Abbott H, Bingham GE. Roles of maximal strength and rate of force development in maximizing muscular power. *Strength Cond J.* 2016;38(1):71–78. doi:10.1519/SSC.0000000000000193

61. Haff GG, Nimphius S. Training principles for power. *Strength Cond J.* 2012;34(6):2–12. doi:10.1519/SSC.0b013e31826db467

62. Suchomel TJ, Nimphius S, Bellon CR, Stone MH. The importance of muscular strength: Training considerations. *Sport Med.* 2018;48(4):765–785. doi:10.1007/s40279-018-0862-z

63. Maestroni L, Read P, Bishop C, Turner A. Strength and power training in rehabilitation: Underpinning principles and practical strategies to return athletes to high performance. *Sport Med.* 2020;50(2):239–252. doi:10.1007/s40279-019-01195-6

64. Cormie P, McGuigan MR, Newton RU. Developing maximal neuromuscular power: Part 1 – Biological basis of maximal power production. *Sport Med.* 2011;41(1):17–38. doi:10.2165/11537690-000000000-00000

65. Dideriksen JL, Del Vecchio A, Farina D. Neural and muscular determinants of maximal rate of force development. *J Neurophysiol.* 2020;123(1):149–157. doi:10.1152/jn.00330.2019

66. Folland JP, Buckthorpe MW, Hannah R. Human capacity for explosive force production: Neural and contractile determinants. 2014;24(6):894–906. doi:10.1111/sms.12131

67. Van Cutsem M, Duchateau J, Hainaut K. Changes in single motor unit behaviour contribute to the increase in contraction speed after dynamic training in humans. *J Physiol.* 1998;513:295–305. doi:10.1111/j.1469-7793.1998.295by.x

68. Rodríguez-Rosell D, Pareja-Blanco F, Aagaard P, González-Badillo JJ. Physiological and methodological aspects of rate of force development assessment in human skeletal muscle. *Clin Physiol Funct Imaging.* Published online 2018;38(5):743–762. doi:10.1111/cpf.12495

69. Maffiuletti NA, Aagaard P, Blazevich AJ, Folland J, Tillin N, Duchateau J. Rate of force development: physiological and methodological considerations. *Eur J Appl Physiol.* 2016;116(6):1091–1116. doi:10.1007/s00421-016-3346-6

70. Moir GL, Getz A, Davis SE, Marques M, Witmer CA. The inter-session reliability of isometric force-time variables and the effects of filtering and starting force. *J Hum Kinet.* 2019;66(1):43–55. doi:10.2478/hukin-2018-0049

71. Courel-Ibáñez J, Hernández-Belmonte A, Cava-Martínez A, Pallarés JG. Familiarization and reliability of the isometric knee extension test for rapid force production assessment. *Appl Sci.* 2020;10(13):4499. doi:10.3390/app10134499

72. Lesnak J, Anderson D, Farmer B, Katsavelis D, Grindstaff TL. Validity of hand-held dynamometry in measuring quadriceps strength and rate of torque development. *Int J Sports Phys Ther.* 2019;14(2):180–187. doi:10.26603/ijspt20190180

73. Buckthorpe MW, Hannah R, Pain TG, Folland JP. Reliability of neuromuscular measurements during explosive isometric contractions, with special reference to electromyography normalization techniques. *Muscle and Nerve.* 2012;46(4):566–576. doi:10.1002/mus.23322

74. Iacono AD, Valentin S, Sanderson M, Halperin I. The isometric horizontal push test: Test-retest reliability and validation study. *Int J Sports Physiol Perform.* 2020;15(4):581–584. doi:10.1123/ijspp.2019-0357

75. Brady CJ, Harrison AJ, Flanagan EP, Gregory Haff G, Comyns TM. A comparison of the isometric midthigh pull and isometric squat: Intraday reliability, usefulness, and the magnitude of difference between tests. *Int J Sports Physiol Perform.* 2018;13(7):844–852. doi:10.1123/ijspp.2017-0480

76. Laffaye G, Wagner P. Eccentric rate of force development determines jumping performance. *Comput Methods Biomech Biomed Engin.* 2013;16(Suppl. 1):82–83. doi:10.1080/10255842.2013.815839

77. Laffaye G, Wagner PP, Tombleson TIL. Countermovement jump height: Gender and sport-specific differences in the force-time variables. *J Strength Cond Res.* 2014;28(4):1096–1105. doi:10.1519/JSC.0b013e3182a1db03

78. Mclellan CP, Lovell DI, Gass GC. The role of rate of force development on vertical jump performance. *J Strength Cond Res.* 2011;25(2):379–385. doi:10.1519/JSC.0b013e3181be305c

79. Andersen LL, Aagaard P. Influence of maximal muscle strength and intrinsic muscle contractile properties on contractile rate of force development. *Eur J Appl Physiol.* 2006;96(1):46–52. doi:10.1007/s00421-005-0070-z

80. Andersen LL, Andersen JL, Zebis MK, Aagaard P. Early and late rate of force development: Differential adaptive responses to resistance training? *Scand J Med Sci Sport.* 2010;20(1):e162–169. doi:10.1111/j.1600-0838.2009.00933.x

81. Junge N, Morin J-B, Nybo L. Leg extension force-velocity imbalance has negative impact on sprint performance in ball-game players. *Sport Biomech.* 2023;22(8): 1027–10404. doi:10.1080/14763141.2020.1775877

82. Ishøi L, Aagaard P, Nielsen MF, et al. The influence of hamstring muscle peak torque and rate of torque development for sprinting performance in football players: A cross-sectional study. *Int J Sports Physiol Perform.* 2019;14(5):665–673. doi:10.1123/ijspp.2018-0464

83. Dai B, Mao D, Garrett WE, Yu B. Anterior cruciate ligament injuries in soccer: Loading mechanisms, risk factors, and prevention programs. *J Sport Heal Sci.* 2014;3(4): 299–306. doi:10.1016/j.jshs.2014.06.002

84. Buckthorpe MW, Roi GS. The time has come to incorporate a greater focus on rate of force development training in the sports injury rehabilitation process. *Muscles Ligaments Tendons J.* 2017;7(3):435. doi:10.11138/MLTJ/2017.7.3.435

85. Nielsen JL, Arp K, Villadsen ML, Christensen SS, Aagaard P. Rate of force development remains reduced in the knee flexors 3 to 9 months after anterior cruciate ligament reconstruction using medial hamstring autografts: A cross-sectional study. *Am J Sports Med.* 2020;48(13):3214–3223. doi:10.1177/0363546520960108

86. Grazioli R, Lopez P, Andersen LL, et al. Hamstring rate of torque development is more affected than maximal voluntary contraction after a professional soccer match. *Eur J Sport Sci.* 2019;19(10):1336–1341. doi:10.1080/17461391.2019.1620863

87. Peñailillo L, Blazevich A, Numazawa H, Nosaka K. Rate of force development as a measure of muscle damage. *Scand J Med Sci Sport.* 2015;25(3):417–427. doi:10.1111/sms.12241

88. Akehi K, Palmer TB, Conchola EC, et al. Changes in knee extension and flexion maximal and rapid torque characteristics during a collegiate women's soccer season. *J Strength Cond Res.* 2020;36(5):1389–1395. doi:10.1519/jsc.0000000000003607

89. Zebis MK, Andersen LL, Ellingsgaard H, Aagaard P. Rapid hamstring/quadriceps force capacity in male vs. female elite soccer players. *J Strength Cond Res.* 2011;25(7): 1989–1993. doi:10.1519/JSC.0b013e3181e501a6

90. Ruschel C, Haupenthal A, Jacomel GF, et al. Validity and reliability of an instrumented leg-extension machine for measuring isometric muscle strength of the knee extensors. *J Sport Rehabil.* 2015;24(2):1–4. doi:10.1123/jsr.2013-0122

91. Lopes JSS, Micheletti JK, Machado AF, et al. Test-retest reliability of knee extensors endurance test with elastic resistance. *PLoS One.* 2018;13(8):1–12. doi:10.1371/journal.pone.0203259

92. James LP, Roberts LA, Haff GG, Kelly VG, Beckman EM. Validity and reliability of a portable isometric mid-thigh clean pull. *J Strength Cond Res.* 2017;31(5):1378–1386. doi:10.1519/JSC.0000000000001201

93. Keogh C, Collins DJ, Warrington G, Comyns T. Intra-trial reliability and usefulness of isometric mid-thigh pull testing on portable force plates. *J Hum Kinet.* 2020;71(1): 33–45. doi:10.2478/hukin-2019-0094

94. Brady C, Comyns T, Harrison A, Warrington G. Focus of attention for diagnostic testing of the force-velocity curve. *Strength Cond J.* 2017;39(1):57–70. doi:10.1519/SSC.0000000000000271

95. Oranchuk DJ, Switaj ZJ, Zuleger BM. The addition of a "Rapid Response" neuromuscular activation to a standard dynamic warm-up improves isometric force and rate of force development. *J Aust Strength Cond.* 2017;25(4):19–24.

96. Haff GG, Ruben RP, Lider J, Twine C, Cormie P. A comparison of methods for determining the rate of force development during isometric midthigh clean pulls. *J Strength Cond Res*. 2015;29(2):386–395. doi:10.1519/JSC.0000000000000705

97. Comfort P, Dos'Santos T, Beckham GK, Stone MH, Guppy SN, Haff GG. Standardization and methodological considerations for the isometric midthigh pull. *Strength Cond J*. 2019;41(2):57–79. doi:10.1519/SSC.0000000000000433

98. McGuigan MR, Winchester JB. The relationship between isometric and dynamic strength in college football players. *J Sport Sci Med*. 2008;7(1):101–105. doi:10.1249/01.mss.0000322664.81874.75

99. Kawamori N, Rossi SJ, Justice BD, et al. Peak force and rate of force development during isometric and dynamic mid-thigh clean pulls performed at various intensities. *J Strength Cond Res*. 2006;20(3):483–491. doi:10.1519/18025.1

9

ASSESSMENT AND QUANTIFICATION OF EXTERNAL LOAD

Moisés de Hoyo Lora and
Miguel Ángel Campos Vázquez

9.1 Introduction

As part of efforts to increase performance and minimize injury occurrence, many football teams employ fitness and sport science personnel who engage in the monitoring of training load (TL) on a daily basis [1]. The quantification and monitoring of TL is therefore an important aspect of football player management [2] and has the potential to provide practitioners and coaches with an objective framework for evidence-based decisions [2]. This process is particularly important in a team sport environment, where practitioners need to employ different strategies to assess how similar training loads might affect each player individually [3]. TL encompasses both external and internal dimensions, with external training loads representing the physical work performed during the training session or competition and internal training loads being the associated biochemical (physical and physiological) and biomechanical stress responses [2].

Developments in technology and analytical methods have led to new possibilities in the applied environment, and practitioners now have the ability to monitor TL using global positioning systems (GPS), inertial measurement units (IMUs), local positioning systems (LPS), and video-based optical tracking systems [4, 5]. Each of these athlete-tracking technologies has its own advantages and disadvantages. For instance, video-based optical systems and LPS are a non-invasive instrument, but clubs often consider installing this technology only in the stadiums, so it is not possible to monitor training sessions in the team's training ground [5]. On the other hand, GPS is the most popular technology used by professional team sports and sport scientists [6]. GPS devices provide a portable solution to monitor football players and supplying practitioners with an estimate of the external load experienced by players [7, 8]. However, the accuracy of GPS devices in stadiums

DOI: 10.4324/9781032637006-9

with high walls or roofs can be compromised by poor signal quality [9]. Finally, IMUs such as accelerometers (to detect movements), gyroscopes (to measure rotation), and magnetometers (to measure orientation) allow the practitioners to have access in both indoor and outdoor conditions, to a valid count of impacts, collisions, and specific parameters such as PlayerLoad and BodyLoad developed from specific algorithms [10]. Nevertheless, the main location for the attachment of the device (the trunk, between the scapulae) could determine the data obtained, underestimating the acceleration of segments at locations inferior to the trunk [9]. The integration of GPS and IMUs in the devices provides practitioners with a plethora of external load variables [10]. Using such technology within training and competition enables coaches to not only understand the distinct game requirements of various playing positions but to also recognize the conditioning needs for the individual roles within the team [11, 12].

In this sense, over recent years, we have seen a large growth in interest on football external load research [13–16], and time-motion analysis has been used extensively to evaluate the movement patterns during football matches [13, 15–19]. Thus, the player's activity during competitive games has shown that football players cover 9–12 km during a match. Of this, 8–12% is high-intensity running or sprinting [18, 19]. The practical value of such analyses is that well-chosen running performance indicators can help coaches develop a training program with specific training drills, which mimics the physiological conditions imposed by the game [20]. One of the main aims of staff working in elite football is the periodization of training [12]. This presents itself in the form of the training day and the weekly microcycle [12].

9.2 Main variables used in time-motion analysis

A wide range of GPS metrics is currently available from which coaches can be objectively informed and subsequently adjust training programs. The extent of activity performed by the players is commonly quantified using arbitrary (player-independent) speed zones [4]. Normally, to simplify and summarize time-motion analysis results, locomotor categories have been used that are defined as a range of velocities [15, 21, 22], a mean velocity (> 3 different means reported) [23], or various subjective descriptions of locomotor activities (e.g., walking, jogging, striding, and sprinting) [24–26]. More recently, some authors have simplified the terminology by using low-, moderate-, high-, and very high-intensity running classifications [27, 28]. Presently, there are no consistent definitions for velocity ranges, making comparisons between studies problematic [29]. According this, players' activities have been coded into the following categories and speed thresholds: standing (0–0.6 km· h^{-1}), walking (0.7–7.1 km· h^{-1}), jogging (7.2–14.3 km· h^{-1}), running (14.4–19.7 km· h^{-1}), and high-speed running (19.8–25.1 km· h^{-1}) and sprinting (> 25.1 km· h^{-1}). High-intensity running consisted of running, high-speed running, and sprinting (running speed > 14.4 km· h^{-1}).

Very high-intensity running consisted of high-speed running and sprinting (running speed > 19.8 km· h⁻¹) [13,18,30].

On the other hand, several studies have shown a relevant limitation in estimating high-intensity efforts during short duration movements using these speed thresholds [20]. Normally, when short distances are covered at maximal-intensity running starting from a low speed, these tasks do not achieve the sprinting velocity threshold and are undetected [29, 31, 32]. In this sense, a few football-specific movements can cause significant physical stress on the players despite a low distance and/or speed, which might underestimate the external loads during a football match when only looking at the results from a time-motion analysis.

Based on the aforementioned argument, absolute speed values exclude short accelerations in the analysis [33]. Thus, Varley and Aughey [32] showed that football players perform eight times as many accelerations as reported sprints per match. Moreover, of maximal accelerations, ~98% commenced from a starting velocity lower than that considered high-velocity running in the literature, while ~85% did not reach the high-velocity running threshold [32]. Likewise, accelerations are more energetically demanding than constant velocity running [18, 19, 34]. Even when these accelerations start from a low running speed, players experienced a high metabolic load [34, 35]. Therefore, measuring methods that capture accelerations would markedly strengthen match analyses and should be considered by professionals [33]. Thus, Bradley et al. [13] defined two acceleration thresholds: (a) moderate, from 2.5 to 4.0 m·s⁻², and (b) high, > 4.0 m·s⁻². Subsequently, Akenhead et al. [36] specified these parameters as (a) low, from 1 to 2 m·s⁻², (b) moderate, from 2 to 3 m·s⁻², and (c) high, > 3 m·s⁻² [36]. By contrast, Varley and Aughey [32] used an absolute value of > 2.78 m s⁻².

Recently, reports in team sports have shown that metabolic power can estimate power output and energetic costs of intermittent running and competitive match play [35, 37–39]. These investigations provide an additional insight to previous studies that have employed traditional time-motion analyses of activity demands of training and match play. Metabolic power represents the net metabolic demands incurred by locomotion [40], and it can be calculated multiplying instantaneous energy cost by running speed [35]. Thus, the corresponding energy cost can be estimated on the basis of the biomechanical equivalence between accelerated/decelerated running on flat terrain and constant speed running uphill/downhill [41]. This approach allows one to (i) estimate the time course of the instantaneous metabolic power requirement of any given player and (ii) infer therefrom the overall energy expenditure of any given time window of a football drill or match [41]. Metabolic power seems to be a more accurate way of estimating training intensity because it takes into account the speed and acceleration that the player shows at each moment, instead of considering them separately [35]. Regarding this approach, the most common parameters used are estimation of average metabolic power (W·kg⁻¹; P_{met}) and total energy expenditure (kJ·kg⁻¹), as well as distance (m) and energy produced above the high-power threshold

(>25 W·kg^{-1}; HP) [6]. Besides, metabolic power in the intermittent activity can be expressed as a rate of oxygen demand, showing the following equivalence: 1 w·kg^{-1} ~ 2.87 ml·kg^{-1}·kg^{-1} [42]. This equivalence could be especially useful to estimate oxygen consumption in game-based tasks (Figure 9.1).

Normally, calculations are provided for equivalent distance (ED), which represents the equivalent steady-state distance required to match the estimated energy expenditure during exercise. Additionally, the authors have used Equivalent Distance Index (EDI), representing the ratio between ED and total distance [37, 38]. Gaudino et al. [43] identified that depending on playing position, HP distance was between 62 and 84% greater than high-speed running distances during games. As a result, the authors cautioned that high-speed running may neglect the contribution of accelerated running and therefore underestimate the true energetic cost of training activities [43]. Despite the increasing use of metabolic power in the monitoring process, this approach presents some limitations. For instance, metabolic power considers only the running performance, neglecting many other typical activities performed by the players during the football matches, such as jumping, kicking the ball, or tackling [35]. Besides, other authors concluded that the energy expenditure was underestimated during intermittent movements (shuttle running) and in circuit drills and overestimated at a constant speed [44–46]. Thus, practitioners need to take into account all these limitations when using metabolic power in a daily basis.

Finally, the integration of triaxial accelerometers into the GPS devices provides the opportunity to analyze new load parameters, such as three axes acceleration recorded during sports movements, measured in arbitrary units [47]. For instance, PlayerLoad, which quantifies the sum of the individual triaxial accelerometer vectors [14], or dynamic stress load (DSL), which is the total of weighted impacts at a magnitude above 2 g including both collisions and step impacts while running and can be a valid metric to monitor the athlete's fatigue in a quick way [48].

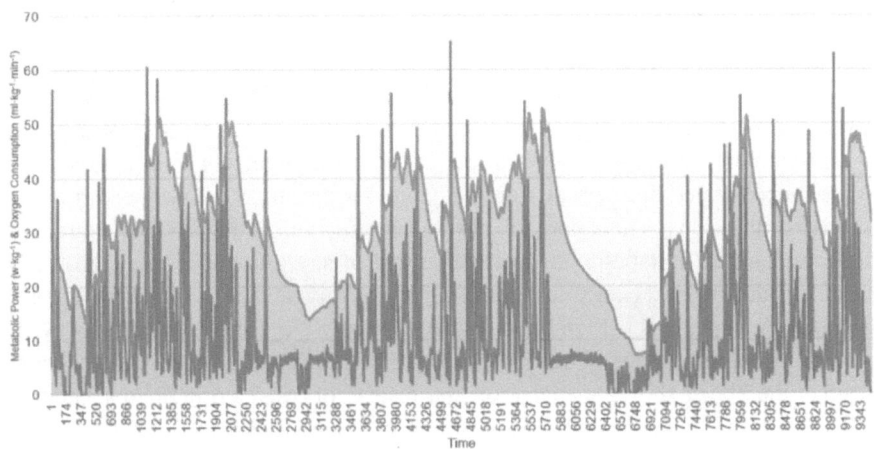

FIGURE 9.1   Evolution of metabolic power (foreground line) and oxygen consumption (background line) during a 5 versus 5 small-sided game (3 × 4 min, 2 min rest period).

9.3 Peak match demands

Historically, practitioners have reported absolute match demands as totals (e.g., total distance) or averages (e.g., relative distance: distance travelled per minute) for the whole and/or half-match [10]. This method of analysis provides some indication of the total external load that players are exposed to during match play. However, due to the intermittent nature of the competition, players are usually exposed to high-intensity periods that widely overcome the average physical demands of the game [12, 49]. Thus, whole match values may not be sensitive enough to detect the most intense periods of a match [49]. These high-intensity periods are known in scientific literature as peak match demands [10], the most demanding passages of play [12], worst-case scenarios [50], or simply maximum intensity periods, and it should be taken into account when designing training drills in order to avoid players underprepared to cope with match demands and or players at a high injury risk [50].

Practitioners are advised to take into account different aspects related with the quantification of peak match demands, such as the analysis method used (segmental or rolling average), the duration of the selected time windows, or the criterion variables analyzed [10]. Accordingly, the maximum intensity periods could be defined as periods of play whose duration is determined by the practitioner, and in which the intensity has been greater (in relation to the time window used) regarding the criterion variable used in the analysis (Figure 9.2).

Several studies have aimed to identify the peak match demands using different arbitrary time windows ranging from 1 to 10 minutes in professional football players [12, 49], elite youth football players [51, 52], and female football players [53]. Initially, researchers used segmental analysis, splitting the total match into fixed periods from the start to the end of the match (e.g., for 5-min blocks, a match would be split from 0 to 5, 5 to 10, and 10 to 15 min). However, the use of the rolling average method is currently considered more accurate for quantifying peak match

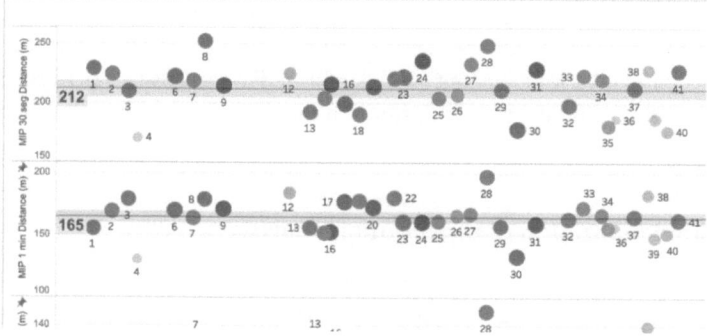

FIGURE 9.2 Evolution of maximum intensity periods (MIP) using total distance as criterion variable (m·min-1) along competitive season, for a professional center forward. Grey zone (mean ± 95% confidence interval). 1, 2, 3,... 1st, 2nd, 3rd round.

demands [32, 54] as this method detects the exact period in which the player is at peak intensity (e.g., from the period 1′23″–6′23″ for time window of 5 min). The use of different time windows to analyze match demands allows training drills to be assessed relative to the peak running intensities achieved during competition (e.g., time window of 5 min as a reference for 5 × 5 small-sided game formats). Thus, future studies could identify time durations shorter than 1 minute (e.g., 6 seconds and 30 seconds) to use as a reference to certain drills that are usually performed in sets of duration less than 1 minute (e.g., 1 × 1 drills and or repeated sprints drills).

The most demanding passages of play values are defined based on the criterion variable and are position-dependent [12, 49]. Besides, the performance in this maximum-intensity periods is associated with different contextual variables such as match location, match outcome, match half, or congested calendars [52, 54, 55]. Also, different criterion variables have been used to analyze peak match demands in football players, such as total distance, high-speed distance, average acceleration, or average metabolic power [10], and researchers conclude that the peaks in running intensity increase as the length of the moving average decreased [49]. For example, peak match demands to midfielders range from 204 to 140 m·min⁻¹ when total distance is used as the criterion variable for time windows of 1 and 10 min, respectively [12]. Additionally, it should be taken into account that due to the stochastic and multidimensional nature of the game, when the players reach their peak values in any criterion variable (e.g., distance covered), they perform other activities that must be considered when designing the training task, such as accelerations-decelerations or high-speed running [12].

It is important to note from a practical perspective that peak intensity periods refer to an isolated event that occurs during the game. As a consequence, a possible high match-to-match variability along the season in peak match demands is expected, especially for shorter time windows. However, players are exposed frequently to other periods in which the intensity required is not maximum but near to maximum. Consequently, conditioning for peak match demands should be only a part of the overall periodized training program [56], and practitioners should consider not only the magnitude of peak match demands but also the number of passages that players may experience during match play [54]. In fact, the training practice should take into account all the intermediate intensities between the average and peak match demands [56] through the use of different game formats and other types of tasks [57].

9.4 Individualization of time-motion analysis

Typically monitoring systems adopt arbitrary speed thresholds to determine the intensity distribution of the task, and in particular there has been a focus on 'high-intensity' running to quantify the external load of players. Since opposing players compete on an absolute basis, using arbitrary speed thresholds to quantify "high-intensity" running enables practitioners and coaches to make inter-player contrasts [58].

Despite the inherent information available from distance covered within arbitrary speed zones, this method is biased by the potential players' diversity within a team (e.g., fitness, age, training experience, and injury history), consequently masking individual capacities and thus neglecting external TL imposed on the individual player [59]. However, as the exercise-intensity continuum is player-dependent, the use of individualized (player-dependent) speed zones has recently therefore been proposed for quantifying external TL, reducing the confounding effect of between-player variation in physical capacity [59, 60]. Without an individualized approach to physical match analysis, the true energetic demands of a training or match stimulus are unknown, and the practitioner is unable to administer a player-specific approach to performance monitoring and training prescription [61].

The use of high-intensity activity is one of the most appropriate measures of match physical performance [61]. Thus, it is important that the method used for measuring when a player is active in the high-intensity "zone" be accurate. This is important in both applied and research settings. For example, many sport scientists track the distance run at high intensity from match to match for an individual player as an indication of their match physical performance. They also compare the high-intensity distance between players to "rank" their physical performance during a given match. However, it appears that in both applied and research settings, the speed criteria used to define where high-intensity running begins, normally, are based on absolute and therefore "player-independent" speeds.

In this sense, the first step should be to choose the criterion for setting the individual thresholds. Thus, maximal aerobic speed (MAS) is very strongly correlated to maximal oxygen uptake and, in conjunction with maximal sprinting speed (MSS), allows calculation of the anaerobic speed reserve (ASR; Figure 9.3) that accounts for the transition from high-speed running to sprinting [60]. Indeed, a combined approach to quantifying external TL data that incorporates fitness data from field-based tests to estimate players' MAS (e.g., 30–15 Intermittent Fitness Test) and MSS provides a more accurate definition of speed zones than a single fitness component [60].

Regarding acceleration efforts, the situation is very similar. Previous studies have proposed absolute acceleration thresholds to analyze this parameter during matches. However, these absolute thresholds do not consider the speed where players start to accelerate and the individual maximum acceleration capability. Thus, it is necessary to consider that the capacity to accelerate is greater when accelerations are initiated from a standing position or from a low velocity than any other velocities [63]. Based on this argument, it is important to consider that absolute acceleration thresholds are hypothesized to underestimate actions if the initial speed is high or even overestimate these actions when the initial running speed is low [63]. Further, Terje et al. [64] suggested that this underestimation might be different according to player positions and, thus, to find a solution to this problem. According to this, Sonderegger et al. [63] designed a regression model in order to relate initial speed and maximal individual acceleration. In this sense, recently,

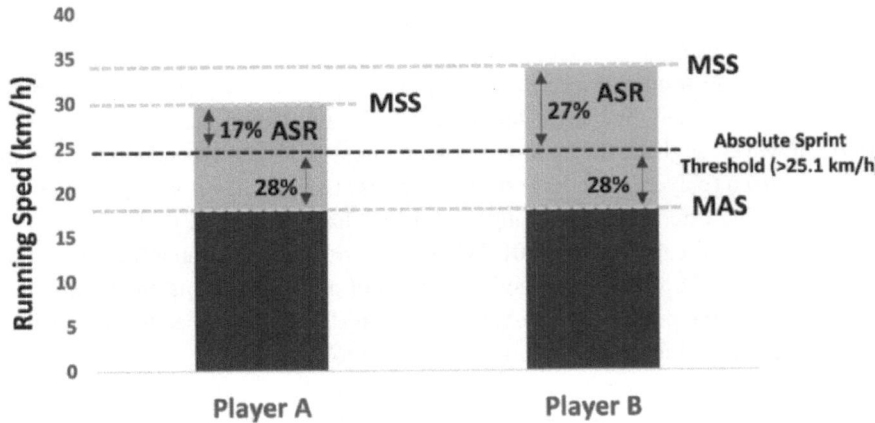

FIGURE 9.3 Illustration of the importance of individual thresholds for two athletes possessing similar Maximal Aerobic Speed (MAS), but different Maximal Sprinting Speed (MSS). During a training session, if we use an absolute sprint threshold (> 25.1 km/h), Player B with a greater Anaerobic Speed Reserve (ASR) will work at a lower percentage of his ASR, and will therefore achieve a lower exercise load compared with Player B (adapted from Buchheit and Laursen [62]).

our group published a study using this regression model and individual maximum acceleration capability [20]. Regarding the acceleration distribution according to initial speed, our results showed that 37.81 ± 23.73 % of total high-intensity accelerations were initiated from 0 to 7 km·h^{-1}, the 17.12 ± 19.41% from 7.1 to 14.3 km·h^{-1}, and 42.95 ± 25.74 % ≥ 14.4 km·h^{-1}. The high-intensity accelerations that started above 14 km·h^{-1} were the most common actions during the match. These results contrast with those obtained in other studies, suggesting that the 98% of the accelerations in a match start from 0 to 7 km·h^{-1} [32]. Again, these differences can be attributed to the absolute threshold used (2.78 m/s^2), which were suggested to both underestimate efforts with high initial running speed and overestimate those actions performed at low initial running speeds.

9.5 Relationship between external load and injury incidence

Top-level football players sustain two injuries per season, resulting in 50 injuries within a squad of 25 players [65]. Injury is multifactorial in nature with inherent risk factors that are both nonmodifiable (e.g., age and sex) and modifiable (e.g., strength and flexibility) [66]. The manipulation of modifiable risk factors provides coaches and sport scientists with opportunities that may reduce the risk of injury [67]. TL is one such modifiable risk factor that has garnered considerable research interest of late [68]. In this sense, these injuries occur when an athlete is exposed to a given workload [69]. Thus, each training or competition bout performed has the potential for athletic injury, indicating that inappropriate workload exposure can increase injury risk [70]. According to Selye's General Adaptation Syndrome, training stimuli below the optimum are insufficient to produce adaptations [71]. Conversely, stimuli above the optimum may lead to overtraining, which is largely associated with a higher incidence of injury [72]. Hence, an appropriate balance between training, competition, and recovery is required to attain peak performance and injury avoidance [73]. According to this, understanding and monitoring the training programs of football players are vital to ensure that the optimal training load is implemented [74]. Ultimately, this will potentially increase positive training adaptations and reduce the prevalence of injury in football [75]. The introduction of GPS into sports has led to many studies which objectively quantify training loads [76].

Traditionally, workload-injury investigations focused on this relationship between absolute workloads and injury [76–79]. Thus, for example, Bowen et al. observed and elevated risk of injury with a very high 3-weekly accumulation of accelerations in elite youth football players [76]. In this line, Colby et al. examined the relationship between accumulated GPS and accelerometer-derived loads and injury in Australian football players [79]. During pre-season and in-season, 3-weekly workloads were indicative of a greater injury risk. Ultimately, studies must consider the effect of the accumulation of load to fully understand the relationship between injury and workload.

While absolute workloads explore the association of cumulative loads with injury, relative loads compare the load an athlete is currently undergoing (the acute load) to what the athlete is prepared for (the chronic load) [80]. Thus, an important recent development in monitoring training load is the acute:chronic workload ratio (ACWR), a relative measure originating from the original work by Calvert et al., wherein it was known as the "training stress balance," but more recently adapted to be calculated as a ratio by Hulin et al. as opposed to a subtraction [81, 82]. This involves the assessment of the absolute 1-week workload (acute workload) relative to 4-week chronic workload (four-week average acute workload) [70]. A workload index can then be calculated indicating whether the individual's acute workload is greater, less than, or equal to the chronic workload they have been prepared for [70]. In team sports, acute:chronic workload ratio illustrated a range of 0.8–1.3 is considered the "sweet spot" while 1.5 represented the "danger zone" for injury occurrence [83]. Specifically, decreased injury risk was evident with intermediate loads compared to lighter or heavier workloads.

The ACWR can be calculated using (1) the rolling average model (RA) and (2) the exponentially weighted moving average model (EWMA). The RA is calculated by dividing the acute (i.e., rolling seven-day) workload by the chronic workload (i.e., average 28-day) [68]. The EWMA model, as explained by Williams et al., assigns a decreasing weighting for each older load value in order to give greater weighting to the recent load performed by the athlete [84]. There is much debate as to the best model of calculating ACWR with some suggestions that the RA model fails to account for the decaying nature of fitness and fatigue [84, 85]. Instead, the more sensitive EWMA model may be more suitable for modeling training loads [86]. Thus, for example, Bowen et al. reported a significantly increased risk of injury with high ACWR (1.4–1.9) for high-speed distance when the chronic workload was low (< 938 m) [76]. Moreover, recent evidence suggests that higher ACWR combined with low cumulative chronic workloads and rapid increases in player load (week-to-week changes, i.e., a "spike" in workload expose the athlete to load that they may not be prepared for), predisposing the athlete to a higher risk of injury [70, 82, 87–89]. It seems then the assessment of the ACWR, for high and low chronic loads, may provide a more comprehensive prediction of injury risk than absolute workload alone. Evidence of this has been recently demonstrated in A-League football, where meters per minute in the one and four weeks prior to injury were significantly higher than the seasonal average [90].

In contrast to the idea that higher workloads contribute to higher injury incidence, high workloads may contribute to well-developed physical qualities, thereby reducing injury risk [50, 91, 92]. In this sense, gradually increasing the exposure to moderate-to high training loads produced a smaller association to injury risk than exposure to lower training loads [93]. Therefore, appropriate training loads that produce adaptations to enhance their fitness levels and tolerance to physical stress are required [70]. In this case, higher workloads would appear to be protective, while lower workloads may be insufficient to induce adaptations or result in detraining, thereby increasing the risk of injury [70].

Supporting this, the training—injury prevention paradox model has recently been defined and reviewed by Gabbett, who described this chronic workload effect. This 'paradox' of high chronic workloads is their potential preventative effect, as long as week-to-week load changes are kept within ~10% and the ACWR is kept in a moderate range (i.e., training spikes are avoided) [50]. Hulin et al. found that elite rugby players who had very high ACWR as well as high chronic workloads had the largest risk of injury. However, they also demonstrated that as long as ACWR workload ratios were kept within a moderate zone (0.8–1.3), high chronic workloads were associated with the lowest risks of injuries, other than in the case of players with very low (< 2 SD) ACWR [88].

9.6 The use of GPS technology in daily and microcycle planning

In football, the daily monitoring of training and match load can help coaches plan, structure, evaluate, and therewith optimize their training process [3]. In this sense, it has been noted that periodized approaches to elite-level football training may facilitate longitudinal progressive training adaptations and concurrently reduce injury risk [94, 95]. Regardless of its relative importance in the final competitive performance, accumulated TL has been shown to be related to both positive and negative changes in physical fitness performance relevant to match play and injury occurrence [96]. Nonetheless, team periodization strategies are relatively unknown in football [96]. Thus, it is normal practice in football to design a first phase (i.e., preseason) of 3–5 weeks as a means of preparation for the rest of the season [97]. Then, a much longer second phase consisting of the competitive season is carried out (i.e., in-season) [97]. However, little research has systematically attempted to describe the distribution of weekly TL across the different periods of the season in professional football players [7, 98].

Using GPS technology in both training and official matches is an effective tool for monitoring the accumulative player load during a microcycle. In this sense, accumulative weekly load has been examined in English [7, 98, 99], Dutch [100], and Spanish League players [96, 97, 101]. The tactical role of a player seems to be a powerful determinant of their physical match performance, so it is imperative that the conditioning stimulus has a positional element to it [102]. Casamichana et al. [101] showed that during official matches, central backs and midfielders (~300–400 m) cover less HSR than fullbacks and wingers (~600–800 m). Thus, it is very common to express these accumulative training load data against the match reference since this facilitates the interpretation of the data, and hence the training prescription as well as the communication between practitioners, coaches, and players (i.e., 3.5 times the total distance or 1.8 times the sprint distance in a match).

The management of training load is traditionally considered in weekly microcycles consisting of one game per week (i.e., Saturday-to-Saturday schedule), though it is noteworthy that elite football players often play two (e.g., Sunday-to-Saturday) or three (e.g., Sunday-Wednesday-Saturday) games in a 7-day period. This is largely due to involvement in numerous competitions (i.e., domestic league/cup competitions and European competitions) and periods of intense fixture schedules such as the winter period [103]. Such scenarios place considerable demands on sports scientists to monitor and manage training load to ensure optimal match-day performance and recovery [7, 103]. According to this, several studies have found that during a typical week, the last 2 days before the match (MD-2 and MD-1) have usually the lowest load [7, 12, 98, 100, 101]. These findings revealed how a tapering approach may be adopted to reduce the TL close to match day. Owen et al. proposed that a reduced TL should be implemented latterly within the training week to ensure that fatigue accumulation is managed accordingly and tapered to facilitate optimal preparation for subsequent match performance [95].

These studies showed the highest training load on the first (MD-4) and second training of the week (MD-3) [7, 101]. However, Malone et al. found no differences in training load between the first three training sessions of the week [98]. Owen et al. [95] observed a reduced TL (i.e., both volume and intensity markers) in MD-4 compared to MD and MD-3 for percentage of sprint distance (%SpD) and percentage of sprint distance per minute (%SpD·min^{-1}), which is usually due to the fact that in MD-4 small-sided games are usually used, where the acceleration and deceleration profiles are more frequent, and players do not have enough distance to develop high-speed distances. Altogether, these results indicate that differences exist in the distribution of training load between high-level football teams, especially in the middle (MD-5, MD-4, and MD-3) of a full training week [100]. Furthermore, findings from Owen et al. indicated that it is possible to maintain a uniformed and structured mesocycle while inducing variation of the TL output during microcycle periods among elite professional players [95].

Interestingly, when comparing external loads across various European leagues, starters consistently display higher accumulative demands than nonstarters [7, 97, 100, 101], with match time being the major determinant of this difference. Recently, Anderson et al. [7] distinguished starter (starting ≥60% of games), fringe (starting 30–60% of games), and nonstarter (starting < 30% of games) players and found significant differences in external TL (i.e., running, high-speed running, sprinting, duration of total activity, and total distance) between these groups during the training sessions in five different in-season periods. In another study, Casamichana et al. [101] demonstrated that the 0-min and < 60-min groups were lower for most external loading variables in comparison to > 60-min and 90-min groups, with very little difference between the 90-min and the > 60-min group. The data demonstrated that HSR and SPR weekly accumulation was double for the 90-min versus the 0-min group. Despite this, the 0-min group still reached an average weekly accumulation value of one match for HSR and SP. Interestingly, Stevens et al. reported values of 1.5 and 0.5 for HSR and SPR for substitutes in one and two matches per week, respectively [100]. This finding could potentially justify the practices employed by some elite clubs that split the squad for MD+1 work based on greater or less than < 60-min played in previous official matches [12]. For instance, professional teams use a MD+1 recovery session for players completing > 60 min, as opposed to MD+1 complementary, that is for players completing < 60 min and is a compensatory session in an attempt to replicate loading during an official match [12]. Martin-Garcia et al. reported that acceleration and deceleration demand during a MD+1 session exceeded 80% of that performed in an official match [12]. However, in this study, the results revealed for this type of session does not seem to provide sufficient overload to develop HSR and SP capabilities as these external load variables only reach 20–30% of match play demands [12].

In this sense, different authors have shown that the requirement to continually perform high force eccentric actions such as changes in direction, accelerations, and decelerations seems particularly damaging to the muscle and increase the injury incidence [104]. Thus, the management of compensatory training sessions for nonstarter players is a key factor in football fitness programs. In this sense, it is common to include a small HSR and SP dose after the match for substitute players using different intermittent drills, such as pitch running without the ball or position-specific circuits, with the aim to compensate for the decrease of these stimuli during microcycles with two or three matches [105]. This is especially important as a relationship between weekly HSR and SP load and the probability of injury seems to be U-shaped whereby a moderate amount seems to have a protective effect [106].

References

1. McCall A, Davison M, Andersen TE, Beasley I, Bizzini M, Dupont G, et al. Injury prevention strategies at the FIFA 2014 World Cup: Perceptions and practices of the physicians from the 32 participating national teams. *Br J Sports Med* [Internet]. 2015 May;49(9):603–608.

2. McLaren SJ, Macpherson TW, Coutts AJ, Hurst C, Spears IR, Weston M. The relationships between internal and external measures of training load and intensity in team sports: A meta-analysis. *Sport Med* [Internet]. 2018 Mar 29;48(3):641–658.

3. Borresen J, Lambert MI. Quantifying training load: A comparison of subjective and objective methods. *Int J Sports Physiol Perform* [Internet]. 2008 Mar;3(1):16–30.

4. Akenhead R, Nassis GP. Training load and player Monitoring in High-Level Football: Current Practice and Perceptions. *Int J Sports Physiol Perform* [Internet]. 2016 July;11(5):587–593.

5. Pino-Ortega J, Oliva-Lozano JM, Gantois P, Nakamura FY, Rico-González M. Comparison of the validity and reliability of local positioning systems against other tracking technologies in team sport: A systematic review. *Proc Inst Mech Eng Part P J Sport Eng Technol.* 2022;236(2):73–82.

6. Malone JJ, Lovell R, Varley MC, Coutts AJ. Unpacking the black box: Applications and considerations for using GPS devices in sport. *Int J Sports Physiol Perform* [Internet]. 2017 Apr;12(s2):S2-18–S2-26.

7. Anderson L, Orme P, Di Michele R, Close GL, Morgans R, Drust B, et al. Quantification of training load during one-, two- and three-game week schedules in professional soccer players from the English Premier League: Implications for carbohydrate periodisation. *J Sports Sci* [Internet]. 2016 July 2;34(13):1250–1259.

8. Buchheit M, Simpson BM. Player-tracking technology: Half-full or half-empty glass? *Int J Sports Physiol Perform* [Internet]. 2017 Apr;12(s2):S2-35–S2-41.

9. Murray A, Varley MC. Technology in soccer. In: Curtis R, Benjamin C, Huggins R, Casa DJ, editors. Elite Soccer Players Maximizing Performance and Safety [Internet]. 1st ed. Routledge; 2020. p. 442.

10. Whitehead S, Till K, Weaving D, Jones B. The use of microtechnology to quantify the peak match demands of the football codes: A systematic review. *Sport Med* [Internet]. 2018 Nov 7;48(11):2549–2575.

11. Carling C. Interpreting physical performance in professional soccer match-play: Should we be more pragmatic in our approach? *Sport Med* [Internet]. 2013 Aug 11;43(8):655–663.

12. Martín-García A, Gómez Díaz A, Bradley PS, Morera F, Casamichana D. Quantification of a professional football team's external load using a microcycle structure. *J Strength Cond Res* [Internet]. 2018 Dec;32(12):3511–3518.

13. Bradley PS, Sheldon W, Wooster B, Olsen P, Boanas P, Krustrup P. High-intensity running in English FA Premier League soccer matches. *J Sports Sci* [Internet]. 2009 Jan;27(2):159–168.

14. Casamichana D, Castellano J, Castagna C. Comparing the physical demands of friendly matches and small-sided games in semiprofessional soccer players. *J Strength Cond Res* [Internet]. 2012 Mar;26(3):837–843.

15. Di Salvo V, Baron R, Tschan H, Calderon Montero F, Bachl N, Pigozzi F. Performance characteristics according to playing position in elite soccer. *Int J Sports Med* [Internet]. 2007 Mar;28(3):222–227.

16. Torreño N, Munguía-Izquierdo D, Coutts A, de Villarreal ES, Asian-Clemente J, Suarez-Arrones L. Relationship between external and internal loads of professional soccer players during full matches in official games using global positioning systems and heart-rate technology. *Int J Sports Physiol Perform* [Internet]. 2016 Oct;11(7):940–946.

17. Carling C, Bradley P, McCall A, Dupont G. Match-to-match variability in high-speed running activity in a professional soccer team. *J Sports Sci* [Internet]. 2016 Dec 16; 34(24):2215–2223.

18. Rampinini E, Coutts A, Castagna C, Sassi R, Impellizzeri F. Variation in top level soccer match performance. *Int J Sports Med* [Internet]. 2007 Dec;28(12):1018–1024.

19. Vigne G, Gaudino C, Rogowski I, Alloatti G, Hautier C. Activity profile in elite Italian soccer team. *Int J Sports Med* [Internet]. 2010 May 18;31(05):304–310.

20. de Hoyo M, Sañudo B, Suárez-Arrones L, Carrasco L, Joel T, Domínguez-Cobo S, et al. Analysis of the acceleration profile according to initial speed and positional role in elite professional male soccer players. *J Sports Med Phys Fitness* [Internet]. 2018 Nov;58(12):1774–1780.

21. Burgess DJ, Naughton G, Norton KI. Profile of movement demands of national football players in Australia. *J Sci Med Sport* [Internet]. 2006 Aug;9(4):334–341.

22. Cunniffe B, Proctor W, Baker JS, Davies B. An evaluation of the physiological demands of elite rugby union using global positioning system tracking software. *J Strength Cond Res* [Internet]. 2009 July;23(4):1195–1203.

23. Impellizzeri F, Marcora S, Castagna C, Reilly T, Sassi A, Iaia F, et al. Physiological and performance effects of generic versus specific aerobic training in soccer players. *Int J Sports Med* [Internet]. 2006 June;27(6):483–492.

24. Krustrup P, Mohr M, Bangsbo J. Activity profile and physiological demands of top-class soccer assistant refereeing in relation to training status. *J Sports Sci* [Internet]. 2002 Jan 9;20(11):861–871.

25. Gabbett TJ. Changes in physiological and anthropometric characteristics of rugby league players during a competitive season. *J Strength Cond Res* [Internet]. 2005;19(2):400.

26. Spencer M, Rechichi C, Lawrence S, Dawson B, Bishop D, Goodman C. Time-motion analysis of elite field hockey during several games in succession: A tournament scenario. *J Sci Med Sport* [Internet]. 2005 Dec;8(4):382–391.

27. Coutts AJ, Duffield R. Validity and reliability of GPS devices for measuring movement demands of team sports. *J Sci Med Sport* [Internet]. 2010 Jan;13(1):133–135.

28. Rampinini E, Impellizzeri FM, Castagna C, Coutts AJ, Wisløff U. Technical performance during soccer matches of the Italian Serie A league: Effect of fatigue and competitive level. *J Sci Med Sport* [Internet]. 2009 Jan;12(1):227–233.

29. Dwyer DB, Gabbett TJ. Global positioning system data analysis: Velocity ranges and a new definition of sprinting for field sport athletes. *J Strength Cond Res* [Internet]. 2012 Mar;26(3):818–824.

30. Mohr M, Krustrup P, Bangsbo J. Match performance of high-standard soccer players with special reference to development of fatigue. *J Sports Sci* [Internet]. 2003 Jan;21(7):519–528.

31. Haugen T, Buchheit M. Sprint running performance monitoring: Methodological and practical considerations. *Sport Med* [Internet]. 2016 May 14;46(5):641–656.

32. Varley M, Aughey R. Acceleration profiles in elite Australian soccer. *Int J Sports Med* [Internet]. 2012 Aug 15;34(01):34–39.

33. Haugen TA, Tønnessen E, Hisdal J, Seiler S. The role and development of sprinting speed in soccer. *Int J Sports Physiol Perform* [Internet]. 2014 May;9(3):432–441.

34. di Prampero PE. Sprint running: A new energetic approach. *J Exp Biol* [Internet]. 2005 July 15;208(14):2809–2816.

35. Osgnach C, Poser S, Bernardini R, Rinaldo R, di Prampero PE. Energy cost and metabolic power in elite soccer. *Med Sci Sport Exerc* [Internet]. 2010 Jan;42(1):170–178.

36. Akenhead R, Hayes PR, Thompson KG, French D. Diminutions of acceleration and deceleration output during professional football match play. J Sci Med Sport [Internet]. 2013 Nov;16(6):556–561.

37. Kempton T, Sirotic AC, Rampinini E, Coutts AJ. Metabolic power demands of rugby league match play. *Int J Sports Physiol Perform* [Internet]. 2015 Jan;10(1):23–28.
38. Coutts AJ, Kempton T, Sullivan C, Bilsborough J, Cordy J, Rampinini E. Metabolic power and energetic costs of professional Australian football match-play. *J Sci Med Sport* [Internet]. 2015 Mar;18(2):219–224.
39. Malone S, Solan B, Collins K, Doran D. The metabolic power and energetic demands of elite Gaelic football match play. *J Sports Med Phys Fitness*. 2017;57(5):543–549.
40. Polglaze T, Hoppe MW. Metabolic power: A step in the right direction for team sports. *Int J Sports Physiol Perform* [Internet]. 2019 Mar;14(3):407–411.
41. di Prampero P, Osgnach C. Metabolic power in team sports – Part 1: An update. *Int J Sports Med* [Internet]. 2018 July 14;39(08):581–587.
42. Osgnach C, di Prampero P. Metabolic power in team sports – Part 2: Aerobic and anaerobic energy yields. *Int J Sports Med* [Internet]. 2018 July 14;39(08):588–595.
43. Gaudino P, Iaia F, Alberti G, Strudwick A, Atkinson G, Gregson W. Monitoring training in elite soccer players: Systematic bias between running speed and metabolic power data. *Int J Sports Med* [Internet]. 2013 Apr 2;34(11):963–968.
44. Stevens TGA, De Ruiter CJ, Van Maurik D, Van Lierop CJW, Savelsbergh GJP, Beek PJ. Measured and estimated energy cost of constant and shuttle running in soccer players. *Med Sci Sport Exerc* [Internet]. 2015 June;47(6):1219–1224.
45. Brown DM, Dwyer DB, Robertson SJ, Gastin PB. Metabolic power method: Underestimation of energy expenditure in field-sport movements using a global positioning system tracking system. *Int J Sports Physiol Perform* [Internet]. 2016 Nov;11(8):1067–1073.
46. Hader K, Mendez-Villanueva A, Palazzi D, Ahmaidi S, Buchheit M. Metabolic power requirement of change of direction speed in young soccer players: Not all is what it seems. McCrory JL, editor. *PLoS One* [Internet]. 2016 Mar 1;11(3):e0149839.
47. Gómez-Carmona CD, Bastida-Castillo A, Ibáñez SJ, Pino-Ortega J. Accelerometry as a method for external workload monitoring in invasion team sports. A systematic review. Cortis C, editor. *PLoS One* [Internet]. 2020 Aug 25;15(8):e0236643.
48. Beato M, De Keijzer KL, Carty B, Connor M. Monitoring fatigue during intermittent exercise with accelerometer-derived metrics. *Front Physiol* [Internet]. 2019 June 26;10:780.
49. Delaney JA, Thornton HR, Rowell AE, Dascombe BJ, Aughey RJ, Duthie GM. Modelling the decrement in running intensity within professional soccer players. *Sci Med Footb* [Internet]. 2018 Apr 3;2(2):86–92.
50. Gabbett TJ. The training—injury prevention paradox: Should athletes be training smarter and harder? *Br J Sports Med* [Internet]. 2016 Mar;50(5):273–280.
51. Duthie GM, Thornton HR, Delaney JA, Connolly DR, Serpiello FR. Running intensities in elite youth soccer by age and position. *J Strength Cond Res* [Internet]. 2018 Oct;32(10):2918–2924.
52. Castellano J, Martin-Garcia A, Casamichana D. Most running demand passages of match play in youth soccer congestion period. *Biol Sport* [Internet]. 2020;37(4):367–373.
53. Muñiz-González J, Giráldez-Costas V, González-García J, Romero-Moraleda B, Campos-Vázquez MÁ. Positional differences in the most demanding conditional phases in female football competition. *RICYDE Rev Int Ciencias del Deport*. 2020;60(16): 199–213.
54. Oliva-Lozano JM, Martín-Fuentes I, Fortes V, Muyor JM. Differences in worst-case scenarios calculated by fixed length and rolling average methods in professional soccer match-play. *Biol Sport* [Internet]. 2021;38(3):325–331.

55. Casamichana D, Castellano J, Diaz AG, Gabbett TJ, Martin-Garcia A. The most demanding passages of play in football competition: A comparison between halves. *Biol Sport* [Internet]. 2019;36(3):233–240.

56. Riboli A, Esposito F, Coratella G. The distribution of match activities relative to the maximal intensities in elite soccer players: Implications for practice. *Res Sport Med*. 2022;30(5):463–474.

57. Martin-Garcia A, Castellano J, Diaz AG, Cos F, Casamichana D. Positional demands for various-sided games with goalkeepers according to the most demanding passages of match play in football. *Biol Sport* [Internet]. 2019;36(2):171–180.

58. Abt G, Lovell R. The use of individualized speed and intensity thresholds for determining the distance run at high-intensity in professional soccer. *J Sports Sci* [Internet]. 2009 July;27(9):893–898.

59. Rago V, Brito J, Figueiredo P, Krustrup P, Rebelo A. Application of individualized speed zones to quantify external training load in professional soccer. *J Human Kinet* [Internet]. 2020 Mar 31;72(1):279–289.

60. Hunter F, Bray J, Towlson C, Smith M, Barrett S, Madden J, et al. Individualisation of time-motion analysis: A method comparison and case report series. *Int J Sports Med* [Internet]. 2014 Sep 26;36(01):41–48.

61. Lovell R, Abt G. Individualization of time–motion analysis: A case-cohort example. *Int J Sports Physiol Perform* [Internet]. 2013 July;8(4):456–458.

62. Buchheit M, Laursen P. High-intensity interval training, solutions to the programming puzzle: Part I: cardiopulmonary emphasis. *Sport Med*. 2013;43(5):313–338.

63. Sonderegger K, Tschopp M, Taube W. The challenge of evaluating the intensity of short actions in soccer: A new methodological approach using percentage acceleration. Lucía A, editor. *PLoS One* [Internet]. 2016 Nov 15;11(11):e0166534.

64. Dalen T, Jørgen I, Gertjan E, Geir Havard H, Ulrik W. Player load, acceleration, and deceleration during forty-five competitive matches of elite soccer. *J Strength Cond Res* [Internet]. 2016 Feb;30(2):351–359.

65. Ekstrand J, Hagglund M, Walden M. Injury incidence and injury patterns in professional football: The UEFA injury study. *Br J Sports Med* [Internet]. 2011 June 1;45(7):553–558.

66. Meeuwisse W. Assessing causation in sport injury: A multifactorial model. *Clin J Sport Med*. 1994;44(3):166–170.

67. Eckard TG, Padua DA, Hearn DW, Pexa BS, Frank BS. The relationship between training load and injury in athletes: A systematic review. *Sport Med* [Internet]. 2018 Aug 26;48(8):1929–1961.

68. Griffin A, Kenny IC, Comyns TM, Lyons M. The association between the acute: Chronic workload ratio and injury and its application in team sports: A systematic review. *Sport Med* [Internet]. 2020 Mar 5;50(3):561–580.

69. Windt J, Zumbo BD, Sporer B, MacDonald K, Gabbett TJ. Why do workload spikes cause injuries, and which athletes are at higher risk? Mediators and moderators in workload–injury investigations. *Br J Sports Med* [Internet]. 2017 July;51(13):993–994.

70. Bowen L, Gross AS, Gimpel M, Bruce-Low S, Li F-X. Spikes in acute: Chronic workload ratio (ACWR) associated with a 5–7 times greater injury rate in English Premier League football players: A comprehensive 3-year study. *Br J Sports Med* [Internet]. 2020 June;54(12):731–738.

71. Selye H. The general adaptation syndrome and the diseases of adaptation. *J Clin Endocrinol Metab* [Internet]. 1946 Feb;6(2):117–230.

72. Gabbett TJ, Ullah S. Relationship between running loads and soft-tissue injury in elite team sport athletes. *J Strength Cond Res* [Internet]. 2012 Apr;26(4):953–960.

73. Gabbett TJ, Domrow N. Relationships between training load, injury, and fitness in sub-elite collision sport athletes. *J Sports Sci* [Internet]. 2007 Nov;25(13):1507–1519.

74. Seyle H. The general adaptation syndrome and the diseases of adaptation. *J Clin Endocrinol Metab* [Internet]. 1946 Feb;6(2):117–230.

75. Rogalski B, Dawson B, Heasman J, Gabbett TJ. Training and game loads and injury risk in elite Australian footballers. *J Sci Med Sport* [Internet]. 2013 Nov;16(6):499–503.

76. Bowen L, Gross AS, Gimpel M, Li F-X. Accumulated workloads and the acute: Chronic workload ratio relate to injury risk in elite youth football players. *Br J Sports Med* [Internet]. 2017 Mar;51(5):452–459.

77. Gabbett TJ. Influence of training and match intensity on injuries in rugby league. *J Sports Sci* [Internet]. 2004 May;22(5):409–417.

78. Killen NM, Gabbett TJ, Jenkins DG. Training loads and incidence of injury during the preseason in professional rugby league players. *J Strength Cond Res* [Internet]. 2010 Aug;24(8):2079–2084.

79. Colby MJ, Dawson B, Heasman J, Rogalski B, Gabbett TJ. Accelerometer and GPS-derived running loads and injury risk in elite Australian footballers. *J Strength Cond Res* [Internet]. 2014 Aug;28(8):2244–2252.

80. Andrade R, Wik EH, Rebelo-Marques A, Blanch P, Whiteley R, Espregueira-Mendes J, et al. Is the acute: Chronic workload ratio (ACWR) Associated with risk of time-loss injury in professional team sports? A systematic review of methodology, variables and injury risk in practical situations. *Sport Med* [Internet]. 2020 Sep 22;50(9):1613–1635.

81. Calvert TW, Banister EW, Savage M V., Bach T. A systems model of the effects of training on physical performance. *IEEE Trans Syst Man Cybern* [Internet]. 1976 Feb;SMC-6(2):94–102.

82. Hulin BT, Gabbett TJ, Blanch P, Chapman P, Bailey D, Orchard JW. Spikes in acute workload are associated with increased injury risk in elite cricket fast bowlers. *Br J Sports Med* [Internet]. 2014 Apr;48(8):708–712.

83. Blanch P, Gabbett TJ. Has the athlete trained enough to return to play safely? The acute: Chronic workload ratio permits clinicians to quantify a player's risk of subsequent injury. *Br J Sports Med* [Internet]. 2016 Apr;50(8):471–475.

84. Williams S, West S, Cross MJ, Stokes KA. Better way to determine the acute: Chronic workload ratio? *Br J Sports Med* [Internet]. 2017 Feb;51(3):209–210.

85. Menaspà P. Are rolling averages a good way to assess training load for injury prevention? *Br J Sports Med* [Internet]. 2017 Apr;51(7):618.1–619.

86. Murray NB, Gabbett TJ, Townshend AD, Blanch P. Calculating acute: Chronic workload ratios using exponentially weighted moving averages provides a more sensitive indicator of injury likelihood than rolling averages. *Br J Sports Med* [Internet]. 2017 May;51(9):749–754.

87. Colby MJ, Dawson B, Peeling P, Heasman J, Rogalski B, Drew MK, et al. Multivariate modelling of subjective and objective monitoring data improve the detection of non-contact injury risk in elite Australian footballers. *J Sci Med Sport* [Internet]. 2017 Dec;20(12):1068–1074.

88. Hulin BT, Gabbett TJ, Lawson DW, Caputi P, Sampson JA. The acute: Chronic workload ratio predicts injury: High chronic workload may decrease injury risk in elite rugby league players. *Br J Sports Med* [Internet]. 2016 Feb;50(4):231–236.

89. Stares J, Dawson B, Peeling P, Heasman J, Rogalski B, Drew M, et al. Identifying high risk loading conditions for in-season injury in elite Australian football players. *J Sci Med Sport* [Internet]. 2018 Jan;21(1):46–51.

90. Ehrmann FE, Duncan CS, Sindhusake D, Franzsen WN, Greene DA. GPS and injury prevention in professional soccer. *J Strength Cond Res* [Internet]. 2016 Feb;30(2):360–367.

91. Emery CA. Injury prevention in paediatric sport-related injuries: A scientific approach. *Br J Sports Med* [Internet]. 2010 Jan 1;44(1):64–69.

92. Gastin PB, Meyer D, Huntsman E, Cook J. Increase in injury risk with low body mass and aerobic-running fitness in elite Australian football. *Int J Sports Physiol Perform* [Internet]. 2015 May;10(4):458–463.

93. Malone S, Owen A, Newton M, Mendes B, Collins KD, Gabbett TJ. The acute: Chonic workload ratio in relation to injury risk in professional soccer. *J Sci Med Sport* [Internet]. 2017 June;20(6):561–565.

94. Mallo J, Dellal A. Injury risk in professional football players with special reference to the playing position and training periodization. *J Sports Med Phys Fitness* [Internet]. 2012 Dec;52(6):631–638.

95. Owen AL, Lago-Penñs C, Gómez MÁ, Mendes B, Dellal A. Analysis of a training mesocycle and positional quantification in elite European soccer players. *Int J Sport Sci Coach* [Internet]. 2017 Oct 23;12(5):665–676.

96. Los Arcos A, Mendez-Villanueva A, Martínez-Santos R. In-season training periodization of professional soccer players. *Biol Sport* [Internet]. 2017;2:149–155.

97. Azcárate U, Yanci J, Los Arcos A. Influence of match playing time and the length of the between-match microcycle in Spanish professional soccer players' perceived training load. *Sci Med Footb* [Internet]. 2018 Jan 2;2(1):23–28.

98. Malone JJ, Di Michele R, Morgans R, Burgess D, Morton JP, Drust B. Seasonal training-load quantification in elite English Premier League soccer players. *Int J Sports Physiol Perform* [Internet]. 2015 May;10(4):489–497.

99. Owen AL, Djaoui L, Newton M, Malone S, Mendes B. A contemporary multi-modal mechanical approach to training monitoring in elite professional soccer. *Sci Med Footb* [Internet]. 2017 Sep 2;1(3):216–221.

100. Stevens TGA, de Ruiter CJ, Twisk JWR, Savelsbergh GJP, Beek PJ. Quantification of in-season training load relative to match load in professional Dutch Eredivisie football players. *Sci Med Footb* [Internet]. 2017 May 4;1(2):117–125.

101. Casamichana D, Martín-García A, Gómez Díaz A, S Bradley P, Castellano J. Accumulative weekly load in a professional football team: With special reference to match playing time and game position. *Biol Sport* [Internet]. 2021;39(1):115–124.

102. Ade J, Fitzpatrick J, Bradley PS. High-intensity efforts in elite soccer matches and associated movement patterns, technical skills and tactical actions. Information for position-specific training drills. *J Sports Sci* [Internet]. 2016 Dec 16;34(24):2205–2214.

103. Morgans R, Orme P, Anderson L, Drust B, Morton JP. An intensive winter fixture schedule induces a transient fall in salivary IgA in English Premier League soccer players. *Res Sport Med* [Internet]. 2014 Oct 2;22(4):346–354.

104. de Hoyo M, Cohen DD, Sañudo B, Carrasco L, Álvarez-Mesa A, del Ojo JJ, et al. Influence of football match time–motion parameters on recovery time course of muscle damage and jump ability. *J Sports Sci* [Internet]. 2016 July 17;34(14):1363–1370.

105. Ade JD, Harley JA, Bradley PS. Physiological Response, Time–motion characteristics, and reproducibility of various speed-endurance drills in elite youth soccer players: Small-sided games versus generic running. *Int J Sports Physiol Perform* [Internet]. 2014 May;9(3):471–479.

106. Malone S, Owen A, Mendes B, Hughes B, Collins K, Gabbett TJ. High-speed running and sprinting as an injury risk factor in soccer: Can well-developed physical qualities reduce the risk? *J Sci Med Sport* [Internet]. 2018 Mar;21(3):257–262.

10

ASSESSMENT AND QUANTIFICATION OF INTERNAL LOAD

Moisés de Hoyo Lora and Borja Sañudo Corrales

10.1 Introduction

Monitoring football players' training load (TL) is essential for determining whether they are adapting to their training program, understanding individual responses to training, assessing fatigue and the associated need for recovery, and minimizing the risk of nonfunctional overreaching, injury, and illness [1]. Excessive amounts of training can lead to overload of the system's capacity and increased risk of injury and illness. Otherwise, insufficient training may annihilate the performance benefits. It is thus generally accepted that players should be challenged adequately through appropriate periodization of their activities, allowing optimal recovery between bouts of activity to achieve the desired physiological adaptations of the system [2].

In line with this, Calvert et al. suggested in the Banister's model that performance at any given time point is determined by two main components: a fitness response and a fatigue response [3]. The fitness response involves the physiological adaptation to training, which is the long-term positive effect and will eventually result in an improvement in performance. The fatigue response is a shorter-term negative effect caused by the training-induced fatigue, resulting in a decrease in performance [3]. Therefore, authors suggest that, in its simplest form, performance at any time in a training program can be defined as the fitness gains in response to training minus the level of fatigue (Performance = Fitness − Fatigue). We can see that for a given training load, there are simultaneous fitness (+) and fatigue (−) responses, while when fatigue is greater than fitness, the player is in a negative performance state. However, as fatigue dissipates at the quicker rate, performance increases until the player is in a positive performance state (Figure 10.1).

DOI: 10.4324/9781032637006-10

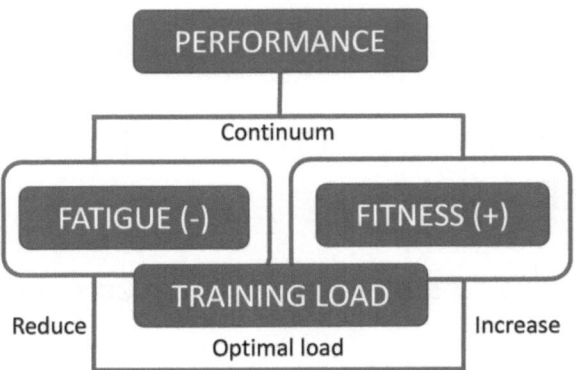

FIGURE 10.1 Conceptual Banister's model of the dose–response relationship (adapted from Calvert et al. [3]).

The training process starts with the training plan in which a certain training dose (or training load) is prescribed by the coach. One of the first steps in the setup of a successful training monitoring system is to quantify the dose of training and matches. The activities performed by the player represent an external load (ETL); yet, the abovementioned physiological adaptations come about because of internal load (ITL), primarily in the form of biochemical stresses [2]. Besides biochemical stresses, the activities performed by the athlete also lead to mechanical stresses on the different tissues that comprise the musculoskeletal system, i.e., on cartilage, bone, muscle, and tendon tissue [2]. Vanrenterghem et al. [2] suggested a novel conceptual model in which the physiological and biomechanical load adaptation pathways are considered separately, as schematically presented in Figure 10.2. Albeit oversimplified, for physiological load adaptations, one could seek analogy in the workings of a car engine, where the key focus is on the consumption of fuel and oxygen. Sticking with this car analogy, the biomechanical load adaptations could be represented by the suspension system, where the key focus is on keeping the mechanical properties intact.

Common measures of ITL (Figure 10.3) include subjective measures (self-reported) of rating of perceived exertion (RPE), session rating of perceived exertion (sRPE), and well-being questionary and objective measures of heart rate (HR), heart rate variability (HRV), blood lactate, oxygen consumption, creatine kinase, hormonal response, joint range of motion (ROM), sleep quality, and skin temperature [4].

10.2 Subjective measurements

Subjective measures of TL, and in particular sRPE, are recommended as a primary measure of TL in systematic reviews of the literature [5, 6]. Subjective measures may also be more sensitive and consistent than objective measures [7], and sRPE

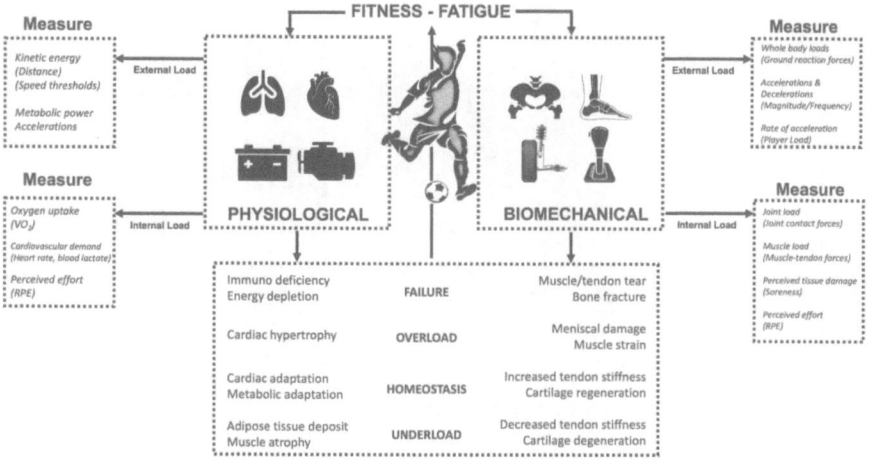

FIGURE 10.2 Player load monitoring outlining the cyclical nature in which physiological and biomechanical load leads to adaptation of the biological system as a whole, as proposed by Vanrenterghem et al. [2].

has been reported as the most commonly assessed TL variable in most sports [8]. Besides sRPE, there are other subjective methods of assessing players' response to training, e.g., visual analog scales and perceived wellness/stress questionnaires [9]. Although sRPE may give a better representation of overall load on the player, it should not be interpreted as a representation of physiological or biomechanical load [9].

To examine different components of training stress, sport scientists may also consider differential RPE [9]. Differential RPE refines how players rate different components of training/performance and requires separate scores for combinations of breathlessness (bRPE), leg muscle exertion (lRPE), upper body exertion (uRPE), and technical/cognitive exertion (tRPE) and in some cases match exertion (mRPE) [10–12]. With these components, differential RPE seems to encompass perceptions of separate physiological (bRPE) and biomechanical load (lRPE), while also accounting for mental load (tRPE) [9]. As an example, Barrett et al. [10] observed positional differences following football match play for bRPE, lRPE, and tRPE. Full backs had substantially higher dRPE than any other position, with all players reporting increased tRPE when playing teams at the top of the league. Differential RPE may also enhance measurement precision and sensitivity and improve within-athlete reliability compared to traditional global sRPE scores [2, 12]. Practically, separate scores (e.g., bRPE, lRPE, and tRPE) may be averaged to give a global RPE score if desired [9].

On the other hand, the importance of managing athlete fatigue has led to an increase in interest in monitoring player loads, particularly in terms of the measures, which may offer insights into whether the player is adapting positively or

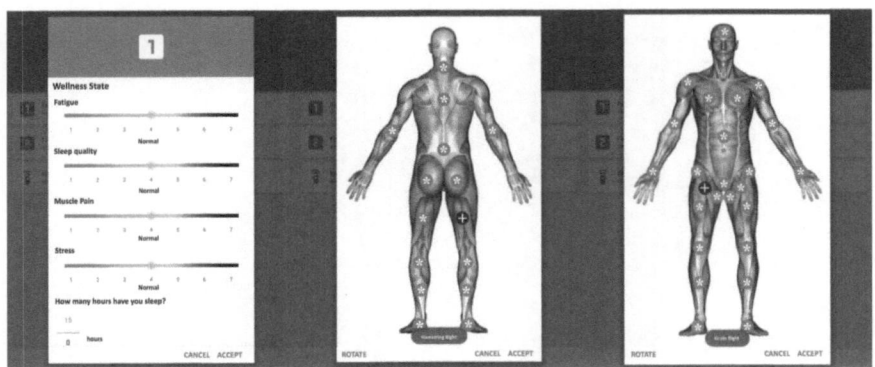

FIGURE 10.3 Perceived wellness questionnaire.

negatively to the collective stresses of training and competition [13]. In this sense, recent surveys on fatigue monitoring in high-performance sport demonstrate that athlete self-report measures are used extensively for assessing the overall wellbeing of team sport athletes [14].

For example, different Australian Football League (AFL) and English Premier League (EPL) research studies have shown custom psychometric scales to be sensitive to daily, within-weekly, and seasonal changes in training load [15–17]. Indeed, daily wellness questionary (fatigue, sleep quality, stress, mood, and muscle soreness. See Figure 10.3) were significantly correlated with daily TL in a pre-season camp and competitive period in AFL and EPL players, respectively [16, 18]. Further, importance of this type of information and relationship with injury/illness has been observed in Rugby League. In this study, fluctuations in athlete self-report measures between macrocycles were shown to provide useful insights into possible illness risk in players [19].

10.3   Blood biomarkers

The demands of competitive football, including sprints, accelerations, decelerations, changes of direction, jumps, and direct contacts with opposing players, have a powerful eccentric component [20], producing potential concomitant homeostatic perturbations including metabolic (i.e., muscle glycogen depletion), mechanical (i.e., muscle damage), and oxidative stress (i.e., production of reactive oxygen and nitrogen species) [21]. The magnitude of all these disturbances increases within the first 24 hours after exercise or competition, peaks between 24 and 48 hours, and thereafter subsides and returns to baseline after 72–96 hours [21–24]. Together with a decline in performance, muscle damage and increased levels of intramuscular enzymes such as creatine kinase (CK) and inflammatory markers are reported following football competition [21–24].

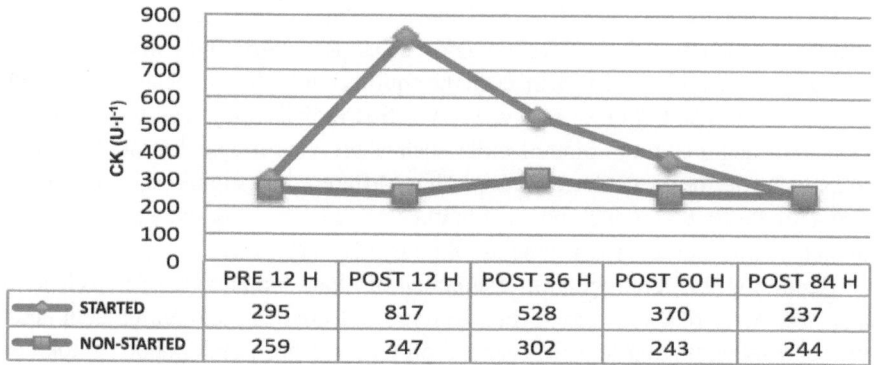

	PRE 12 H	POST 12 H	POST 36 H	POST 60 H	POST 84 H
STARTED	295	817	528	370	237
NON-STARTED	259	247	302	243	244

FIGURE 10.4   CK evolution after an official football match in started (line with dia-
monds) and non-started players (line with squares).

The increase in plasma concentration/activity of certain intracellular proteins (e.g., Mb and CK) has been widely used as indirect markers of tissue damage [25]. Increased Mb contents immediately after [22, 23] and in CK activity throughout the 72–96 hours of the recovery period of a match (CK) with semi-professional [21–23, 26] and professional players [24] have been reported. In this line, Figure 10.4 shows an example of CK evolution after a football match.

The production of inflammatory mediators' post-game or workout is one of the fundamental features of adaptation to training. This favorable effect of inflammation may be explained by the "stress-response" hormesis theory [27], whereby low levels of stress can be beneficial through induction of adaptive mechanisms, increasing the tolerance against future stress incidents (e.g., enhanced resistance to fatigue during a future exercise bout). However, prolonged production of inflammatory mediators can exert negative effects on muscle repair and growth by impeding muscle protein synthesis and overwhelming the endogenous defense mechanisms of the body (e.g., anti-oxidant resources), resulting in chronic systemic inflammation. Interestingly, it has been shown that the recovery time between successive games during a three-game weekly microcycle may not be adequate for the restoration of normal homeostasis and the resolution of the inflammatory response [28, 29]. The long-term consequences of a lack of recovery may leave many players in an energy-depleted state, both emotionally and physically, and could result in an increased risk for injury [30]. According to this, IL-6 is produced in larger amounts than any other cytokine, prompting its use as a global measure of inflammation [31]. IL-6 peaks immediately after the cessation of exercise and then rapidly returns to baseline values after 24 hours [24, 28, 32]. C-reactive protein and uric acid have been found to be more sensitive markers of inflammation after football match play [24, 26, 28]. Indeed, increases of up ~50% 48 hours post-match have been observed in elite football players [26]. Furthermore, in a similar study in elite football players, uric acid peaked 72 hours after a match [28].

High-intensity exercise also upregulates oxidative stress responses due to an increased production of reactive oxygen species (ROS) that challenge the systems scavenging ROS [33]. Disturbances in the equilibrium of free radicals such as ROS and the antioxidant defense in favor of the free radicals may lead to progressive change or degradation of biomolecules such as proteins and nucleic acids, leading to exercise performance deterioration. Thus, different investigations have reported that a single football match elicits a marked increase in oxidative stress and anti-oxidant status markers for as long as 48 hours [24, 34].

According this, the regular measurement of blood biomarkers of muscle damage (e.g., CK), oxidative stress (biomarkers of pro-oxidant and antioxidant activity), and inflammation (e.g., C-reactive protein and pro-inflammatory cytokines) may be used to make inferences about the athletes underlying physiology and recovery before and after a game. By examining these markers, it may be possible to draw some conclusion about the extent of damage to the muscle as a result of the game and provide the practitioner with "actionable" data to promote recovery in the interval between successive matches.

10.4 Endocrine response

Regarding the endocrine response, the official football match altered the catabolic/anabolic-related hormonal homeostasis toward a predominant catabolic response during the first 48 hours of the recovery period [34]. Thus, adrenal hormones cortisol and testosterone have been shown to increase up to 50% during 48 hours post-competition in team sports [28]. Alterations in systemic cortisol and testosterone concentrations have been applied as systemic indicators of over-reaching in scientific research [34]. Salivary cortisol is a hormonal marker that is highly responsive to exercise and is directly related to the catabolic activity [35]. Cortisol has recently been suggested as a relevant indicator to monitor recovery in football, in response to the induced stress [36]. Increased levels of salivary cortisol, as a result of accumulated stress, can negatively impact mucosal immunity, subsequently increasing the risk of illness [37]. Moreover, cortisol has also been implicated in the regulation of the acute inflammatory response following exercise by increasing neutrophils and suppressing lymphocytes and natural killer cells [38]. In fact, cortisol increase following two football matches within a 2-day frame was correlated with changes in neutrophil count [38]. This cortisol action may be expressed through the upregulation of immunoglobin M and adhesion molecule activity [38]. Moreover, cortisol level increase is probably controlled by interlukin 6 (IL-6), which coincides with the simultaneous post-game rise of IL-6 observed by Mohr et al. [28].

On the other hand, different authors have suggested that congested fixture periods are associated with perturbations in mucosal immunity [39]. In addition, an elevation of injury incidence [37, 40] has been related with a greater reduction in mean relative immunoglobulin A (IgA) salivary concentration following an intensive competition period compared with a less competitive period in rugby union. Moreover, the decrease in absolute salivary IgA concentrations was associated with a corresponding increase in salivary cortisol [37]. Moreover, Morgans et al. observed in football players salivary IgA reductions during a taper phase and a period of international competition [39, 41].

10.5 Heart rate

10.5.1 Heart rate: intensity zones

Several studies have evaluated this measure, mostly in absolute (min) and relative values (%min). However, there are differences regarding the division of the zones themselves. Wrigley et al. [42] delimited HR assessment in six zones using the maximum HR (HR_{max}) as reference: < 50% HR_{max}, 51–60% HR_{max}, 61–70% HR_{max}, 71–80% HR_{max}, 81–90% HR_{max}, and > 90% HR_{max}. Other authors such as Abade et al. [43] proposed an HR analysis into four zones: < 75% HR_{max}, 75–84.9% HR_{max}, 85–89.9% HR_{max}, and ≥ 90% HR_{max}. Akenhead et al. [44], Campos-Vazquez et al. [45], and Stevens et al. [46] only analyzed the activity time above 90% HR_{max}.

10.5.2 TRIMP methods

Banister training impulse (TRIMP) was established to quantify the internal load of a training session [47]. This method considers the intensity and exercise duration, using a coefficient, which relates HR and blood lactate during incremental exercise. The total load value, TRIMP, is expressed in arbitrary units (AU).

Banister's TRIMP = D × (factor A × ΔHR × $\exp^{(factor\ B\ \times\ \Delta HR)}$), where:

D = duration of the training session in minutes.
For men: Factor A = 0.64 and Factor B = 1.92.
For women: Factor A = 0.86 and Factor B = 1.67.
ΔHR ratio = (HR_{ex} – HR_{rest})/ (HR_{max} – HR_{rest}), in which
HR_{ex} is the average heart rate of the exercise session,
HR_{rest} is the resting heart rate,
HR_{max} is the maximal heart rate.

Silva et al. [48] observed a high correlation between Banister TRIMP and accelerations and high-intensity repeated efforts (high-intensity bursts) during official games. The second method is commonly known as the Edwards' TRIMP or the summated heart rate zones' score method, originally introduced by Edwards [49], calculated as the product of the cumulated training duration (in minutes) for five heart rate zones multiplied by a coefficient relative to each zone (i.e., 50–60%

HRmax = 1; 60–70% HRmax = 2; 70–80% HRmax = 3; 80–90% HRmax = 4; 90–100% HRmax = 5). The Edwards TL formula is as follows:

Edwards' TRIMP = D in zone 1 × 1 + D in zone 2 × 2 + D in zone 3 × 3 + D in zone 4 × 4 + D in zone 5 × 5

Other authors have developed methods for quantifying the ITL that could provide more specific and individual responses [50]. Lucía's TRIMP [51] justifies the evaluation of TL according to ventilatory thresholds (VT). This method has been less stated and evaluated in the scientific literature and is based on individually determined lactate thresholds and the onset of blood lactate [La] accumulation. In this method, the activity time, in minutes, spent in each of three heart rate zones (zone 1: below the ventilator threshold; zone 2: between the ventilator threshold and the respiratory compensation point; zone 3: above the respiratory compensation point) is multiplied by the respective coefficient (k = 1 for zone 1, k = 2 for zone 2, and k = 3 for zone 3) and added to obtain a total load value, expressed in AU. The Lucia's TL formula is as follows:

Lucia's TRIMP = D in zone 1 × 1 + D in zone 2 × 2 + D in zone 3 × 3

Stagno TRIMP directly evaluates the blood lactate profile instead of using a generic equation that reflects a hypothetical profile, obtaining a standard curve of response to increased exercise intensity [52]. Five HR zones are then defined around the lactate threshold and onset of blood lactate accumulation (OBLA), 65–71%HR_{max}, 72–78%, 79–85%, 86–92%, and 93–100%, with the respective weights 1.25, 1.71, 2.54, 3.61, and 5.16. The activity time, in minutes, in each HR zone is multiplied by the respective weighting to determine the ITL, expressed in AU.

Individualized TRIMP ($TRIMP_i$) uses a weighting factor to the physiological response of each athlete to exercise [53]. To evaluate this factor, all athletes are subjected to a maximum test to determine the individual blood lactate concentration profile—blood lactate concentrations were plotted against running speeds and fractional HR elevation, and individual blood lactate concentration profiles were identified via exponential interpolation:

$$TRIMP_i = D \times [(HR_{mean} - HR_{rest})/(HR_{max} - HR_{rest})] \times yi,$$

where yi reflects the profile of the standard curve of blood lactate response to increased exercise intensity. The yi values are calculated for each subject. The TL is expressed in AU.

10.6 Heart rate variability

Cardiac autonomic response can be used to monitor the cardiovascular adjustments made after exercise [54–57], which are mediated by the autonomic nervous system

(ANS) [58], via measures of HR. Heart rate variability (HRV) has been defined as the time variation between consecutive heartbeats [59]. In this sense, resting HRV is an objective physiological marker that has been used as an indicator of recovery status in various athletic populations [60]. HRV reflects neural control of the heart via sympathetic and parasympathetic innervations [54]. Thus, HRV reflects the reaction capacity of the heart to different physiological demands [59].

The basic principle of HRV monitoring is to make inferences on possible changes in the cardiac ANS status with training, while using repeated HRV measures over the time [55]. Since ANS activity is highly sensitive to environmental conditions (e.g., noise, light, and temperature) [61], it is important that precautions be taken to standardize recording conditions in order to isolate the training-induced effects on ANS [55]. Currently, the best practice for athletes tends to be short-term (5–10 min) measurements of HRV upon awakening in the morning [60, 62]. While both supine and standing recordings are often used in the literature [63], the supine condition is better tolerated by athletes in the field [55].

According to all HRV guidelines and publications in the literature, there are several methods for the assessment of cardiac autonomic function by the examination of sympathetic–parasympathetic balance. Thus, the most commonly used methods are time domain and spectral analyses; nonlinear methods such as entropy and symbolic analyses have also gained some interest more recently [55]. Each index captures a different feature of the ANS, with some indices more likely to reflect cardiac sympathetic activity and others cardiac parasympathetic activity [55]. In practice, however, when it comes to selecting the more appropriate HRV indices to monitor athletes in the field, time domain indices (e.g., rMSSD [square root of the mean of the sum of the squares of differences between adjacent normal R-R intervals] or SD1 [standard deviation of instantaneous beat-to-beat R–R interval variability measured from Poincaré plots], both reflecting parasympathetic modulation) are the most attractive ones [55]. Recently, the Stress Score (SS) has been proposed to reflect sympathetic activity in football players using Poincaré plots [59].

Vagal-related time domain parameters of HRV have recently received greater attention than more traditional spectral analyses due to their superior reliability and assessment capture over short periods of time [64, 65]. Sensitivity to changes in training load and performance has mainly been observed [66, 67]. In elite football players, LnrMSSD appeared to decrease, albeit transiently, in response to high-speed running distance [18]. Different research studies suggest that the weekly mean of lnRMSSD (lnRMSSDmean) provides a better reflection of the training status than once per week recordings [62, 68]. The coefficient of variation of lnRMSSDmean (lnRMSSDcv) represents daily fluctuation, with higher CV values being associated with lower fitness and greater training stress and vice versa [69]. Thus, it appears that monitoring lnRMSSDmean and lnRMSSDcv values throughout training will provide important information pertaining to fatigue and adaptation [54].

On the other hand, the Poincaré plot analysis is a nonlinear method that reflects sympathetic–parasympathetic fluctuations [59]. To plot it, all consecutive RR intervals are inserted in a two-dimensional dispersion plot in such a way that every

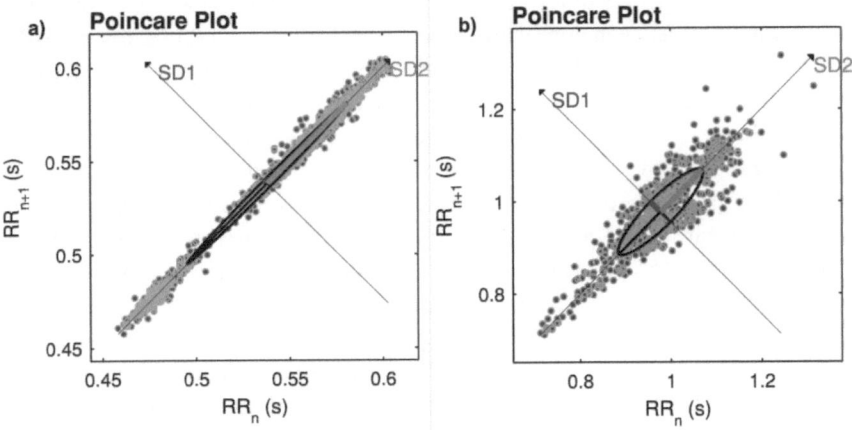

FIGURE 10.5 Poincaré Plot: (a) after 10 min of high-intensity training; (b) after 8 hours of sleep. The SD1 axis is reduced after a fatiguing training and recovery a normal length after 8 hours of sleep.

RR interval point represented against the previous point. Thus, a Poincaré plot (Figure 10.5) shows a qualitative picture of the variations between RR intervals and can be adjusted to an ellipse [70]. The transversal axis (SD1) reflects short time changes in the RR intervals and is directly linked to parasympathetic activity [59]. However, the longitudinal axis (SD2) is inversely proportional to sympathetic activity [59].

The SD1:SD2 ratio is normally used to assess the interaction between parasympathetic and sympathetic activity [59]. Naranjo et al. [59] defined two new indices to help in the interpretation of the Poincaré plot. These indices were SS, expressed as the inverse of the SD2 diameter multiplied by 1000 (with the aim of obtaining a value directly proportional to the sympathetic activity over the sinus node), and the sympathetic–parasympathetic ratio (S/PS ratio), expressed as the ratio between SS and SD1. Its aim is to obtain a real relationship between sympathetic and parasympathetic activity that reflects the autonomic balance via the HRV. Naranjo et al. [71] analyzed these values according to the percentile distribution proposed by the authors [59]; it was observed that an SS of 10 and an S/PS ratio of 0.5 mark the limit of the values obtained in football players of this level and that values of 8 and 0.2, respectively, would indicate a possible alert.

10.7 Neuromuscular response

Different research studies have observed that some players, although potentially dependent on playing standard, may still not be 100% recovered in the 72 hours following a competitive match [72]. Participation in a single match leads to acute and residual fatigue, characterized by a decline in physical performance over the following hours and days [24]. The magnitude of these disturbances increases within the first 24 hours after exercise or competition, peaks between 24 and 48 hours, and thereafter subsides and returns to baseline after 72–96 hours [21–24]. Players demonstrate a dramatic decline in high-intensity running toward the end of a game, causing marked impairment in repeated sprint ability (RSA), intense intermittent exercise, countermovement jump (CMJ), and strength performance [28]. According to this, authors such as de Hoyo et al. [21] observed a decrease in CMJ height and concentric and eccentric force in U-19 football players 24 and 48 hours after the game.

Moreover, in football, players may participate in 50–80 games during a season and in most top leagues, it is a normal procedure for teams to compete in three games per week during several periods within a season. Thus, only 3–4 days of recovery are allowed between successive games, which may be insufficient to restore normal homeostasis [24, 26, 32]. However, the majority of studies investigating recovery aspects from football match-play have only followed the response in a single game. In this sense, Mohr et al. [28] examined the effects of a three-game microcycle on recovery of performance in professional male footballers. Authors observed that high-intensity running during game 2 was 7–14% less compared to games 1 and 3. In this line, the performance in the RSA test declined by 2–9%, 3 days post-game, with game 2 causing the greatest performance impairment.

10.8   Other methods

Other methods included in the control of ITL are the thermography, tensiomyography, and range of motion [73]. Regarding thermography, this is characterized by the use of a camera which can detect radiation and produce thermal images called thermograms [73]. The thermograms contain temperature data that can be analyzed by specific software, which provides temperature of a region of interest [74, 75]. Different studies have analyzed the use of this technique to control ITL following aerobic [76], anaerobic [77], and resistance exercises [78]. Figure 10.6 shows an example of thermal response in the posterior chain to different types of training sessions.

To monitor acute effects of muscle fatigue on mechanical properties of muscle contraction without the assessment itself causing additional fatigue, surface mechanomyographic (MMG) methods have been applied [79]. An alternative and easy-to-handle MMG method was introduced named Tensiomyography™ (TMG) about 20 years ago [80, 81]. TMG is a non-invasive method that measures radial deformation of the skeletal muscle, and in turn its contractile properties, in response to an external electrical stimulus [82]. The device incorporates a high-precision displacement sensor (4 μm) which is placed perpendicularly with a slight pre-tension (0.2 N/ cm2) onto the surface of the muscle belly in order to record the radial deformation of the muscle following electrically evoked stimulation [83].

TMG obtains different measures, which can be derived from the twitch displacement time curve. Thus, the main parameters used in different researches

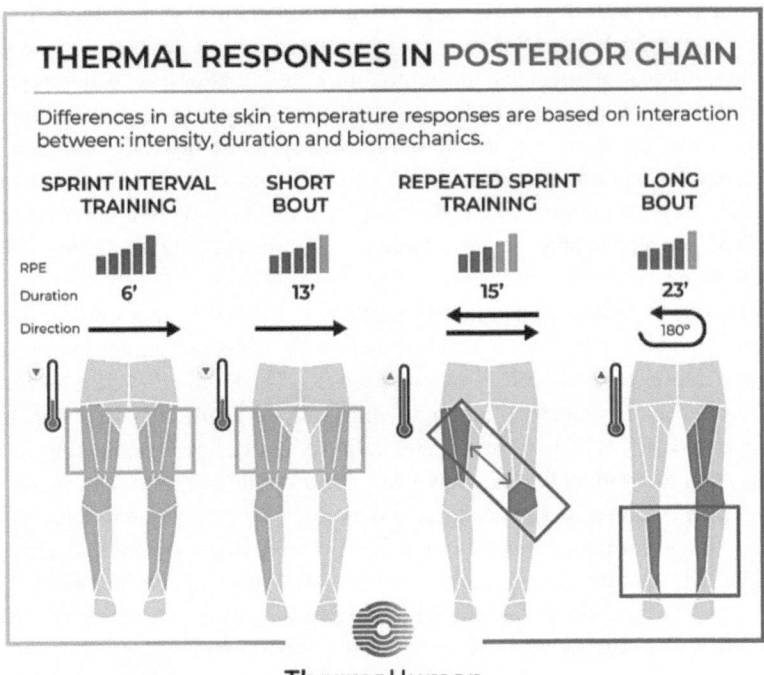

FIGURE 10.6 Thermal responses in posterior chain (with the permission of ®ThermoHuman).

are maximal radial displacement of the muscle belly (Dm, mm), the delay time between the onset of electrical stimulation and 10% of Dm (Td, ms), the contraction time between 10% and 90% of Dm (Tc, ms), and the mean velocity of muscle contraction from the onset of electrical stimulation until 90% of Dm (V90, mm/s) [84]. Some of these TMG variables, such as Dm, Tc, and Td, have been shown to be sensitive to detect muscle fatigue [85, 86]. Moreover, the parameter Dm has been proposed as an indicator of muscle stiffness or muscle contractile force, whereas the parameters Td and Tc have been introduced as measures of muscle response or muscle activation time and speed of force generation, respectively [13, 19, 26, 86–88]. Recently, a novel TMG-derived measurement named "velocity of contraction" (Vc) (i.e., Vc = Dm/Tc+Td) has been proposed to identify acute and chronic changes in neuromuscular performance in non-athletic populations and elite athletes [89, 90]. Pereira et al. [82] showed that the changes in Vc were the same as those observed in performance (SJ and CMJ) assessments after strength and plyometric workouts.

Finally, football match play induces range of motion (ROM) changes that could affect the player's intrinsic modifiable risk factors [91]. Thus, for example, regarding hamstring muscles, strength imbalances, lower strength characteristics, and decreased ROM at the hip, knee, and ankle joints constitute previously reported intrinsic hamstring injury risk factors [92–94] that are all potentially modifiable after a game. In this sense, Small et al. observed a reduced range of knee extension and hip ROM after a multidirectional football-specific fatigue protocol [95]. In this line, Paul et al. [24] observed a negative impact in hip flexibility after a football match.

References

1. Bourdon PC, Cardinale M, Murray A, Gastin P, Kellmann M, Varley MC, et al. Monitoring Athlete Training Loads: Consensus Statement. *Int J Sports Physiol Perform* [Internet]. 2017 Apr;12(s2):S2-161–S2-170. Available from: https://journals.humankinetics.com/view/journals/ijspp/12/s2/article-pS2-161.xml
2. Vanrenterghem J, Nedergaard NJ, Robinson MA, Drust B. Training Load Monitoring in Team Sports: A Novel Framework Separating Physiological and Biomechanical Load-Adaptation Pathways. *Sport Med* [Internet]. 2017 Nov 10;47(11):2135–2142. Available from: https://link.springer.com/10.1007/s40279-017-0714-2
3. Calvert TW, Banister EW, Savage MV, Bach T. A Systems Model of the Effects of Training on Physical Performance. *IEEE Trans Syst Man Cybern* [Internet]. 1976 Feb;SMC-6(2):94–102. Available from: https://ieeexplore.ieee.org/document/5409179/
4. Griffin A, Kenny IC, Comyns TM, Lyons M. The Association Between the Acute: Chronic Workload Ratio and Injury and its Application in Team Sports: A Systematic Review. *Sport Med* [Internet]. 2020 Mar 5;50(3):561–580. Available from: https://link.springer.com/10.1007/s40279-019-01218-2
5. Drew MK, Finch CF. The Relationship Between Training Load and Injury, Illness and Soreness: A Systematic and Literature Review. *Sport Med* [Internet]. 2016 June 28;46(6):861–883. Available from: https://link.springer.com/10.1007/s40279-015-0459-8
6. McLaren SJ, Macpherson TW, Coutts AJ, Hurst C, Spears IR, Weston M. The Relationships Between Internal and External Measures of Training Load and Intensity in Team Sports: A Meta-Analysis. *Sport Med* [Internet]. 2018 Mar 29;48(3):641–658. Available from: https://link.springer.com/10.1007/s40279-017-0830-z
7. Saw AE, Main LC, Gastin PB. Monitoring the Athlete Training Response: Subjective Self-reported Measures Trump Commonly Used Objective Measures: A Systematic Review. *Br J Sports Med* [Internet]. 2016 Mar;50(5):281–291. Available from: https://bjsm.bmj.com/lookup/doi/10.1136/bjsports-2015-094758
8. Burgess DJ. The Research Doesn't Always Apply: Practical Solutions to Evidence-Based Training-Load Monitoring in Elite Team Sports. *Int J Sports Physiol Perform* [Internet]. 2017 Apr;12(s2):S2-136–S2-141. Available from: https://journals.humankinetics.com/view/journals/ijspp/12/s2/article-pS2-136.xml
9. Coyne JOC, Gregory Haff G, Coutts AJ, Newton RU, Nimphius S. The Current State of Subjective Training Load Monitoring—A Practical Perspective and Call to Action. *Sport Med* [Internet]. 2018 Dec 20;4(1):58. Available from: https://sportsmedicine-open.springeropen.com/articles/10.1186/s40798-018-0172-x
10. Barrett S, McLaren S, Spears I, Ward P, Weston M. The Influence of Playing Position and Contextual Factors on Soccer Players' Match Differential Ratings of Perceived Exertion: A Preliminary Investigation. *Sports* [Internet]. 2018 Feb 12;6(1):13. Available from: https://www.mdpi.com/2075-4663/6/1/13

11. Weston M, Siegler J, Bahnert A, McBrien J, Lovell R. The Application of Differential Ratings of Perceived Exertion to Australian Football League Matches. *J Sci Med Sport* [Internet]. 2015 Nov;18(6):704–708. Available from: https://linkinghub.elsevier.com/retrieve/pii/S1440244014001716

12. McLaren SJ, Smith A, Spears IR, Weston M. A Detailed Quantification of Differential Ratings of Perceived Exertion During Team-sport Training. *J Sci Med Sport* [Internet]. 2017 Mar;20(3):290–295. Available from: https://linkinghub.elsevier.com/retrieve/pii/S1440244016301165

13. Thorpe RT, Atkinson G, Drust B, Gregson W. Monitoring Fatigue Status in Elite Team-Sport Athletes: Implications for Practice. *Int J Sports Physiol Perform* [Internet]. 2017 Apr;12(s2):S2-27–S2-34. Available from: https://journals.humankinetics.com/view/journals/ijspp/12/s2/article-pS2-27.xml

14. Taylor K-L, Chapman DW, Cronin JB, Newton MJ, Gill N. Fatigue Monitoring in High Performance Sport: A Survey of Current Trends. *J Aust Strength Cond*. 2012;20(1):12–23.

15. Gastin PB, Meyer D, Robinson D. Perceptions of Wellness to Monitor Adaptive Responses to Training and Competition in Elite Australian Football. *J Strength Cond Res* [Internet]. 2013 Sep;27(9):2518–2526. Available from: https://journals.lww.com/00124278-201309000-00021

16. Gallo TF, Cormack SJ, Gabbett TJ, Lorenzen CH. Self-Reported Wellness Profiles of Professional Australian Football Players During the Competition Phase of the Season. *J Strength Cond Res* [Internet]. 2017 Feb;31(2):495–502. Available from: https://journals.lww.com/00124278-201702000-00028

17. Buchheit M, Racinais S, Bilsborough JC, Bourdon PC, Voss SC, Hocking J, et al. Monitoring Fitness, Fatigue and Running Performance During a Pre-season Training Camp in Elite Football Players. *J Sci Med Sport* [Internet]. 2013 Nov;16(6):550–555. Available from: https://linkinghub.elsevier.com/retrieve/pii/S1440244012011322

18. Thorpe RT, Strudwick AJ, Buchheit M, Atkinson G, Drust B, Gregson W. Monitoring Fatigue During the In-Season Competitive Phase in Elite Soccer Players. *Int J Sports Physiol Perform* [Internet]. 2015 Nov;10(8):958–964. Available from: https://journals.humankinetics.com/view/journals/ijspp/10/8/article-p958.xml

19. Thornton HR, Delaney JA, Duthie GM, Scott BR, Chivers WJ, Sanctuary CE, et al. Predicting Self-Reported Illness for Professional Team-Sport Athletes. *Int J Sports Physiol Perform* [Internet]. 2016 May;11(4):543–550. Available from: https://journals.humankinetics.com/view/journals/ijspp/11/4/article-p543.xml

20. Nédélec M, McCall A, Carling C, Legall F, Berthoin S, Dupont G. Recovery in Soccer. *Sport Med* [Internet]. 2012 Dec;42(12):997–1015. Available from: https://content.wkhealth.com/linkback/openurl?sid=WKPTLP:landingpage&an=00007256-201242120-00002

21. de Hoyo M, Cohen DD, Sañudo B, Carrasco L, Álvarez-Mesa A, del Ojo JJ, et al. Influence of Football Match Time–Motion Parameters on Recovery Time Course of Muscle Damage and Jump Ability. *J Sports Sci* [Internet]. 2016 July 17;34(14):1363–1370. Available from: https://www.tandfonline.com/doi/full/10.1080/02640414.2016.1150603

22. Magalhães J, Rebelo A, Oliveira E, Silva JR, Marques F, Ascensão A. Impact of Loughborough Intermittent Shuttle Test Versus Soccer Match on Physiological, Biochemical and Neuromuscular Parameters. *Eur J Appl Physiol* [Internet]. 2010 Jan 16;108(1):39–48. Available from: https://link.springer.com/10.1007/s00421-009-1161-z

23. Ascensão A, Rebelo A, Oliveira E, Marques F, Pereira L, Magalhães J. Biochemical Impact of a Soccer Match — Analysis of Oxidative Stress and Muscle Damage Markers Throughout Recovery. *Clin Biochem* [Internet]. 2008 July;41(10–11):841–851. Available from: https://linkinghub.elsevier.com/retrieve/pii/S0009912008001616

24. Ispirlidis I, Fatouros IG, Jamurtas AZ, Nikolaidis MG, Michailidis I, Douroudos I, et al. Time-course of Changes in Inflammatory and Performance Responses Following a Soccer Game. *Clin J Sport Med* [Internet]. 2008 Sep;18(5):423–431. Available from: https://journals.lww.com/00042752-200809000-00010

25. Brancaccio P, Maffulli N, Limongelli FM. Creatine Kinase Monitoring in Sport Medicine. *Br Med Bull* [Internet]. 2007 Feb 6;81–82(1):209–230. Available from: https://academic.oup.com/bmb/article-lookup/doi/10.1093/bmb/ldm014

26. Fatouros IG, Chatzinikolaou A, Douroudos II, Nikolaidis MG, Kyparos A, Margonis K, et al. Time-Course of Changes in Oxidative Stress and Antioxidant Status Responses Following a Soccer Game. *J Strength Cond Res* [Internet]. 2010 Dec;24(12): 3278–3286. Available from: https://journals.lww.com/00124278-201012000-00012

27. Margaritelis N V., Theodorou AA, Baltzopoulos V, Maganaris CN, Paschalis V, Kyparos A, et al. Muscle Damage and Inflammation After Eccentric Exercise: Can the Repeated Bout Effect Be Removed? *Physiol Rep* [Internet]. 2015 Dec;3(12):e12648. Available from: https://doi.wiley.com/10.14814/phy2.12648

28. Mohr M, Draganidis D, Chatzinikolaou A, Barbero-Álvarez JC, Castagna C, Douroudos I, et al. Muscle Damage, Inflammatory, Immune and Performance Responses to Three Football Games in 1 Week in Competitive Male Players. *Eur J Appl Physiol* [Internet]. 2016 Jan 16;116(1):179–193. Available from: https://link.springer.com/10.1007/s00421-015-3245-2

29. Owen AL. Biochemical Response Comparisons of a Competitive Microcycle Vs. Congested Fixture Periods in Elite Level European Champions League Soccer Players. *J Complement Med Altern Healthc* [Internet]. 2019 Aug 5;10(1). Available from: https://juniperpublishers.com/jcmah/JCMAH.MS.ID.555778.php

30. Ekstrand J. A Congested Football Calendar and the Wellbeing of Players: Correlation Between Match Exposure of European Footballers Before the World Cup 2002 and Their Injuries and Performances during that World Cup. *Br J Sports Med* [Internet]. 2004 Aug 1;38(4):493–497. Available from: https://bjsm.bmj.com/lookup/doi/10.1136/bjsm.2003.009134

31. Tidball JG. Inflammatory Processes in Muscle Injury and Repair. *Am J Physiol Integr Comp Physiol* [Internet]. 2005 Feb;288(2):R345–R353. Available from: https://www.physiology.org/doi/10.1152/ajpregu.00454.2004

32. Andersson H, Raastad T, Nilsson J, Paulsen G, Garthe I, Kadi F. Neuromuscular Fatigue and Recovery in Elite Female Soccer. *Med Sci Sport Exerc* [Internet]. 2008 Feb;40(2): 372–80. Available from: https://journals.lww.com/00005768-200802000-00024

33. Michailidis Y, Karagounis LG, Terzis G, Jamurtas AZ, Spengos K, Tsoukas D, et al. Thiol-based Antioxidant Supplementation Alters Human Skeletal Muscle Signaling and Attenuates its Inflammatory Response and Recovery After Intense Eccentric Exercise. *Am J Clin Nutr* [Internet]. 2013 July 1;98(1):233–245. Available from: https://academic.oup.com/ajcn/article/98/1/233/4578325

34. Silva JR, Ascensão A, Marques F, Seabra A, Rebelo A, Magalhães J. Neuromuscular Function, Hormonal and Redox Status and Muscle Damage of Professional Soccer Players After a High-level Competitive Match. *Eur J Appl Physiol* [Internet]. 2013 Sep 10;113(9):2193–2201. Available from: https://link.springer.com/10.1007/s00421-013-2633-8

35. Banfi G, Dolci A. Free Testosterone/Cortisol Ratio in Soccer: Usefulness of a Categorization of Values. *J Sports Med Phys Fitness* [Internet]. 2006 Dec;46(4):611–616. Available from: https://www.ncbi.nlm.nih.gov/pubmed/17119528

36. Romagnoli M, Sanchis-Gomar F, Alis R, Risso-Ballester J, Bosio A, Graziani RL, et al. Changes in Muscle Damage, Inflammation, and Fatigue-related Parameters

in Young Elite Soccer Players after a Match. *J Sports Med Phys Fitness* [Internet]. 2016 Oct;56(10):1198–1205. Available from: https://www.ncbi.nlm.nih.gov/pubmed/26558831

37. Cunniffe B, Griffiths H, Proctor W, Davies B, Baker JS, Jones KP. Mucosal Immunity and Illness Incidence in Elite Rugby Union Players across a Season. *Med Sci Sport Exerc* [Internet]. 2011 Mar;43(3):388–397. Available from: https://journals.lww.com/00005768-201103000-00003

38. Malm C, Ekblom O, Ekblom B. Immune System Alteration in Response to Two Consecutive Soccer Games. *Acta Physiol Scand* [Internet]. 2004 Feb;180(2):143–155. Available from: https://doi.wiley.com/10.1046/j.0001-6772.2003.01232.x

39. Morgans R, Orme P, Anderson L, Drust B, Morton JP. An Intensive Winter Fixture Schedule Induces a Transient Fall in Salivary IgA in English Premier League Soccer Players. *Res Sport Med* [Internet]. 2014 Oct 2;22(4):346–54. Available from: https://www.tandfonline.com/doi/full/10.1080/15438627.2014.944641

40. Bengtsson H, Ekstrand J, Waldén M, Hägglund M. Muscle Injury Rates in Professional Football Increase With Fixture Congestion: An 11-Year Follow-Up of the Uefa Champions League Injury Study. *Br J Sports Med* [Internet]. 2014 Apr 11;48(7):566-567. Available from: https://bjsm.bmj.com/lookup/doi/10.1136/bjsports-2014-093494.19

41. Morgans R, Owen A, Doran D, Drust B, Morton JP. Prematch Salivary Secretory Immunoglobulin A in Soccer Players From the 2014 World Cup Qualifying Campaign. *Int J Sports Physiol Perform* [Internet]. 2015 Apr;10(3):401–413. Available from: https://journals.humankinetics.com/view/journals/ijspp/10/3/article-p401.xml

42. Wrigley R, Drust B, Stratton G, Scott M, Gregson W. Quantification of the Typical Weekly In-season Training Load in Elite Junior Soccer Players. *J Sports Sci* [Internet]. 2012 Nov;30(15):1573–1580. Available from: https://www.tandfonline.com/doi/abs/10.1080/02640414.2012.709265

43. Abade EA, Gonçalves B V., Leite NM, Sampaio JE. Time–Motion and Physiological Profile of Football Training Sessions Performed by Under-15, Under-17, and Under-19 Elite Portuguese Players. *Int J Sports Physiol Perform* [Internet]. 2014 May;9(3):463–470. Available from: https://journals.humankinetics.com/view/journals/ijspp/9/3/article-p463.xml

44. Akenhead R, Harley JA, Tweddle SP. Examining the External Training Load of an English Premier League Football Team With Special Reference to Acceleration. *J Strength Cond Res* [Internet]. 2016 Sep;30(9):2424–2432. Available from: https://journals.lww.com/00124278-201609000-00008

45. Campos-Vazquez MA, Toscano-Bendala FJ, Mora-Ferrera JC, Suarez-Arrones LJ. Relationship Between Internal Load Indicators and Changes on Intermittent Performance After the Preseason in Professional Soccer Players. *J Strength Cond Res* [Internet]. 2017 June;31(6):1477–1485. Available from: https://journals.lww.com/00124278-201706000-00003

46. Stevens TGA, de Ruiter CJ, Twisk JWR, Savelsbergh GJP, Beek PJ. Quantification of In-season Training Load Relative to Match Load in Professional Dutch Eredivisie Football Players. *Sci Med Footb* [Internet]. 2017 May 4;1(2):117–125. Available from: https://www.tandfonline.com/doi/full/10.1080/24733938.2017.1282163

47. Banister EW. Modeling elite athletic performance. In: *Physiological Testing of the High-Performance Athlete*. Champaign, IL: Human Kinetics Publishers; 1991, pp. 403–424.

48. Silva P, Santos E Dos, Grishin M, Rocha JM. Validity of Heart Rate-Based Indices to Measure Training Load and Intensity in Elite Football Players. *J Strength Cond*

Res [Internet]. 2018 Aug;32(8):2340–2347. Available from: https://journals.lww. com/00124278-201808000-00028

49. Edwards S. High performance training and racing. In: Edwards S, editor. *The heart rate monitor book*. Sacramento: Feet Fleet Press; 1993, pp. 113–123.

50. Miguel M, Oliveira R, Loureiro N, García-Rubio J, Ibáñez SJ. Load Measures in Training/Match Monitoring in Soccer: A Systematic Review. *Int J Environ Res Public Health* [Internet]. 2021 Mar 8;18(5):2721. Available from: https://www.mdpi. com/1660-4601/18/5/2721

51. Lucia A, Hoyos J, Santalla A, Earnest C, Chicharro JL. Tour de France versus Vuelta a España: Which Is Harder? *Med Sci Sport Exerc* [Internet]. 2003 May;35(5):872–878. Available from: https://journals.lww.com/00005768-200305000-00023

52. Stagno KM, Thatcher R, van Someren KA. A Modified TRIMP to Quantify the In-season Training Load of Team Sport Players. *J Sports Sci* [Internet]. 2007 Apr;25(6):629–634. Available from: https://www.tandfonline.com/doi/abs/10.1080/02640410600811817

53. Manzi V, Iellamo F, Impellizzeri F, D'ottavio S, Castagna C. Relation between Individualized Training Impulses and Performance in Distance Runners. *Med Sci Sport Exerc* [Internet]. 2009 Nov;41(11):2090–2096. Available from: https://journals.lww. com/00005768-200911000-00017

54. Flatt AA, Esco MR, Nakamura FY. Individual Heart Rate Variability Responses to Preseason Training in High Level Female Soccer Players. *J Strength Cond Res* [Internet]. 2017 Feb;31(2):531–538. Available from: https://journals.lww.com/00124278-201702000-00032

55. Buchheit M. Monitoring Training Status with HR Measures: Do All Roads Lead to Rome? *Front Physiol* [Internet]. 2014;5. Available from: https://journal.frontiersin.org/ article/10.3389/fphys.2014.00073/abstract

56. Rabbani A, Clemente FM, Kargarfard M, Chamari K. Match Fatigue Time-Course Assessment Over Four Days: Usefulness of the Hooper Index and Heart Rate Variability in Professional Soccer Players. *Front Physiol* [Internet]. 2019 Feb 19;10. Available from: https://www.frontiersin.org/article/10.3389/fphys.2019.00109/full

57. Muñoz-López A, Naranjo-Orellana J. Individual versus Team Heart Rate Variability Responsiveness Analyses in a National Soccer Team During Training Camps. *Sci Rep* [Internet]. 2020 Dec 16;10(1):11726. Available from: https://www.nature.com/articles/ s41598-020-68698-5

58. Borresen J, Lambert MI. Quantifying Training Load: A Comparison of Subjective and Objective Methods. *Int J Sports Physiol Perform* [Internet]. 2008 Mar;3(1):16–30. Available from: https://journals.humankinetics.com/view/journals/ijspp/3/1/article-p16.xml

59. Orellana JN, Torres B de la C, Cachadiña ES, de Hoyo M, Cobo SD. Two New Indexes for the Assessment of Autonomic Balance in Elite Soccer Players. *Int J Sports Physiol Perform* [Internet]. 2015 May;10(4):452–457. Available from: https://journals. humankinetics.com/view/journals/ijspp/10/4/article-p452.xml

60. Stanley J, Peake JM, Buchheit M. Cardiac Parasympathetic Reactivation Following Exercise: Implications for Training Prescription. *Sport Med* [Internet]. 2013 Dec 3;43(12):1259–1277. Available from: https://link.springer.com/10.1007/s40279-013-0083-4

61. Achten J, Jeukendrup AE. Heart Rate Monitoring: applications and limitations. *Sport Med* [Internet]. 2003;33(7):517–538. Available from: https://link.springer.com/10.2165/ 00007256-200333070-00004

62. Plews DJ, Laursen PB, Stanley J, Kilding AE, Buchheit M. Training Adaptation and Heart Rate Variability in Elite Endurance Athletes: Opening the Door to Effective

Monitoring. *Sport Med* [Internet]. 2013 Sep 13;43(9):773–781. Available from: https://link.springer.com/10.1007/s40279-013-0071-8

63. Schmitt L, Regnard J, Desmarets M, Mauny F, Mourot L, Fouillot J-P, et al. Fatigue Shifts and Scatters Heart Rate Variability in Elite Endurance Athletes. Zirlik A, editor. *PLoS One* [Internet]. 2013 Aug 12;8(8):e71588. Available from: https://dx.plos.org/10.1371/journal.pone.0071588

64. Al Haddad H, Laursen P, Chollet D, Ahmaidi S, Buchheit M. Reliability of Resting and Postexercise Heart Rate Measures. *Int J Sports Med* [Internet]. 2011 Aug 13;32(08):598–605. Available from: https://www.thieme-connect.de/DOI/DOI?10.1055/s-0031-1275356

65. Esco MR, Flatt AA. Ultra-short-term Heart Rate Variability Indexes at Rest and Post-exercise in Athletes: Evaluating the Agreement With Accepted Recommendations. *J Sports Sci Med* [Internet]. 2014 Sep;13(3):535–541. Available from: https://www.ncbi.nlm.nih.gov/pubmed/25177179

66. Borresen J, Lambert MI. Changes in Heart Rate Recovery in Response to Acute Changes in Training Load. *Eur J Appl Physiol* [Internet]. 2007 Sep 18;101(4):503–511. Available from: https://link.springer.com/10.1007/s00421-007-0516-6

67. Manzi V, Castagna C, Padua E, Lombardo M, D'Ottavio S, Massaro M, et al. Dose-response Relationship of Autonomic Nervous System Responses to Individualized Training Impulse in Marathon Runners. *Am J Physiol Circ Physiol* [Internet]. 2009 June;296(6):H1733–H1740. Available from: https://www.physiology.org/doi/10.1152/ajpheart.00054.2009

68. Le Meur Y, Pichon A, Schaal K, Schmitt L, Louis J, Gueneron J, et al. Evidence of Parasympathetic Hyperactivity in Functionally Overreached Athletes. *Med Sci Sport Exerc* [Internet]. 2013 Nov;45(11):2061–2071. Available from: https://journals.lww.com/00005768-201311000-00006

69. Buchheit M, Mendez-Villanueva A, Quod MJ, Poulos N, Bourdon P. Determinants of the Variability of Heart Rate Measures During a Competitive Period in Young Soccer Players. *Eur J Appl Physiol* [Internet]. 2010 July 14;109(5):869–878. Available from: https://link.springer.com/10.1007/s00421-010-1422-x

70. Tulppo MP, Makikallio TH, Takala TE, Seppanen T, Huikuri H V. Quantitative Beat-to-beat Analysis of Heart Rate Dynamics During Exercise. *Am J Physiol Circ Physiol* [Internet]. 1996 July 1;271(1):H244–H252. Available from: https://www.physiology.org/doi/10.1152/ajpheart.1996.271.1.H244

71. Naranjo J, De la Cruz B, Sarabia E, De Hoyo M, Domínguez-Cobo S. Heart Rate Variability: a Follow-up in Elite Soccer Players Throughout the Season. *Int J Sports Med* [Internet]. 2015 July 3;36(11):881–886. Available from: https://www.thieme-connect.de/DOI/DOI?10.1055/s-0035-1550047

72. Julian R, Page RM, Harper LD. The Effect of Fixture Congestion on Performance During Professional Male Soccer Match-Play: A Systematic Critical Review with Meta-Analysis. *Sport Med* [Internet]. 2021 Feb 17;51(2):255–273. Available from: https://link.springer.com/10.1007/s40279-020-01359-9

73. Moreira DG, Costello JT, Brito CJ, Adamczyk JG, Ammer K, Bach AJE, et al. Thermographic Imaging in Sports and Exercise Medicine: A Delphi Study and Consensus Statement on the Measurement of Human Skin Temperature. *J Therm Biol* [Internet]. 2017 Oct;69:155–162. Available from: https://linkinghub.elsevier.com/retrieve/pii/S0306456517302073

74. Costello JT, McInerney CD, Bleakley CM, Selfe J, Donnelly AE. The Use of Thermal Imaging in Assessing Skin Temperature Following Cryotherapy: A Review. *J Therm*

Biol [Internet]. 2012 Feb;37(2):103–110. Available from: https://linkinghub.elsevier.com/retrieve/pii/S030645651100163X

75. Selfe J, Hardaker N, Thewlis D, Karki A. An Accurate and Reliable Method of Thermal Data Analysis in Thermal Imaging of the Anterior Knee for Use in Cryotherapy Research. *Arch Phys Med Rehabil* [Internet]. 2006 Dec;87(12):1630–1635. Available from: https://linkinghub.elsevier.com/retrieve/pii/S0003999306013311

76. Priego Quesada JI, Martínez Guillamón N, Cibrián Ortiz de Anda RM, Psikuta A, Annaheim S, Rossi RM, et al. Effect of Perspiration on Skin Temperature Measurements by Infrared Thermography and Contact Thermometry During Aerobic Cycling. *Infrared Phys Technol* [Internet]. 2015 Sep;72:68–76. Available from: https://linkinghub.elsevier.com/retrieve/pii/S1350449515001632

77. Adamczyk JG, Dariusz B, Siewierski M. Thermographic Evaluation of Lactate Level in Capillary Blood During Post-exercise Recovery. *Kinesiol Int J Fundam Appl Kinesiol.* 2014;46(2):186–193.

78. Ferreira JJA, Mendonça LCS, Nunes LAO, Andrade Filho ACC, Rebelatto JR, Salvini TF. Exercise-Associated Thermographic Changes in Young and Elderly Subjects. *Ann Biomed Eng* [Internet]. 2008 Aug 10;36(8):1420–1427. Available from: https://link.springer.com/10.1007/s10439-008-9512-1

79. Tosovic D, Than C, Brown JMM. The Effects of Accumulated Muscle Fatigue on the Mechanomyographic Waveform: Implications for Injury Prediction. *Eur J Appl Physiol* [Internet]. 2016 Aug 3;116(8):1485–1494. Available from: https://link.springer.com/10.1007/s00421-016-3398-7

80. Dahmane R, Valenčič V, Knez N, Eržen I. Evaluation of the Ability to Make Non-invasive Estimation of Muscle Contractile Properties on the Basis of the Muscle Belly Response. *Med Biol Eng Comput* [Internet]. 2001 Jan;39(1):51–55. Available from: https://link.springer.com/10.1007/BF02345266

81. Kersevan K, Valencic V, Djordjevic S, Simunic B. The Muscle Adaptation Process as a Result of Pathological Changes or Specific Training Procedures. *Cell Mol Biol Lett* [Internet]. 2002;7(2):367–369. Available from: https://www.ncbi.nlm.nih.gov/pubmed/12097988

82. Pereira LA, Ramirez-Campillo R, Martín-Rodríguez S, Kobal R, Abad CCC, Arruda AFS, et al. Is Tensiomyography-Derived Velocity of Contraction a Sensitive Marker to Detect Acute Performance Changes in Elite Team-Sport Athletes? *Int J Sports Physiol Perform* [Internet]. 2020 Jan 1;15(1):31–37. Available from: https://journals.humankinetics.com/view/journals/ijspp/15/1/article-p31.xml

83. Lohr C, Schmidt T, Medina-Porqueres I, Braumann K-M, Reer R, Porthun J. Diagnostic Accuracy, Validity, and Reliability of Tensiomyography to Assess Muscle Function and Exercise-induced Fatigue in Healthy Participants. A Systematic Review With Meta-analysis. *J Electromyogr Kinesiol* [Internet]. 2019 Aug;47:65–87. Available from: https://linkinghub.elsevier.com/retrieve/pii/S1050641118304176

84. Raeder C, Wiewelhove T, Simola RÁDP, Kellmann M, Meyer T, Pfeiffer M, et al. Assessment of Fatigue and Recovery in Male and Female Athletes After 6 Days of Intensified Strength Training. *J Strength Cond Res* [Internet]. 2016 Dec;30(12):3412–3427. Available from: https://journals.lww.com/00124278-201612000-00018

85. García-Manso JM, Rodríguez-Matoso D, Sarmiento S, de Saa Y, Vaamonde D, Rodríguez-Ruiz D, et al. Effect of High-load and High-volume Resistance Exercise on the Tensiomyographic Twitch Response of Biceps Brachii. *J Electromyogr Kinesiol* [Internet]. 2012 Aug;22(4):612–619. Available from: https://linkinghub.elsevier.com/retrieve/pii/S1050641112000077

86. García-manso JM, Rodríguez-Ruiz D, Rodríguez-Matoso D, de Saa Y, Sarmiento S, Quiroga M. Assessment of muscle fatigue after an ultra-endurance triathlon using tensiomyography (TMG). *J Sports Sci* [Internet]. 2011 Mar;29(6):619–625. Available from: https://www.tandfonline.com/doi/abs/10.1080/02640414.2010.548822

87. de Paula Simola RÁ, Harms N, Raeder C, Kellmann M, Meyer T, Pfeiffer M, et al. Assessment of Neuromuscular Function After Different Strength Training Protocols Using Tensiomyography. *J Strength Cond Res* [Internet]. 2015 May;29(5):1339–1348. Available from: https://journals.lww.com/00124278-201505000-00024

88. Hunter AM, Galloway SD, Smith IJ, Tallent J, Ditroilo M, Fairweather MM, et al. Assessment of Eccentric Exercise-induced Muscle Damage of the Elbow Flexors by Tensiomyography. *J Electromyogr Kinesiol* [Internet]. 2012 June;22(3):334–341. Available from: https://linkinghub.elsevier.com/retrieve/pii/S1050641112000119

89. Loturco I, Pereira LA, Kobal R, Kitamura K, Ramírez-Campillo R, Zanetti V, et al. Muscle Contraction Velocity: A Suitable Approach to Analyze the Functional Adaptations in Elite Soccer Players. *J Sports Sci Med* [Internet]. 2016 Sep;15(3):483–491. Available from: https://www.ncbi.nlm.nih.gov/pubmed/27803627

90. Wiewelhove T, Raeder C, de Paula Simola RA, Schneider C, Döweling A, Ferrauti A. Tensiomyographic Markers Are Not Sensitive for Monitoring Muscle Fatigue in Elite Youth Athletes: A Pilot Study. *Front Physiol* [Internet]. 2017 June 16;8. Available from: https://journal.frontiersin.org/article/10.3389/fphys.2017.00406/full

91. Wollin M, Thorborg K, Pizzari T. The Acute Effect of Match Play on Hamstring Strength and Lower Limb Flexibility in Elite Youth Football Players. *Scand J Med Sci* Sports [Internet]. 2017 Mar;27(3):282–288. Available from: https://doi.wiley.com/10.1111/sms.12655

92. Witvrouw E, Danneels L, Asselman P, D'Have T, Cambier D. Muscle Flexibility as a Risk Factor for Developing Muscle Injuries in Male Professional Soccer Players. *Am J Sports Med* [Internet]. 2003 Jan 30;31(1):41–46. Available from: https://journals.sagepub.com/doi/10.1177/03635465030310011801/

93. Bradley PS, Portas MD. The Relationship Between Preseason Range of Motion and Muscle Strain Injury in Elite Soccer Players. *J Strength Cond Res* [Internet]. 2007;21(4):1155. Available from: https://nsca.allenpress.com/nscaonline/?request=get-abstract&doi=10.1519%2FR-20416.1

94. Henderson G, Barnes CA, Portas MD. Factors Associated With Increased Propensity for Hamstring Injury in English Premier League Soccer Players. *J Sci Med Sport* [Internet]. 2010 July;13(4):397–402. Available from: https://linkinghub.elsevier.com/retrieve/pii/S1440244009001789

95. Small K, McNaughton L, Greig M, Lovell R. The Effects of Multidirectional Soccer-specific Fatigue on Markers of Hamstring Injury Risk. *J Sci Med Sport* [Internet]. 2010 Jan;13(1):120–125. Available from: https://linkinghub.elsevier.com/retrieve/pii/S144024400800162X

11

TYPOLOGY AND SEVERITY OF FOOTBALL INJURIES

Data from incidence studies

Sergio Tejero García and Beatriz Martínez Sañudo

11.1 Injuries in professional soccer players. Incidence and epidemiology

The injury incidence in professional soccer players ranges from 2.48 to 9.4 injuries per 1000 hours of exposure [1–4]. In competition, the rate is higher (8.7–65.9 injuries per 1000 hours of exposure) than training (1.37–5.8 injuries per a 1000 hours of exposure) [5, 6].

Ekstrand et al. reported 2,908 muscle injuries (53% during competition and 47% during training). The most frequent injury types were strains, contusions, and sprains [4, 7–10]. It is also observed that more severe injuries occurred during matches.

The thigh was the most frequently injured part [11, 12], and in two studies, the hamstrings were the most affected location [4, 11]. Most thigh injuries were strains, with a higher incidence in the posterior portion, even so quadriceps strains led to a longer recuperation than hamstring injuries. Other common injury locations were the groin, knee, and ankle. Fractures represented only a small percentage of all injuries, but most of them imply prolonged lack of activity.

Reinjuries: Failure of the natural process of muscle fibers to completely recover to their normal elasticity, creating a scar tissue, and continued efforts over the zone when the player returns to full activity produce higher rates of reinjury. Reinjuries are more common during training than in matches. Walden et al. found a rate of 15.3% (101 of 658) of reinjuries, and over two-thirds (63%) of those were overuse injuries. The most frequently reinjured body part was the hamstrings, and 16% of the muscle injuries were reinjuries. Reinjuries required more time of recovery than new injuries [3].

DOI: 10.4324/9781032637006-11

11.2 Risk factors in football injuries

Factors can be divided into two groups: intrinsic (personal factors) and extrinsic (environmental factors).

Intrinsic factors: these factors are not possible to modify.

- Age: most of the studies agreed the risk of injury increases with age [13]. Studies report that football produces a low risk of injury in the preadolescent and adolescent age groups. Sullivan et al. found an injury rate of less than 1% in a group of players younger than 12. McCarroll et al. reported on injury rates for football players aged 10 years and under (1.9%), 12 and under (3.1%), and 14 and under (5.3%). It is important to remark that preadolescent and adolescent players could have specific injuries different to adults because of their bone particularities. In this group, we can observe that ligaments are stronger than bones, producing traction apophysitis like Osgood Schlatter or Sever, and avulsions in some mechanisms like hyperflexion of the hip (avulsion of ASIS) or knee torsion (avulsion of tibial spines). Younger players have also lower risk of reinjury [14].
- Maturity status: Bone age is not always the same as the individual's age that would correspond with the mean. Sometimes, the bone age is higher than the mean (early maturing players), and the higher incidence of tendinopathies, groin strains, and re-injuries sustained have been observed in these players; meanwhile, in those whose bone age is lower than the mean (late mature players), a higher incidence of osteochondral disorders and major injuries can be appreciated. In normal maturing players, there is a higher incidence of tendinopathies (players over 27 years old) and osteochondral injuries [15].
- Gender: Knee injury is the most prevalent injury in female players, which is probably in relation to higher laxity in women. ACL injury is the most common major injury with a 4.6% of incidence in the studies by Giza et al. [16]. In this study, they also rated 1.93 injuries per 1000 hours that indicate that women players suffered less injuries than male. This question generates controversy because studies in the 1980s and 1990s have reported a greater injury rate in women [17, 18].

Extrinsic factors: these factors can be modifiable.

- Match: Injury rates during matches are higher than training in all age groups of players. This could be explained because the higher speed and intensity in competition increase the body contact and tackling and also a higher muscle fatigue and overload [19].
- Playing position: The playing position influences the risk of injury. Midfielders had significantly more injuries, especially in thighs [20]. The distance covered during a competitive game increases the risk of knee and ankle injury, and acceleration/deceleration mechanism is considered to be a higher risk factor to suffer a musculoskeletal injury. Upper extremity injuries are reported to be up to five

times more prevalent in goalkeepers than in outfield players, attaining a high rate of more than 18% of all injuries among professional goalkeepers [21, 22].

- Time of match: Most injuries occur in the beginning of the first half and toward the end of the second half. They occur in the beginning because of an insufficient warming up and the initial intensity at the beginning of a match. Fatigue has been matched with the loss of elasticity and eccentric strength [23]. Toward the end of the match, muscle fatigue results in muscle overload and loss of concentration executing wrong technical patterns, increasing the risk of injury [24].
- Season: Injuries in preseason are most frequent than in-season [25]. September is the predominant month for injuries, whereas June had the least number of injuries.
- Double burden: Overuse injuries ranged for 27–33% of the injury incidences. Inklaar et al. [26] noted that two-thirds of the injuries in youth football players were traumatic, whereas one-third were overuse injuries. These findings highlight the role of injury prevention programs in avoiding risk factors and mechanisms that produce traumatic and overuse injuries [27]. Overuse injuries are occasioned by repetitive stress without enough time to obtain a successful regenerative process. Physical stress and recovery are considered the most relevant factors in relation to overuse injuries [28].
- Training: Each player is different from others, and fitness tests are important to identify the physical capacity of players. Player exposure has been discussed as a possible risk factor for injuries in football, but few studies are available [29]. Ekstrand et al. found that teams with superior average training suffered the lowest injury rate [30].
- Playing on uneven surfaces: playing in hard surfaces with high friction and inappropriate footwear would lead to injury. Incorrect footwear can lead to slipping. In synthetic turf, the higher frictional forces will produce more torque when twisting, these overloads can produce injuries in player [31], but studies have not shown differences in the rate of injury between artificial turf and natural grass [32].

11.3 Injury location

The most common injury mechanisms were tackling, running, being tackled, shooting, twisting and turning, and jumping and landing. Tackling is a defense skill used to try to steal the ball. The lower extremities are often injured during tackling as players cannot respond quickly enough to avoid rapid and unpredictable movement.

The most common injury types were strains, sprains, and contusions. The thigh is the most frequently injured body part, and hamstrings are the most affected location as mentioned above. Fractures represented only a small percentage of all injuries.

- *Head and face injuries.*

   a Concussion: Is defined as an immediate and post-traumatic temporally reversible brain injury, which produces alterations of consciousness, blurred vision, loss of memory, etc. These injuries are more characteristic between goalkeepers and strikers. It is important for players to know symptoms of concussion to warn their trainer or physician for restriction in their activity. They could return to play if no loss of consciousness, no or minimal head-ache which does not worsen with exertion, no or resolved amnesia, and no other post-concussive symptoms.

b   Cumulative head trauma: The consequences of repeated sub-concussive head trauma from heading the ball have been raised as an important health issue for football players [21]. Possible solutions include the use of a softer ball for younger players, strengthening of the neck muscula-ture to reduce the force of impact, and training to perform the head shot patterns.

c   Eye injuries: Significant eye injuries due to the ball impact do occur with a lesser incidence and severity than in other sports because of the big size of the ball. Eyes and orbit injuries may be due to the impact of the football ball, fingers, elbows, heads, and knees. These injuries could produce hyphemia, vitreous hemorrhages, or corneal injuries. Eyebrow wounds are also frequent due to the bone rim in this zone.

d   Nasal injuries: The most common nasal injuries include fractures and epistaxis. The semiology of nasal bone fracture includes bone crepitus, deformity, epistaxis, dorsal nasal swelling and tenderness, and ecchymosis. Some of these fractures could need precise surgical care.

•   *Upper member injuries.*

It is considered that these injuries are uncommon in the football practice excluding the goalkeepers, but it is not certainly true. Football is a contact sport which involves a higher percentage of upper member direct and indirect trauma in each match produced by the contact with the grass over the upper limbs. Following 57 male professional European football teams from 16 countries between the years 2001 and 2011, Ekstrand and colleagues showed that 90% of upper extremity injuries are traumatic, and only 10% are related to overuse. The incidence in match play in some studies was almost seven times higher than in training [21]. We can find some injuries like

e   Clavicle fracture: It is a common injury in teenagers and also in young foot-ball players when they fall with their arms outstretched. The middle third fractures are the most frequent, and usually surgery is not necessary. The distal third fractures usually require surgical care.

f   Shoulder dislocation: In some series is the most frequent injury in the upper extremity. The first episode usually is a high-energy mechanism with humeral abduction and external rotation combining against a force of exter-nal rotation and horizontal extension. Shoulder dislocation has lay-off time on average of 1.5 months. It is important in training programs to be optimal for the prevention of upper extremity injuries and shoulder injuries. There is controversy over the treatment of first-time shoulder dislocations and may support early surgical intervention.

g Acromioclavicular joint sprain: ACJ injury is commonly the result of a direct fall on the shoulder with the arm adducted or extended. ACJ sprain is a mild injury in football players, excepting the goalkeepers, who are severely affected by this injury with long periods of lack of activity. There are six types of ACJ sprain, and the types I, II, and III are the most common. In I and II degrees, the treatment consists of rest, ice, analgesics, nonsteroid drugs, and the use of a sling to reduce pain. In severe degrees of acromioclavicular sprain (types IV, V, and VI), surgery must be required, although some controversy exists between surgery or orthopedic strategies for treating III degree dislocations.

h Elbow dislocation/sprain, joint fracture, and olecranon bursitis: The most common elbow injuries in the Ekstrand cohort were elbow medial collateral ligament (MCL) sprain and olecranon bursitis. The MCL is the primary stabilizer of the valgus stress, and MCL sprain occurs when the elbow is subjected to a valgus force beating the normal ligament elasticity [33].

Olecranon bursitis is characterized by the occupation of the elbow bursa with serous, sanguineous, or purulent fluid. Nonpurulent bursitis must be treated conservative, only doing needle aspiration of the bursa if there is a septic suspicion.

Elbow dislocations are further classified into simple (no associated fractures) and complex (associated with fractures). Simple dislocations are usually treated with early mobilization after closed reduction; there is a low risk of relapse. The complex type of elbow fracture dislocation has higher complication and re-dislocation rates and requires surgical treatment in most cases. The "terrible triad" of the elbow (posterior elbow dislocation, radial head fracture, and coronoid fracture) represents a specific complex elbow dislocation scenario that is difficult to manage because of conflicting aims of ensuring elbow stability, while maintaining early range of motion.

i Wrist fracture: Distal radius fractures in football usually occur as a result of a fall on with the wrist in extension and will usually be comminuted, displaced, and intra-articular compared with low-impact sports. Surgical management of open reduction and internal fixation with plate is needed, which will allow for rapid start of early mobilization and return to play.

j Fractures of the metacarpal and phalanx in the hand: Phalangeal fractures and metacarpal fractures are the most common fractures of the hand in sports in general (being the fifth ray the most affected), but for the outfield player, it does not suppose a long absence.

Another common hand injury found in football goalkeepers and involving the base of the thumb is the "skier's thumb" or "gamekeeper's thumb," that is, the complete tear of the ulnar collateral ligament (UCL) of the first metacarpophalangeal (MCP) joint as a result of an acute radial or valgus stress on the thumb. Sometimes, there exists a bone avulsion of the ligament insertion. On examination, swelling and tenderness over the thumb UCL are observed. A Stener lesion is an abnormality that occurs when the thumb adductor muscle aponeurosis interposes between the two ends of the ruptured UCL, preventing UCL healing by immobilization alone. Stener lesion needs surgery to be repaired.

k Scaphoid fracture: Is the most common carpal bone fracture that typically occurs when the player falls on an outstretched hand. Casting the patient with a nondisplaced scaphoid waist fracture has been the traditional treatment; however, stiffness and weakness can occur with long-term casting. Surgical treatment, which was traditionally indicated for displaced or proximal pole fractures, is currently also considered for nondisplaced scaphoid waist fractures in professional athletes. This treatment allows a faster return to professional sport, which must be considered when healing is at least 50% of the one to avoid nonunion or the avascular necrosis. Outfield players can return to play with a protective cast or brace until full healing is observed on radiography.

l Scapholunate dissociation: Tension injuries occur on the palmar aspect of the wrist with disruption or attenuation of the supporting ligaments or interosseous membranes. This provides scapholunate tears or scapholunate dissociation, injuries commonly associated with other contact sports. Surgical treatment is necessary when scapholunate ligaments are disrupted completely in order to avoid wrist osteoarthritis in the future.

• *Upper limb injuries.*

m Muscle strains: Are frequent injuries that commonly occur in the pelvis and thigh region, affecting mainly the adductors, quadriceps, and hamstrings. Strains vary greatly in their severity and may occur because of an acute overload of the muscle tendon unit or from repetitive stress. A mild strain does not present swelling or deformity, mild tenderness on palpation, and preservation of strength. More severe injuries may result in significant swelling and ecchymoses, weakness, and possible muscle defect. Treatment initially consists of ice and compression to minimize swelling and inflammation, analgesics, and relative rest, depending on the severity of the injury. A stretching and progressive strengthening program helps return to activity and will decrease risk of recurrent injury [34].

n Groin sprains: In relation to the age and previous injuries. The most common cause of groin pain in football players is musculotendinous strain of the adductor group. This muscle group is predisposed to acute and overuse strains because of its implication in the game of football. Some studies have described a relationship between less hip adductor flexibility and higher maximal average power in the groin strain group [13].

o Apophysitis or apophyseal avulsion fractures may occur in the skeletally immature athlete. Sites of injury include the adductor, hamstring, hip flexor, and sartorius attachments, producing sometimes the avulsion of structures like the lower anterior iliac spine or iliac crest. For minimal or nondisplaced avulsion fractures, non-weight bearing or protected weight bearing is recommended until walking is pain-free. For displacements bigger than 2 centimeters of the lower anterior iliac, spine surgery is required.

p Pubalgia: Is an inflammatory injury of the pubic symphysis and the neighbor structures because of a muscle imbalance between the abdominal musculature and the adductors, which is associated with pelvic instability, as has been thought classically. Currently, there is a hypothesis regarding pubalgia in which the asymmetric shortening of one hamstring compared to the other can provoke a shear mechanism in the pubic symphysis. Other factors involved in manifestation of the symptoms may be in relationship with the repeated kicking movements, which produce an overload on the abdominal musculature, hamstrings, hip flexors, and adductors. The incidence of this type of injury in football players varies between 0.5% and 28%. The symptomatology that characterizes this pathology is a progressive pain in the region of the pubic symphysis, which may irradiate to the abdomen, perineum, and adductors. The pain may worsen with flexion of the trunk and fast changes in direction during running and kicking movements. In some cases, the injury could progress avoiding the football players' performance and their activity, including training. In professional football players, excessive numbers of games and overloading during training sessions could worsen this problem. The treatment for pubalgia is essentially rest, ice, physiotherapy, analgesics, nonsteroidal anti-inflammatory drugs, and corticoid infiltrations which are adjuvant treatments. However, in 5–10% of the cases, there is no improvement and surgical treatment is indicated due to the association of the mechanical dilation of the internal inguinal ring (sport hernia) [35].

q Thigh: In adults, muscle injury may represent approximately 30% of all injuries and be responsible for up to 15% of time off during the season [20]. Injuries are most frequent in the three major muscle groups in this order: quadriceps, hamstrings, and adductors, representing more than 97% of all thigh muscle injuries. The anatomic site of injury is related to severity with proportionally more severe injuries among hamstring injuries.

r Hamstring sprains: The players who incurred hamstring strains usually have previous injuries, and age is an important factor in this group of injuries.

s Knee injuries:

   Knee ligament injury: The frequency of medial instability in players with previous knee sprains is significantly higher than among players who never had sprained their knees [13]. The normal knee has a full range of motion between the position of varus-flexion-internal rotation and valgus-flexion-external rotation. The majority of knee injuries occur when stress limits are exceeded in these extreme positions. Medial collateral ligament injuries are caused by a valgus stress; conversely lateral collateral ligament and/or posterolateral corner injuries are caused by varus stress. Anterior cruciate ligament (ACL) injuries are often accompanied by the sensation of an audible "pop," a feeling of instability, and immediate swelling from the hemarthrosis. These injuries occur because of valgus load with external rotation, hyperextension, deceleration with the knee flexed, and varus stress on a flexed knee. The posterior cruciate ligament (PCL) is often injured by force hyperextension.

Other less frequent injuries are combined ligament injuries like the "unhappy triad," which consists of the damage of the MCL, ACL, and medial menisci. Excessive stress in varus can produce an injury of the lateral collateral ligament, posterior cruciate ligament, and popliteus corner. First-degree collateral ligament sprains demonstrate swelling and tenderness over the ligament with no increase in laxity compared with the uninjured knee. Second-degree sprains show variable increase in laxity at 10–20° but stability at full knee extension, mild swelling, and tenderness. Third-degree sprains show laxity at full extension, significant laxity at 20° of flexion, and tenderness. Effusion may be lacking as fluid may track through the complete tear. A third-degree collateral sprain should spark a thorough search for associated ligamentous and capsular injury. At this point, mechanical knee instability could need the surgical reconstruction of all implicated ligaments.

Meniscal injuries: The medial and lateral menisci may suffer isolated injury or be injured in conjunction with ligamentous injury. A frequent mechanism is that of a twisting stress to a loaded leg. The player usually localizes pain over the affected joint line. Subjective symptoms of clicking, catching, or locking are common as is a small-to-moderate effusion.

Patellofemoral injuries: Patellar dislocations are more commonly seen in younger football players. The player will explain a history of a sensation of the patella shifting out of place, and in the most part of cases, the patella suffers a spontaneous relocation. It can recidivate in a percentage of players with risk of osteochondral injury in each dislocation.

Overuse injuries in the knee: Very common. These include quadriceps and patellar tendinitis, iliotibial band syndrome, and patellofemoral syndrome. Appropriate treatments include activity modification, ice, analgesics, or nonsteroidal anti-inflammatories for control of pain and inflammation and aggressive physical therapy.

Strained calf muscle: The gastrocnemius and soleus muscles, commonly referred to as the calf muscles, are located on the back of the lower leg. These muscles are particularly vulnerable to strain injuries. In football, they usually happen when a player quickly tries to reach the ball. The middle part of the gastrocnemius muscle is most often injured. Strain injuries in the soleus muscle are also quite common. This type of injury is classified as an overuse injury, which is why players who run a lot of kilometers in each match are at higher risk. Injuries commonly occur as a result of fatigue or overtraining.

u Achilles injury: Rupture of the Achilles tendon requires two pathologic processes: tendinosis and an eccentric contracture of sufficient force to rupture the damaged tendon. This tendinosis is likely more common in older players. Support for this argument comes from an 11-year epidemiological study on Achilles-related injuries in the UEFA, in which the 205 Achilles tendon injuries identified accounted for only 2.5% of all recorded injuries; however, 96% of these were tendinopathies [36].

v Ankle Injuries: The lateral ligament injuries are the most common. The usual mechanism of injury is inversion with the foot in plantar flexion. The ligaments most involved are the anterior talofibular (which is the weakest ligament in the lateral complex) and calcaneal fibular ligament. The severity of sprains varies in three degrees:

First-degree injuries with mild stretching of the ligaments, tenderness, minimal swelling, and possibility to walking.

Second-degree injury is the partial tear of the ligament. Swelling and pain is greater, the patients can bear weight, but they usually are incapable of walking.

Third-degree injuries in which the lateral ligaments are significantly or completely torn with impossibility to load or walking.

Mild injuries must be treated with the POLICE therapy (P-rotection; O-ptimal Load; I-cing; C-omprehensive; E-levation of the limb). The third-degree injuries are reason for controversy because classically surgery was proposed in elite sportsmen, but nowadays there exist new approaches that support the orthopedic treatment. However, 20% of repetitive lateral ankle injuries could lead to sequelae, needing surgical treatment (osteochondral lesions, ankle instabilities, and ankle impingement syndromes, naming this condition footballer's ankle) [37].

A history of a previous ankle sprain is a significant risk factor for a new sprain on the same side. In previously sprained ankles, there was an increased frequency of lateral instability and positive anterior drawer tests compared with ankles without previous injury.

w Medial ankle injuries: The mechanism is eversion with external rotation frequently present. The medial or deltoid ligament sprain may be associated with a syndesmosis damage. This ankle injury presents with tenderness over the medial deltoid ligament with possible syndesmosis tenderness. Passive eversion or passive external rotation of the ankle joint or compression between the fibula and tibia in the middle third of the calf (squeeze maneuver) may recreate medial and/or syndesmosis pain. Significant swelling is usually present, and weight bearing is difficult. Indeed, some players suffer a subtle syndesmotic injury. It needs to be identified, and surgical treatment is necessary to avoid the "giving away" and talus osteochondral lesions.

Furthermore, isolated syndesmotic injuries are increasing the incidence due to better diagnosis methods, as is believed by authors of this chapter.

x Metatharsal stress fractures: Some identified risk factors include age under 25 years, midfielders (they perform many high-speed passes), during pre-season or early season, the nondominant foot or having weak intrinsic foot muscles strength.

y Goalkeeper injuries: The goalkeeper needs a special chapter in football injuries. There is intense body contact with other players on the ground and in the air and when in crowded situations such as corners, he must fight for the ball and receiving contusion injuries such as muscle hematomas, head contusions, or face traumas (including eyes) produced by the elbows, heads, or knees of the other players. Goalkeepers land with the body because their hands are keeping the ball, increasing the risk of body contusions, abrasion, or other injuries produced by trauma, including goalpost trauma. When the ball is kicked directly at the goalkeeper, the ball can knock his fingers and hands, producing sometimes sprains, dislocations, and fractures of the fingers and the hands. The goalkeeper should regularly practice special exercises in agility as a general means of preventing injury. Because his situation is different, he should train individually as well as with the team, concentrating on stretching exercises, specific movements, and quick reactions. He should also be made to train his capacity for concentration [38].

References

1. FIFA. *FIFA Big Count 2006: 270 million people active in football.* 2007. FIFA Communications Division Information Services; Zurich, Switzerland: 2007.
2. Fuller C, Ekstrand J, Junge A, et al. Consensus statement on injury definitions and data collection procedures in studies of football (soccer) injuries. *Br J Sports Med.* 2006; 40(3): p. 193–201.
3. Ekstrand J, Hägglund M, Wald M. Epidemiology of muscle injuries in professional football (soccer). *Am J Sports Med.* 2011; 39(6): p. 1226–1232.
4. Walden M, Hägglund M, Ekstrand J. UEFA champions league study: a prospective study of injuries in professional football during the 2001–2002 season. *Br J Sports Med.* 2005; 39(8): p. 542–546.
5. Eirale C, Hamilton B, Bisciotti G, Grantham J, Chalabi H. Injury epidemiology in a national football team of the Middle East. *Scand J Med Sci Sports.* 2012; 22(3): p. 323–329.
6. Pfirrmann D, Hebst M, Ingelfinger P, et al. Analysis of injury incidences in male professional adult and elite youth soccer players: a systematic review. *J Athl Train.* 2016 May; 51(5): p. 410–424.
7. Hawkins R, Fuller C. A prospective epidemiological study of injuries in four English professional football clubs. *Br J Sports Med.* 1999; 33(3): p. 196–203.
8. Morgan B, Oberlader M. An examination of injuries in Major League Soccer: the inaugural season. *Am J Sports Med.* 2001; 29(4): p. 426–430.
9. Ekstrand J, Hâgglund M, Walden M. Injury incidence and injury patterns in professional football: the UEFA injury study. *Br J Sports Med.* 2011; 45(7): p. 553–558.

10. Eirale C, Farooq A, Smiley F, Tol J, Chalabi H. Epidemiology of football injuries in Asia: a prospective study in Qatar. *J Sci Med Sport.* 2013; 16(2): p. 113–117.
11. Dauty M, Collon S. Incidence of injuries in French professional soccer players. *Int J Sports Med.* 2011; 32(12): p. 965–969.
12. Bjorneboe J, Bahr R, Andersen T. Gradual increase in the risk of match injury in Norwegian male professional football: a 6-year prospective study. *Scand J Med Sci Sports.* 2014; 24(1): p. 189–196.
13. Arnason A, Sigurdsson SB, Gudmunsson A, et al. Risks factors for injuries in Football. *Am J Sports Med.* 2004; 32(1 Suppl):5S–16S.
14. Le Gall F, Carling C, Reilly T, et al. Incidence of injuries in elite French youth soccer players: a 10-season study. *Am J Sports Med.* 2006; 34(6): p. 928–938.
15. Le Gall F, Carling C, Reilly T. Biological maturity and injury in elite youth football. *Scand J Med Sci Sports.* 2007; 17(5).
16. Giza E, Mithofer K, Farrel L. Injuries in women's professional soccer. *Br J Sports Med.* 2005; 39: p. 212–216.
17. Nilsson S, Roaas A. Soccer injuries in adolescents. *Am J Sports Med.* 1987; 6: p. 358–361.
18. Maehulum S, Dahl E, Daljord O. Frequency of injuries in a youth soccer tournament. *Phys Sports Med.* 1986; 14: p. 73–79.
19. Inklaar H. Soccer injuries I: incidence and severity. *Sports Med.* 1994; 18: p. 55–73.
20. Cloke D, Moore O, Shah T, et al. Thigh muscle injuries in youth soccer: predictors of recovery. *Am J Sports Med.* 2012; 40(2): 433–439.
21. Ekstrand J, Hagglund M, Tornqvist H. Upper extremity injuries in male elite football players. *Knee Surg Sports Traumatol Arthrosc.* 2013; 21(7): 1626–1632.
22. Ejnisman B, Barbosa G, Andreoli C, et al. Shoulder injuries in soccer goalkeepers: Review and development of a FIFA 11+ shoulder injury prevention programme. *Open Access J Sports Med.* 2016; 7: p. 75–80.
23. Small K, McNaughton L, Greig M, Lohkamp LR. Soccer fatigue sprinting and hamstring injury risk. *Int J Sports Med.* 2009; 30: p. 573–578.
24. Paul D, Brito J, Nassis G. Injury prevention training in football: Time to consider training under fatigue? *Aspetar Sports Med J.* 2014; 3: p. 578–581.
25. Noya SJ, Gómez-Carmona PM, Gracia ML, et al. Epidemiology of injuries in First Division Spanish football. *J Sports Sci.* 2014; 32(13): p. 1263–1270.
26. Inklaar H, Bol E, Schimikli S, Mosterd W. Injuries in male soccer players: team risk analysis. *Int J Sports Med.* 1996; 17(3): p. 229–234.
27. Van Mechelen W, Hlobil H, Kemper H. Incidence, severity, etiology and prevention of sports injuries: a review of concepts. *Sports Med.* 1992; 14(2): p. 82–99.
28. Kenttä G, Hassmen P. Overtraining and recovery: a conceptual model. *Sports Med.* 1998; 26(1): p. 1–16.
29. Dvorak R. Risk factor analysis for injuries in football players. Possibilities for a prevention program. *Am J Sports Med.* 2000; 28(Suppl 5):S69–74.
30. Ekstran J, Gillquist J, Moller M. Incidence of soccer injuries and their relation to training and team success. *Am J Sports Med.* 1983; 11: p. 63–67.
31. Wong P HY. Soccer injury in the lower extremities. *Br J Sports Med.* 2005; 39(8): p. 473–482.
32. Steffen K, Andersen T, Bahr R. Risk of injury on artificial turf and natural grass in young female football players. *Br J Sports Med.* 2007; 41(Suppl 1): p. 33–37.
33. Marom N, Williams III RJ. Upper extremity injuries in soccer. *Am J Orthoped.* 2018; 47(10). doi: 10.12788/ajo.2018.0091

34. Tucker A. Common soccer injuries: Diagnosis, treatment and rehabilitation. *Sports Med.* 1997; 23(1): p. 21–32.

35. De Queiroz RD, De Carvalho RT, De Queiroz Szeles PR, et al. Return to sport after surgical treatment for pubalgia among professional soccer players. *Rev Brasileira Ortoped (English Edition)* 2014; 49(3): p. 233–239.

36. Gajhede-Knudsen M, Ekstrand J, Magnusson H, Maffulli N. Recurrence of Achilles tendon injuries in elite male football players is more common after early return to play: An 11-year follow-up of the UEFA Champions League injury study. *Br J Sport Med.* 2013; 47(12): 763–768.

37. Mc Dougall A. Footballer's ankle. *Lancet.* 1955; 269(6902): p. 1219–1220.

38. Rae K, Orchard J. The orchard sports injury classification system (OSICS) version 10. *Clin J Sport Med.* 2007 May; 17(3): p. 201–204.

12

IDENTIFICATION OF INJURY RISK FACTORS FOR LOWER EXTREMITY MUSCLE INJURY AND PREVENTIVE TRAINING GUIDELINES

Luis Suárez-Arrones

12.1 Introduction

Muscle injuries are very common in football, representing up to 37% of all-time loss injuries at men's professional level. A football team with a 24/25 players could expect around 15 muscle injuries per season and that muscle injuries accounted for more than one-fourth of all lay-off time from injuries [1]. Injuries to four major muscle groups of the lower extremity (adductors, hamstrings, rectus femoris, and calf) comprise more than 90% of all muscle injuries in professional football [1].

Risk factors are traditionally divided into two main categories: internal player-related risk factors and external environmental risk factors [2]. Intrinsic risk factors such as increased age, career duration, or a previous injury could increase the risk of a future injury, while extrinsic factors like a lack of training, low training-to-match ratio, or playing on a hard surface with high friction seem to increase the injury risk [3]. In addition, risk factors can be divided into modifiable and nonmodifiable factors. Although nonmodifiable risk factors, such as gender or age could be of interest, it is important to study factors which are potentially modifiable in order to try to minimize the risk of injury through training interventions and specific therapies.

In order to establish prevention programs, it is important to identify risk factors associated with the multifactorial etiology of injury [4]. Some intrinsic risk factors identified for lower extremity muscle injury include previous injury [2, 5, 6], older age [3–6], decreased muscle strength, or strength imbalances [7–10], but results from different studies are contradictory.

Extrinsic risk factors have only been scarcely investigated, but match play has consistently been associated with an increased rate of muscle injury [1]. Fatigue may be a component in the occurrence of muscle injury since some studies have

DOI: 10.4324/9781032637006-12

found that muscle injuries occur more frequently toward the end of matches [1, 11, 12]. Finally, it has been shown that various match factors, such as the type of match, match location (home or away), and match result may influence general injury rates in professional football [6, 13, 14], but sub-analyses of lower extremity muscle injuries have not been reported.

A previous study [6] 6,140 injuries presented that 35% were muscle injuries located in the hamstrings (42%), adductors (25%), quadriceps (19%), and calf (14%). The overuse injuries (34%) were more frequent in the adductor muscle in comparison with other locations, and 27% of the injuries were re-injuries with a higher re-injury rate in adductor and hamstring muscles (29% and 30%, respectively) in comparison with calf and quadriceps (21%). The rate of injury during the in-season (competition) period was substantially higher in all the muscle groups, excluding the recto femoris muscle, the injury rate of which was superior during the preseason period.

We will now examine the risk factors and potential preventive strategies for the lower extremity muscles that more frequently are injured in professional football players: adductors (groin/hip), hamstrings, quadriceps (recto femoris), and calf.

12.2 Risk factors for groin/hip and adductor injuries and preventive training guidelines

Groin/hip and adductor injuries are common in sports like football that requires kicking, quick changes of direction, twisting and turning, and rapid accelerations and decelerations. At the elite level, approximately one in five male players incur a groin injury causing time loss each season [15, 16]. Adductor injuries were more common in the dominant (kicking) leg (56%) [6], and the most prominent risk factor for groin/hip injuries was previous injury (with seven times greater risk of sustaining and new groin injury), age, and weak adductor muscles [17]. Two out of three cases of groin injuries in football are adductor-related [15, 16]. Adductor-related groin injuries are the second most common type of muscle injury in football [1], and decreased muscle strength of the hip adductors has been shown to be a risk factor for groin injuries; therefore, strength training of the hip adductors seems relevant in the prevention of the adductor-related groin injuries and muscle strains [17, 18]. In addition, > 20% deficit in eccentric strength of the hip adductor muscles has been observed among players with groin pain [19]. The hip adductor muscle tendinous complex is stressed in football, especially during the kicking activities like strong passes and shooting [20], and increased muscle tendinous strength in the hip adductors protects the structures in the groin when it is exposed to eccentric forces [17]. In addition to this, increasing the adductor strength will contribute to improving the energy absorption in the tissues, decreasing stresses at the tendons and the insertion sites (muscle tendinous complex), and preventing overuse injuries and acute tears. Therefore, strengthening the hip adductors may play an important role in reducing the prevalence and rate of groin injuries in football players.

12.2.1 Guidelines for preventive training

Designing an active prevention program requires identification of the risk of adductor injury, followed by the choice of an active program of specific exercises that improve the coordination of the muscles acting on the pelvis [21]. Therefore, an injury prevention program should include exercises for hip adduction–abduction strengthening and testing in order to decrease the stress on the adductor muscle–tendon unit to prevent overuse injury [17, 18]. Interventions with elite-level football players present evident problems because training interventions using randomized controlled trials are impractical and/or ethically questionable in elite populations; therefore, there is limited information on elite football.

A previous study with healthy male football players showed that 8 weeks of hip adduction strength training performed with simple elastic bands as external load increased maximal eccentric hip adduction strength in football players, compared with a control group that did no strength training [17]. The authors concluded that as decreased hip adduction strength is a risk factor for developing groin injuries, the hip adduction strengthening exercise using elastic bands may have implications as a promising approach toward prevention of groin injuries in football.

With semi-professional football players from Norway, a recent study [22] proposed an adductor strengthening program based only on a simple exercise: the Copenhagen adduction exercise. The adductor strengthening program with 1–3 sessions during preseason and only one session of one set per side during the in-season

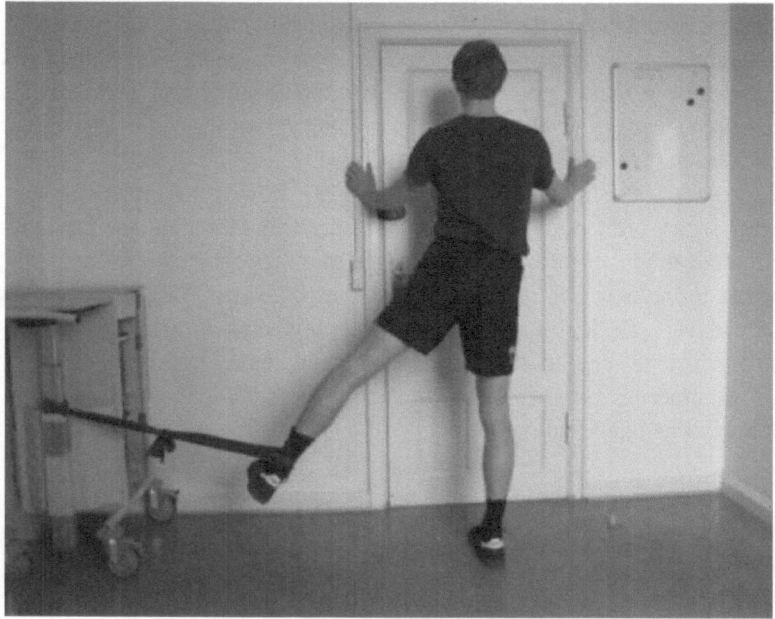

FIGURE 12.1 The intervention exercise with the elastic band (17).

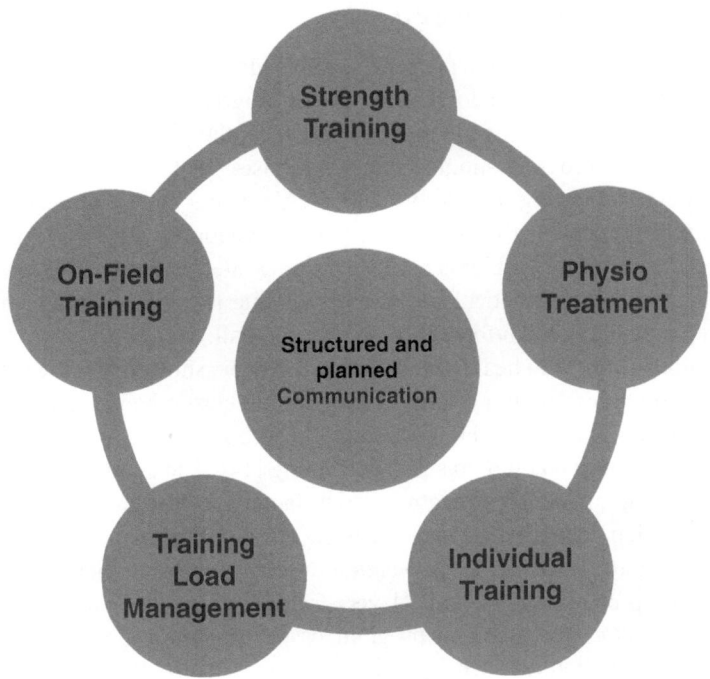

FIGURE 12.2 The Copenhagen adduction exercise with different levels (22).

reduced the prevalence and risk of groin problems in male football players by 41% [22]. An apparent advantage of this exercise is that no equipment is needed; therefore, it can be a good option for amateur football when financial resources are limited. Obviously, with elite players, a greater variety in neuromuscular stimuli for the adductors would be more recommended.

With elite football players, Nuñez et al. [18] showed the effectiveness of two adductor injury-prevention programs using the adductor/abductor ratios and the deficit between legs for design two strength trainings programs for the adductors/abductors throughout the season using a rotatory inertial device in professional football players. Both strength training programs showed a low adductor injury rate in elite professional football players and maintained a good balance in percentage of asymmetries between legs (10%) and for adduction/abduction ratios (0.9) for dominant and nondominant legs.

12.3 Risk factors for hamstring injury and preventive training guidelines

Hamstring muscle tears are the most common injury subtype in male football players and are associated with significant time loss and high financial costs for the player and clubs [23]. The predominant hamstring injury mechanisms in football occur during high-speed running and/or acceleration efforts [24, 25] or during movements with large joint excursions (i.e., stretching-type injury) such as high-kicking, split positions, and glide tackling [24]. Hamstring injuries in football most commonly involve the proximal muscle–tendon unit junction of the biceps femoris long head, accounting for approximately 60–85% of all hamstring injuries [24, 26, 27], and the occurrence of hamstring muscle strains in football is generally believed to be related with the presence of repetitive high force eccentric actions [28], such as the ones observed during high-speed running [29], where the lengthening demands placed on the muscle could exceed the mechanical limits of the tissue. Increasing the eccentric strength of the hamstring muscles has therefore been proposed as a method to prevent hamstring injuries [28].

Awareness of risk factors for hamstring strain injury is an important component of player load management, injury prevention, and return to play decision-making post injury. A previous review has identified that older age and a history of hamstring muscle strain are associated with a greater risk of future hamstring injury [30]. Recently, a systematic review and meta-analysis concluded that older age and a history of hamstring strain injury, ACL injury, and calf strain injury were significant risk factors for a future hamstring strain injury [5]. No influence from leg dominance was found on hamstring injury, and based on Hagglund et al. [6], goalkeepers are less likely to suffer a hamstring injury, while players with previous injury to the quadriceps are also more prone to injury.

12.3.1 Guidelines for preventive training

Since the nature of hamstring injuries is accepted as multifactorial and complex, involving interactions among various factors [31], a more holistic approach for hamstring health is likely needed [32]. In this regard, Buckthorpe et al. [33], in line with an emerging body of evidence-based research, have proposed a holistic approach [32] that translated existing knowledge on hamstring muscle injury risk and applies this to a real-life football context. If the proposed or similar holistic approach is able to objectively and sensibly structure the content and the multiple potential interventions to be applied according to football-specific contents (e.g., coaching style) and associated training loads, multiple risk factors predisposing to hamstring injury [5], and the different injury mechanisms (i.e., sprinting, over-stretching, and shooting), it could conceivably provide flexible programming accounting for both football demands on the team and player and the specific weak points of each player. Contrary to a pre-established "one-size-fits-all," general protocol [24, 34, 35], this approach deals with injury prevention as hypercomplex phenomena connecting several interacting components [32, 33, 36] and often involving the skills and experience of different professionals to deliver the intervention, for example, coaches, fitness coaches, doctors, and physiotherapists.

Preventing hamstring injury strain in elite football players is likely to benefit from a holistic approach with a complex program, which considers multiple risk factors, their inter-relations, and their context alongside other injuries [32, 33, 37]. A recent study showed a prevention strategy, namely, a complex prevention program consisted mainly of six components: (i) strength training including specific exercises for the posterior chain, (ii) control of on-field training, (iii) physiotherapy treatment, (iv) training load management, (v) individual training (weak points), and (vi) club staff communication and individual management of the players [38].

The results of the study showed that the incidence of hamstring injuries was reduced ~3 times during the seasons in which elite football players were exposed to the multicomponent and complex prevention training with individual approaches based on players' needs in comparison to the control seasons without a clearly defined and structured injury prevention intervention [38].

12.4 Risk factors for quadriceps injury and preventive training guidelines

Muscle strain injuries usually occur during eccentric muscle actions. Sprinting and kicking require eccentric rectus femoris action, and in combination with the biarticular nature of this muscle, it is left vulnerable to injury. Recto femoris injuries are more frequent in the dominant leg (63%), goalkeepers had a decreased rate of quadriceps injury, while a previous injury to the quadriceps, adductors, or calf muscles increased the rate of injury [6]. The maximum length of rectus femoris happens during the early swing phase where it is contracted eccentrically and the wind-up phase of kicking where it may be predisposed to injury [39, 40]. The most common mechanism of rectus femoris muscle injury in football is kicking [41], with much of the work performed eccentrically in the early phases. During the ball contact phase of kicking, the rectus is in a relatively shortened state, and muscles need to be in a relatively stretched state to induce a strain injury; therefore, during the ball contact phase, the quadriceps muscles are not in danger of strain injury because they are not lengthened or eccentrically contracted in this moment [39, 42]. During the sprinting mechanism, maximum elongation takes place near 55% of sprint cycle just after the initial contact of the contralateral leg, just in the transition from maximal hip extension to maximum hip and knee flexion; therefore, high angular velocities of the hip and knee during the swing phase of sprinting combined with high eccentric activation make the rectus femoris more prone to injury [29, 39].

Several risk factors have been suggested for recto femoris muscle injuries. Although the incidence of muscle injuries generally increases with age, prospective studies found no association between age and this muscle injury [1, 39, 43]. Increased risk of rectus femoris injury was found in players with a previous injury of the quadriceps muscle. In addition, a recent hamstring strain significantly increases the risk of quadriceps strain due to the altered gait patterns that occur after hamstring muscle strains [39, 43]. Leg dominance could be a risk factor as the majority of rectus femoris muscle injuries involve the dominant leg (60%), whereas only 33% affect the nondominant leg (7% were reported in both legs or the leg dominant was not clear) [1]. Further investigations are required, but while concentric strength is not a risk factor for quadriceps injury, likely eccentric strength differences at preseason were found between those injured compared to uninjured professional football players [10].

12.4.1 Guidelines for preventive training

Intervention scientific articles using preventive strategies for rectus femoris injury prevention in professional soccer are very limited. Therefore, the best prevention strategy is to address known risk factors and injury mechanism biomechanics [39].

Quadriceps muscle flexibility should be a cornerstone of a rectus femoris injury prevention program, at least in soccer [10, 39]. Based on the recommendations by Mendiguchia et al. [39], a lack of hip extension may require the rectus femoris to generate more hip flexion force and fatigue, and a restricted psoas may mechanically irritate the femoral nerve and cause tension further down the neurodynamic chain [39].

In order to minimize the risk of rectus femoris injuries, improving the proximal hip strength and knee extension strength at long muscle length seems to be an essential target. Kicking performance is influenced by both knee extension and hip flexion moments [39, 44, 45]. Previous studies showed a high activation of iliacus and psoas muscles during kicking motion concurrently with the rectus femoris [46]. When the iliopsoas muscle force is reduced by 50%, rectus femoris force is increased to compensate this weakness and may result in an overload in rectus femoris, increasing the risk of injury [47]. Therefore, good function of hip flexor muscles is necessary to prevent quadriceps muscle injuries [39].

The quadriceps muscle is actively lengthened during hip extension and knee flexion, and the knee joint generates more change in the length of the rectus femoris than the hip. Muscle strain injuries are contracted at greater than the optimal length [48], and eccentric exercise is the only training that showed consistent increase in development of optimum length of tension in knee extensors [39]. Eccentric quadriceps strength improves the muscle ability to absorb more energy before failing in minimizing the risk of injury [49]. Chronic exposure to eccentric muscle activity provides an active mechanism of structure adaptations, the force threshold for muscle failure is increased, and a protective effect may take place [49]. Therefore, eccentric exercises involving multiple joints designed to increase the optimum length, sprinting, and deceleration–acceleration exercises should be incorporated in the injury prevention programs in football players [39].

12.5 Risk factors for calf injury and preventive training guidelines

Calf muscle strain injuries are one of the most prevalent soft tissue injuries in the elite competition including elite football [50]. Calf complex is critical during locomotor activities, requiring both explosive power and prolonged endurance [50, 51]. When a football player is running at a speed of 22 km/h, the soleus and gastroc-nemius collectively generate a peak force as high as 12.5 times the bodyweight [52]. Around two-thirds of this force can be attributed to the soleus due to its large physi-ological cross-sectional area. Recent musculoskeletal studies showed that the calf muscles are the dominant contributors to upward and forward acceleration of the body's center of mass (support and propulsion, respectively) for running at a range of steady-state speeds [53] as well as for maximum acceleration sprinting [54].

The injury burden in calf strain injuries varies considerably, from no missed games to a recovery period of up to 95 days [50]. Specific injury characteristics warrant consideration, such as the injury site as well as the presence and severity of connective tissue disruption [50, 51]. Calf injuries have a high mean time to return to sport in the event of any recurrence [55], and one study suggests that they more likely to occur during critical competitive periods, such as the end of the competi-tion season in football [56].

Strong evidence exists for an association between increased age and future calf strain in football and Australian football [6, 43], and these studies also provide strong evidence for a history of previous calf muscle injury and future risk in football. A lim-ited evidence exists for an association between previous adductor, previous ham-string, previous quadriceps, and previous knee injury and future calf strain injuries [6, 43, 57]. Despite a limited number of studies available, other authors suggest that data analysis provides evidence for age and previous calf strain injury as the strong-est risk factors, while previous adductor, hamstring, quadriceps, or knee injury may also influence the likelihood of injury, while factors such as player weight, height, gender, and side dominance can be considered to lack evidence of an association with sustaining a calf muscle injury, but more studies are needed [50].

12.5.1   Guidelines for preventive training

There is limited information related with how to prevent calf strain injuries in football players. As muscle strain injuries occur when the muscle is contracted at greater than the optimal length [48], eccentric exercise is a training that showed consistently increased development of the optimum length of tension in the mus-cles [39]. Therefore, eccentric strength improves the calf muscle's ability to absorb more energy before failing in minimizing the risk of injury. In addition to this, eccentric training increases the fascicle length that is recognized to promote an optimum angle and length [58] shift and improvement in eccentric peak torque [59], which was proposed to be related to an increase in elastic energy storage capacity. The increase in fascicle length is important for improving performance and also for the prevention of injuries such as muscle strain because the muscles can work more efficiently without exposure to overstretching.

In this line, a recent study [60] showed the effects of eccentric calf raise exer-cise (plyometric training) on the fascicle length and muscle thickness of the gastrocnemius medialis muscle. The results revealed that continued stretching of the gastrocnemius medialis muscle during eccentric calf raise exercise enhanced the morphological structures, such as the fascicle length and muscle thickness. Therefore, based on the previous scientific literature, the eccentric training (using in this case the calf raise exercise) may help the muscles to work more efficiently without exposure to overstretching, minimizing the risk of injury (2).

12.6   Perspectives

Preventing muscle strain injuries in football players requires a holistic approach with a complex program, which considers multiple risk factors, their inter-relations, and it is put in context alongside other injuries [32, 33, 37], and football clubs with good internal communication between the staff and the medical team are associated with fewer injuries and greater player availability [61]. Despite that the nature underlying muscle injuries is accepted as multifactorial and complex [32, 33], try to prevent a muscle injury targeting only one factor (i.e. strength or sprinting), it could be a reductionist view, and other potential modifiable risk factors linked in some way to muscle strains such us hip extensors and flexors strength, horizontal strength, deceleration steps, outer ranges strength, hip mobility, hip stabilizers, proximal lumbo-pelvic stability, sprinting performance, sport-specific training load, and or game exposure (as examples) must be considered [38].

References

1. Ekstrand J, Hagglund M, Walden M. Epidemiology of muscle injuries in professional football (soccer). *Am J Sports Med.* 2011; 39(6): 1226–1232.
2. Bahr R, Holme I. Risk factors for sports injuries – a methodological approach. *Br J Sports Med.* 2003; 37(5): 384–392.
3. Arnason A, Sigurdsson SB, Gudmundsson A, Holme I, Engebretsen L, Bahr R. Risk factors for injuries in football. *Am J Sports Med.* 2004; 32(1 Suppl): 5S–16S.
4. Meeuwisse WH, Tyreman H, Hagel B, Emery C. A dynamic model of etiology in sport injury: the recursive nature of risk and causation. *Clin J Sport Med.* 2007; 17(3): 215–219.
5. Green B, Lin M, Schache AG, McClelland JA, Semciw AI, Rotstein A, Cook J, Pizzari T. Calf muscle strain injuries in elite Australian Football players: A descriptive epidemiological evaluation. *Scand J Med Sci Sports.* 2020; 30(1): 174–184.
6. Hagglund M, Walden M, Ekstrand J. Risk factors for lower extremity muscle injury in professional soccer: The UEFA Injury Study. *Am J Sports Med.* 2013; 41(2): 327–335.
7. Croisier JL, Forthomme B, Namurois MH, Vanderthommen M, Crielaard JM. Hamstring muscle strain recurrence and strength performance disorders. *Am J Sports Med.* 2002; 30(2): 199–203.
8. Croisier JL, Ganteaume S, Binet J, Genty M, Ferret JM. Strength imbalances and prevention of hamstring injury in professional soccer players: a prospective study. *Am J Sports Med.* 2008; 36(8): 1469–1475.
9. Engebretsen AH, Myklebust G, Holme I, Engebretsen L, Bahr R. Intrinsic risk factors for groin injuries among male soccer players: a prospective cohort study. *Am J Sports Med.* 2010; 38(10): 2051–2057.

10. Fousekis K, Tsepis E, Poulmedis P, Athanasopoulos S, Vagenas G. Intrinsic risk factors of non-contact quadriceps and hamstring strains in soccer: a prospective study of 100 professional players. *Br J Sports Med,* 2011; 45(9): 709–714.

11. Hawkins RD, Fuller CW. A prospective epidemiological study of injuries in four English professional football clubs. *Br J Sports Med.* 1999; 33(3): 196–203.

12. Woods C, Hawkins RD, Maltby S, Hulse M, Thomas A, Hodson A. The football association medical research programme: an audit of injuries in professional football – analysis of hamstring injuries. *Br J Sports Med.* 2004; 38(1): 36–41.

13. Carling C, Orhant E, LeGall F. Match injuries in professional soccer: inter-seasonal variation and effects of competition type, match congestion and positional role. *Int J Sports Med.* 2010; 31(4): 271–276.

14. Ekstrand J, Walden M, Hagglund M. Risk for injury when playing in a national football team. *Scand J Med Sci Sports.* 2004; 14(1): 34–38.

15. Werner J, Hagglund M, Ekstrand J, Walden M. Hip and groin time-loss injuries decreased slightly but injury burden remained constant in men's professional football: the 15-year prospective UEFA Elite Club Injury Study. *Br J Sports Med.* 2019; 53(9): 539–546.

16. Werner J, Hagglund M, Walden M, Ekstrand J. UEFA injury study: a prospective study of hip and groin injuries in professional football over seven consecutive seasons. *Br J Sports Med.* 2009; 43(13): 1036–1040.

17. Jensen, J., Hölmich, P., Bandholm, T., Zebis, M. K., Andersen, L. L., & Thorborg, K. Eccentric strengthening effect of hip-adductor training with elastic bands in soccer players: a randomised controlled trial. *Br J Sports Med.*2014; 48(4): 332–338.

18. Nunez JF, Fernandez I, Torres A, Garcia S, Manzanet P, Casani P, Suarez-Arrones L. Strength conditioning program to prevent adductor muscle strains in football: does it really help professional football players? *Int J Environ Res Public Health.* 2020; 17(17):6408.

19. Thorborg K, Branci S, Nielsen MP, Tang L, Nielsen MB, Holmich P. Eccentric and isometric hip adduction strength in male soccer players with and without adductor-related groin pain: an assessor-blinded comparison. *Orthop J Sports Med.* 2014; 2(2): 2325967114521778.

20. Charnock BL, Lewis CL, Garrett WE Jr, Queen RM. Adductor longus mechanics during the maximal effort soccer kick. *Sports Biomech.* 2009; 8(3): 223–234.

21. Holmich P, Uhrskou P, Ulnits L, Kanstrup IL, Nielsen MB, Bjerg AM, Krogsgaard K. Effectiveness of active physical training as treatment for long-standing adductor-related groin pain in athletes: randomised trial. *Lancet.* 1999; 353(9151): 439–443.

22. Haroy J, Clarsen B, Wiger EG, Oyen MG, Serner A, Thorborg K, Holmich P, Andersen TE, Bahr R. The adductor strengthening programme prevents groin problems among male football players: a cluster-randomised controlled trial. *Br J Sports Med.* 2019; 53(3): 150–157.

23. Ekstrand J, Walden M, Hagglund M. Hamstring injuries have increased by 4% annually in men's professional football, since 2001: a 13-year longitudinal analysis of the UEFA Elite Club injury study. *Br J Sports Med.* 2016; 50(12): 731–737.

24. Askling C, Karlsson J, Thorstensson A. Hamstring injury occurrence in elite soccer players after preseason strength training with eccentric overload. *Scand J Med Sci Sports.* 2003; 13(4): 244–250.

25. Woods C, Hawkins RD, Maltby S, Hulse M, Thomas A, Hodson A. The football association medical research programme: an audit of injuries in professional football – analysis of hamstring injuries. *Br J Sports Med.* 2004; 38(1): 36–41.

26. Hallen A, Ekstrand J. Return to play following muscle injuries in professional footballers. *J Sports Sci.* 2014; 32(13): 1229–1236.
27. Petersen J, Thorborg K, Nielsen MB, Skjodt T, Bolvig L, Bang N, Holmich P. The diagnostic and prognostic value of ultrasonography in soccer players with acute hamstring injuries. *Am J Sports Med.* 2014; 42(2): 399–404.
28. Opar DA, Williams MD, Timmins RG, Hickey J, Duhig SJ, Shield AJ. Eccentric hamstring strength and hamstring injury risk in Australian footballers. *Med Sci Sports Exerc.* 2015; 47(4): 857–865.
29. Schache AG, Dorn TW, Blanch PD, Brown NA, Pandy MG. Mechanics of the human hamstring muscles during sprinting. *Med Sci Sports Exerc.* 2012; 44(4): 647–658.
30. Opar DA, Williams MD, Shield AJ. Hamstring strain injuries: factors that lead to injury and re-injury. *Sports Med.* 2012; 42(3): 209–226.
31. Mendiguchia J, Martinez-Ruiz E, Edouard P, Morin JB, Martinez-Martinez F, Idoate F, Mendez-Villanueva A. A multifactorial, criteria-based progressive algorithm for hamstring injury treatment. *Med Sci Sports Exerc.* 2017; 49(7): 1482–1492.
32. Oakley AJ, Jennings J, Bishop CJ. Holistic hamstring health: not just the Nordic hamstring exercise. *Br J Sports Med.* 2018; 52(13): 816–817.
33. Buckthorpe M, Gimpel M, Wright S, Sturdy T, Stride M. Hamstring muscle injuries in elite football: translating research into practice. *Br J Sports Med.* 2018; 52(10): 628–629.
34. Arnason A, Andersen TE, Holme I, Engebretsen L, Bahr R. Prevention of hamstring strains in elite soccer: an intervention study. *Scand J Med Sci Sports.* 2008; 18(1): 40–48.
35. Petersen J, Thorborg K, Nielsen MB, Budtz-Jorgensen E, Holmich P. Preventive effect of eccentric training on acute hamstring injuries in men's soccer: a cluster-randomized controlled trial. *Am J Sports Med.* 2011; 39(11): 2296–2303.
36. Buckthorpe M, Wright S, Bruce-Low S, Nanni G, Sturdy T, Gross AS, Bowen L, Styles B, Della Villa S, Davison M, Gimpel M. Recommendations for hamstring injury prevention in elite football: translating research into practice. *Br J Sports Med.* 2019; 53(7): 449–456.
37. Mendez-Villanueva A, Suarez-Arrones L, Rodas G, Fernandez-Gonzalo R, Tesch P, Linnehan R, Kreider R, Di Salvo V. MRI-based regional muscle use during hamstring strengthening exercises in elite soccer players. *PLoS One.* 2016; 11(9): e0161356.
38. Suarez-Arrones L, Nakamura FY, Maldonado RA, Torreno N, Di Salvo V, Mendez-Villanueva A. Applying a holistic hamstring injury prevention approach in elite football: 12 seasons, single club study. *Scand J Med Sci Sports.* 2021; 31(4): 861–874.
39. Mendiguchia J, Alentorn-Geli E, Idoate F, Myer GD. Rectus femoris muscle injuries in football: a clinically relevant review of mechanisms of injury, risk factors and preventive strategies. *Br J Sports Med.* 2013; 47(6): 359–366.
40. Riley PO, Franz J, Dicharry J, Kerrigan DC. Changes in hip joint muscle-tendon lengths with mode of locomotion. *Gait Posture.* 2010; 31(2): 279–283.
41. Woods C, Hawkins RD, Hulse M, Hodson A. The Football Association Medical Research Programme: an audit of injuries in professional football—analysis of preseason injuries. *Br J Sports Med.* 2002; 36(6): 436–441.
42. Lieber RL, Friden J. Mechanisms of muscle injury gleaned from animal models. *Am J Phys Med Rehabil.* 2002; 81(11 Suppl): S70–79.
43. Orchard JW. Intrinsic and extrinsic risk factors for muscle strains in Australian football. *Am J Sports Med.* 2001; 29(3): 300–303.

44. Dorge HC, Anderson TB, Sorensen H, Simonsen EB. Biomechanical differences in soccer kicking with the preferred and the non-preferred leg. *J Sports Sci.* 2002; 20(4): 293–299.

45. Kellis E, Katis A, Gissis I. Knee biomechanics of the support leg in soccer kicks from three angles of approach. *Med Sci Sports Exerc.* 2004; 36(6): 1017–1028.

46. Baczkowski K, Marks P, Silberstein M, Schneider-Kolsky ME. A new look into kicking a football: an investigation of muscle activity using MRI. *Australas Radiol.* 2006; 50(4): 324–329.

47. Lewis CL, Sahrmann SA, Moran DW. Anterior hip joint force increases with hip extension, decreased gluteal force, or decreased iliopsoas force. *J Biomech.* 2007; 40(16): 3725–3731.

48. Brooks JH, Fuller CW, Kemp SP, Reddin DB. Incidence, risk, and prevention of hamstring muscle injuries in professional rugby union. *Am J Sports Med.* 2006; 34(8): 1297–1306.

49. Lindstedt SL, LaStayo PC, Reich TE. When active muscles lengthen: properties and consequences of eccentric contractions. *News Physiol Sci.* 2001; 16: 256–261.

50. Green B, Bourne MN, van Dyk N, Pizzari T. Recalibrating the risk of hamstring strain injury (HSI): a 2020 systematic review and meta-analysis of risk factors for index and recurrent hamstring strain injury in sport. *Br J Sports Med.* 2020; 54(18): 1081–1088.

51. Green B, Pizzari T. Calf muscle strain injuries in sport: a systematic review of risk factors for injury. *Br J Sports Med.* 2017; 51(16): 1189–1194.

52. Komi PV. Relevance of in vivo force measurements to human biomechanics. *J Biomech.* 1990; 23(Suppl 1): 23–34.

53. Hamner SR, Delp SL. Muscle contributions to fore-aft and vertical body mass center accelerations over a range of running speeds. *J Biomech.* 2013; 46(4): 780–787.

54. Debaere S, Delecluse C, Aerenhouts D, Hagman F, Jonkers I. Control of propulsion and body lift during the first two stances of sprint running: a simulation study. *J Sports Sci.* 2015; 33(19): 2016–2024.

55. Carling C, Le Gall F, Orhant E. A four-season prospective study of muscle strain reoccurrences in a professional football club. *Res Sports Med.* 2011; 19(2): 92–102.

56. Mallo J, Dellal A. Injury risk in professional football players with special reference to the playing position and training periodization. *J Sports Med Phys Fitness.* 2012; 52(6): 631–638.

57. Nilstad A, Andersen TE, Bahr R, Holme I, Steffen K. Risk factors for lower extremity injuries in elite female soccer players. *Am J Sports Med.* 2014; 42(4): 940–948.

58. Guex K, Degache F, Morisod C, Sailly M, Millet GP. Hamstring architectural and functional adaptations following long vs. short muscle length eccentric training. *Front Physiol.* 2016; 7: 340.

59. Blazevich AJ, Cannavan D, Coleman DR, Horne S. Influence of concentric and eccentric resistance training on architectural adaptation in human quadriceps muscles. *J Appl Physiol.* 2007; 103(5): 1565–1575.

60. Kudo S, Sato T, Miyashita T. Effect of plyometric training on the fascicle length of the gastrocnemius medialis muscle. *J Phys Ther Sci.* 2020; 32(4): 277–280.

61. Ekstrand J, Lundqvist D, Davison M, D'Hooghe M, Pensgaard AM. Communication quality between the medical team and the head coach/manager is associated with injury burden and player availability in elite football clubs. *Br J Sports Med.* 2019; 53(5): 304–308.

13

FITNESS TESTING AND FUNCTIONAL ASSESSMENT OF FOOTBALL PLAYERS DURING INJURY PERIODS

Francisco Javier Núñez Sánchez and Alberto Torres Campos

13.1 Introduction

An injury, especially in a football player, has a multifactorial nature. The recovery–rehabilitation process to achieve their reincorporation to training and competition must be planned and executed by professionals from different fields of action (doctor, physiotherapist, physical rehabilitator, physical trainer, psychologist, and nutritionist). The moment a football player suffers an injury, regardless of the type of injury suffered, the entire environment that surrounds the football player goes into a real frenzy to estimate when he will be available to the team again. At that precise moment, from the department of "fitness testing and functional assessment" of a club, rather than thinking about when, it is necessary to know exactly what his physical state should be in order to be available to the team again. For this reason, it becomes more important to establish what type of test we will use during the time that he is not injured to determine his current physical state and therefore what he should have in the "return to play" after an injury than the tests usually applied to evaluate injury evolution. Most of the tests applied to the injured football player that we find in the scientific literature are based on an analysis of what happens once he is already injured. From our point of view, this evaluation is already distorted since, once the injury occurs, even the non-injured leg will not show its maximum capacity in any of the tests to which it is subjected. That is why, in this chapter, we propose a player evaluation model that helps us know the state of the injured player compared to what he had when he was healthy; know which muscle chain shows a different behavior from its contralateral, or itself at another time, regardless of whether it is the cause or consequence of the injury produced; propose simple assessments that help test and train efficiently during the rehabilitation process of a lesion regardless of the damaged tissue. At the end of this chapter, we

DOI: 10.4324/9781032637006-13

will also address some considerations to be taken into account in the evaluation of the football player based on the type of tissue damaged in the injury.

13.2 Return to play? Let's focus on the physical condition state in the closest moment before the injury, this is the goal!

The only way to be able to accurately determine the "fitness" that a football player should achieve before the "return to play" is to have been able to record, as exhaustively as possible, the training and competition process developed by himself before the injury. There are two factors that determine the effectiveness of this record in a professional football player: (1) training monitoring must be carried out with instrumentation that allows us to obtain records of the football player's behavior without interfering or decontextualizing the usual training dynamics, or competition (e.g., the quantitative analysis of the movements of the football player with global positioning system or GPS or qualitative analysis of the movements of the football players using video analysis); (2) in the case in which the obtaining of information on the behavior of the football player had to be decontextualized, that such information does not depend on his voluntary nature (e.g., TMG). If the means of obtaining this information depended on the will of the football player, it should be obtained through tests applied with regularity, which are integrated into their usual work dynamics and are not considered something exceptional or casual (e.g., manual muscle testing). All these means of obtaining information remain active when the football player is healthy as well as when he is in a process of recovering from an injury, although in this second option, the "timing" for obtaining data may be modified.

13.2.1 Global positioning system and video analysis

For more than a decade, the GPS provides a valid and reliable quantitative measure of the football players' locomotor profile both in training situations and during competition [1, 2]. As we will see in other chapters, the most analyzed variables are the total distance traveled, the distance traveled at high intensity, peak speed reached, number of sprints, frequency of sprints, and types of accelerations–decelerations and number of accelerations–decelerations of each type. Currently, through the accelerometry of these devices, we can also know if a player in his movements makes greater use of one of his legs with respect to the contralateral [3]. This variable will reflect a different behavior in each player, mainly due to the type of movements that predominate in his movements, but it is relatively stable throughout a season if the player has not suffered any major injury. As an example, if a player presents a habitual imbalance between dominant and nondominant legs of 6%, at a certain moment this imbalance increases to 16% and is maintained throughout the week; this change will not be due to a greater quantitative capacity of the movement, but rather a qualitative modification of it. This modification could be related to the establishment of a new role within the game, but if not, it should serve as an alert system since this qualitative change in movement will almost certainly be related to some kind of annoyance suffered. Hence, it is vital to be able to correlate the quantitative data of the football player locomotor profile with the qualitative analysis of the movements produced, determining predominant movements in the player, laterality, fluidity, and amplitude, and this is not possible if all the interventions of the football player during training and competition are not recorded in video in order to be able to carry out an analysis later. The continuous recording of the player's quantitative and qualitative locomotor profile, both in training and competition situations, will allow us to immediately establish the external load that he should bear to "return to play," which would be the same or even in better conditions than the previous ones, who left him due to injury. Taking into account the latest epidemiological data on the football players injury, we verify that there is a high percentage of new injury (different from the one initially produced) in a period of time not very long after having suffered an injury [4]. Therefore, during the recovery–rehabilitation process, we must also develop said continuous record in order to assess both the quantitative progress and the possible qualitative modifications of its locomotor capacity that the injury is causing and thus be able to anticipate other possible injuries by a change in their movement dynamics.

13.2.2 Tensiomyography (TMG)

TMG is a test that allows us to measure the muscular contractile properties of the football player, in a resting position and without any voluntary action, in a valid and reliable way [1, 2]. The system synchronizes a sensor, with a spring constant of 0.17 N · mm−1, placed perpendicular to the muscle belly to be measured, just at the point where it produces its greatest displacement, with an electrostimulator that contracts the muscle through two adhesive electrodes placed on the muscle surface (10 cm apart) and in line with the direction of the stimulated muscle fibers (Figure 13.1).

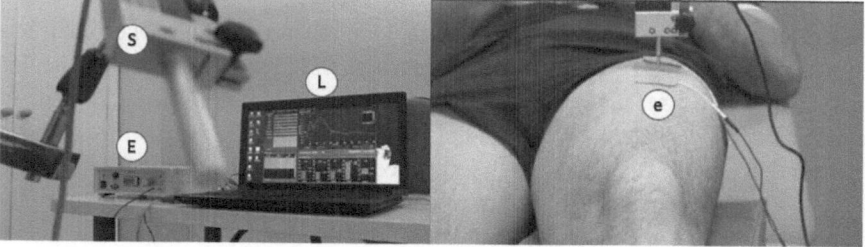

FIGURE 13.1   Tensiomyography. S: sensor; E: electrostimulator; L: laptop; e: adhesive electrodes.

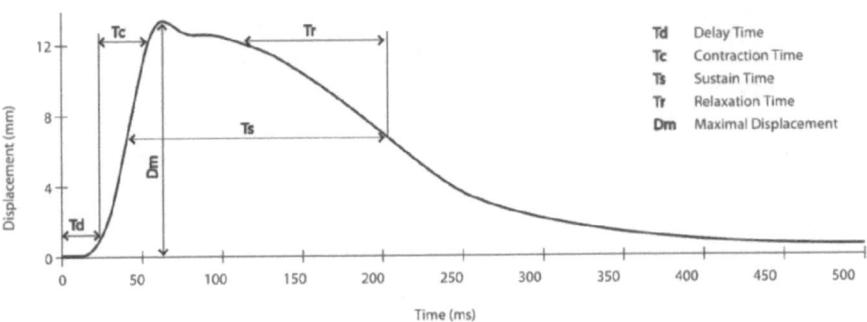

FIGURE 13.2 Numerical variables obtained through the TMG.

The test begins with the transmission of an electrical impulse of 1 millisecond duration and a signal amplitude of 20 mA. The amplitude is increased in 10 mA sequences, until the maximum displacement of the muscle belly is achieved, or a smaller displacement is obtained than the previous stimulation. The analyzed muscle contractile properties analyzed of the stimulation that has a greater displacement are the displacement of the muscle surface, measured in mm (Dm); the contraction time elapsed between 10 and 90% of its maximum displacement, measured in ms (Tc); and the delay time from when the electrical stimulus is applied until it reaches 10% of its maximum displacement, measured in ms (Td) (Figure 13.2).

Previous studies have shown a high level of reliability in the measurement of these variables (ICC. 0.82, CV, 5%) [2]. The passive assessment of the musculature is carried out in four basic positions: (a) lying supine, generating a fixed knee angle of 120° using a foam wedge-shaped cushion, to measure the vastus lateralis, rectus femoris, and vastus medialis of the quadriceps, and tibialis anterior; (b) lying on the side, keeping the upper leg extended and supported by a foam cushion to measure the peroneus longus, while the lower leg remains flexed at the hip and knee level and supported on the table for the measurement of the adductor longus; (c) lying supine to measure the rectus abdominis; (d) lying prone, a semi-circular wedge foam cushion under the ankles, maintaining a constant 30° knee flexion, for the measurement of the lumbar, gluteus maximus, biceps femoris, semitendinosus, and lateral and medial calf muscles (Figure 13.3).

The Dm values, associated with the stiffness of the muscle belly when contracting, together with the Tc, allow us to obtain a map of the player's muscle behavior at rest [2], which after the conditioning period of the initial pre-season, it tends to remain relatively constant throughout the season, showing only variability in those muscles that are directly or indirectly influenced by a modification in the behavior pattern. The reference values for these two variables in the musculature normally measured by TMG in a football player are reflected in Table 13.1.

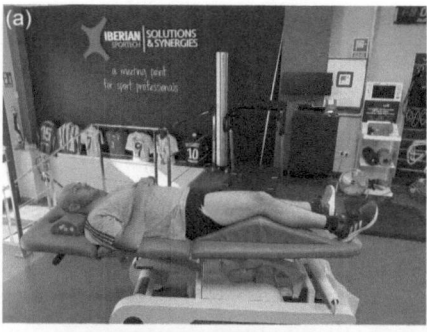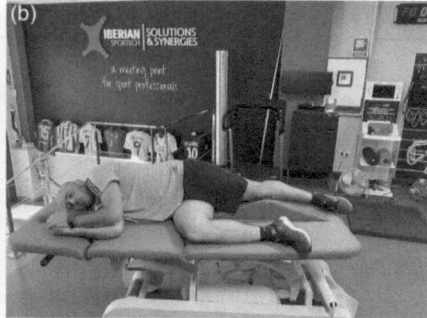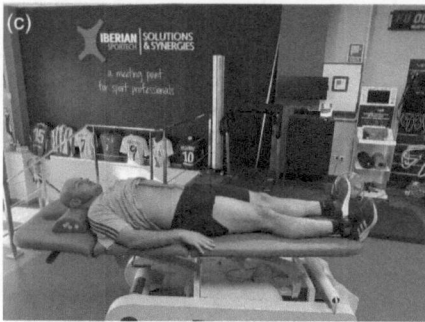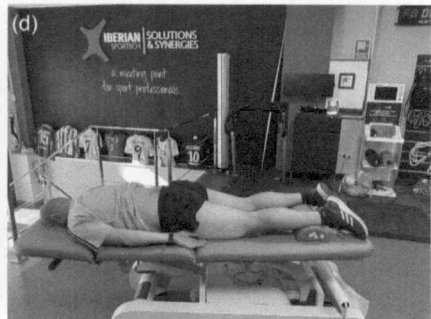

FIGURE 13.3   Player positioning for TMG measurement.

We could interpret that

a An increase in both Dm and Tc shows us a clear detraining of these muscles, either due to disuse or inadequate stimulation.

b A maintenance of Dm values with an increase in Tc would show us a decrease in the contraction speed.

c A maintenance of Tc values with an increase in Dm would show us a decrease in rigidity or muscle tone.

d A reduction in both Dm and Tc could indicate an increase in muscle performance if it occurs in both legs. However, if it only occurs in one leg, it could warn us of a possible risk of muscle injury. We establish that for this to happen there must be differences of around 15% between the values of the same muscles for both legs. The system itself already describes this as "lateral symmetry."

We only use the Td value to assess the long peroneal and anterior tibial muscles, in which a Td value above 27 ms could indicate that these muscles are not very active to face the possible containment of a sprain of the lateral ligaments of the knee and ankle. For the duration of this test (approximately 15 minutes), a TMG assessment

TABLE 13.1 Muscle reference values for TMG analysis in professional soccer players

Zone	Muscle	Tc(ms)	Dm(mm)
Trunk			
Rectus Abdominus			< 8
Erector Spinae			< 8
Hips			
Gluteus Major		< 30	3–6
Adductor Major		< 28	3–6
Thighs			
Vastus Medialis		< 29	5–10
Vastus Lateralis		< 28	3–7
Rectus Femoris		< 30	3–9
Biceps Femoris		< 30	3–6
Semitendinosus		< 40	< 8
Leg			
Gastrocnemius Medialis		< 27	2–4
Gastrocnemius Lateralis		< 30	2–5

is performed every 4 weeks in a healthy player. This period could be shortened in certain injuries where the evolution of contractile capacity is of vital importance for the proper development of the recovery–readaptation processes.

13.2.3 The Manual Muscle Testing (MMT) of the main chains of movement of the football player

The MMT measurement postures used in this chapter have been adapted from Kendall et al. [5]. The MMT consists of a series of tests based on the ability to adapt the force exerted by a muscle chain to the changes in resistance offered, the different directions of movement in which it can participate, and the degree of elongation to which it is subjected in every moment. For this reason, a high knowledge of the football player anatomy and muscle mechanics is required, which allows him to generate force in all his planes and ranges of motion (ROM). Through this type of assessment, we can distinguish the strengths and weaknesses of the same muscle chain in multiple directions and different movements, in a certain degree of its joint range, maintaining a great tension applied at a certain moment or for a long time. The MMT measurement showed a good reliability and validity in the use to test neuromusculoskeletal dysfunction [6]. We consider that if the football player's neuromuscular system works correctly, he will respond immediately and adapt his muscular activity to the demands of the test. However, if, for example, we detect a delay in the recruitment of motor units, it will mean that the neuromuscular system works inadequately. This delay may vary depending on the type of problem or imbalance existing in the neuromuscular system and will affect the force exerted during the test. This MMT is useful both for the evaluation of the state of the healthy football player as well as of the football player with pain, discomfort, overload, or injured, being able to indicate the weakness of the muscles directly involved with the pain, injuries, and musculo-skeletal disorders.

How is an articular muscle assessment performed?

Regardless of the position adopted for the assessment of each muscle chain, during the test, the player will lie on a table, with a voluntary contraction of the muscles of the lumbo-abdominal girdle, and being able to help with the hands to stabilize the position. The evaluator will take the muscle chain to assess the minimum ROM in which the football player can exert force, without making compensatory movements, placing the hand as the limit of muscle shortening. At this time, you are asked to perform force against the hand (muscle shortening), trying to maintain tension against the resistance offered only with the muscles tested. The initial objective is not to "win" the evaluator, but to be able to maintain a minimum isometric tension that allows us to activate the muscles. The evaluator will maintain this position between 7 and 10 seconds, to later ask the player to perform the maximum isometric contraction possible against resistance so as not to be defeated. If compensatory movements are suspected to help the muscles overcome this resistance, the test should be stopped and restarted. If at the beginning of the maximum test the player is overcome by manual resistance, the ROM in which the player can exert force should be decreased and re-test until he finds his strongest and most stable angle. The evaluator must pay attention to the following criteria:

a Place the appropriate position in the joint to prioritize / increase muscle mechanics.
b Properly stabilize the athlete's body.
c Observe the way in which the athlete reaches the test position and how he maintains it.
d View the axis, the lever arm, and the direction of the force.
e Be consistent with the time of holding the position.
f Avoid having a preconceived idea about the muscle response in the test.
g Be careful with the grips and execution of the test to avoid causing pain.
h Take into account the possible contraindications to the performance of the MTT due to the injury, pain, and pathology of the athlete.

Main muscular chains to value in a football player.

The muscle chains usually evaluated are

13.2.4 External rotator muscle chain of the hip in 90° knee flexion

In the prone position on a stretcher, perform an external rotation movement with the leg in knee flexion at 90°, passive, with the contralateral leg in full extension, reaching the maximum possible ROM, which allows us to articulate the hip without compensating with other structures (Figure 13.4).

The compensatory movements that we must avoid in this assessment are

- Hip adduction
- Hip flexion

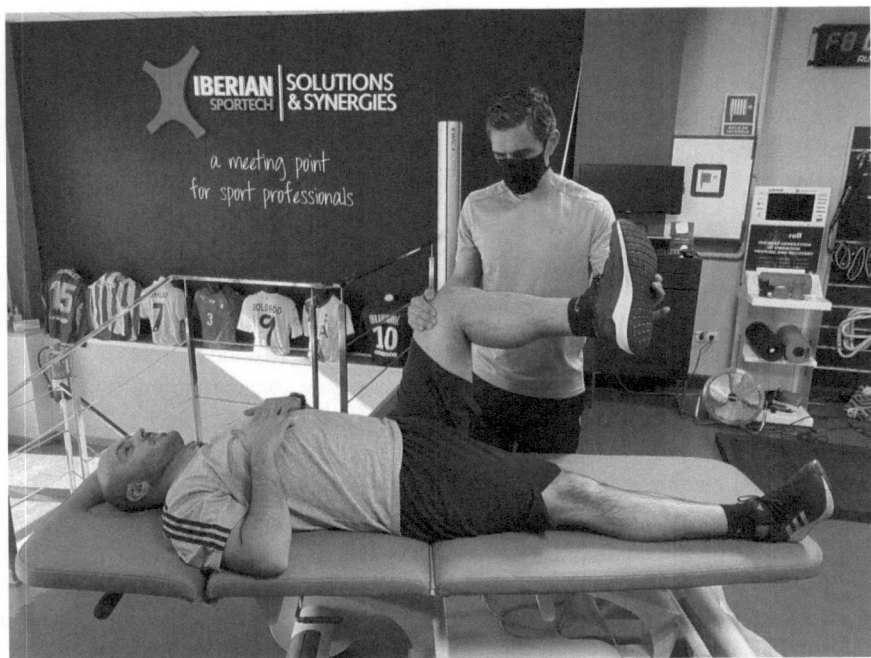

FIGURE 13.4   MTT of the hip external rotator muscle chain [5].

13.2.5 Internal rotator muscle chain of the hip in 90° knee flexion

In the prone position on a stretcher, perform an internal rotation movement with the leg in knee flexion at 90°, passive, with the contralateral leg in full extension, reaching the maximum possible ROM, which allows us to articulate the hip without compensating with other structures (Figure 13.5).

The compensatory movements that we must avoid in this assessment are

– Hip flexion
– Knee flexion

13.2.6 Hip abductor muscle chain

In a supine position on a stretcher, perform a passive abduction movement with the contralateral leg in full extension, reaching the maximum ROM possible, which allows us to articulate the hip without compensating with other structures (Figure 13.6).

The compensatory movements that we must avoid in this assessment are

– External hip rotation
– Hip flexion – Knee flexion
– Hip abduction not assessed
– Hip flexion not valued

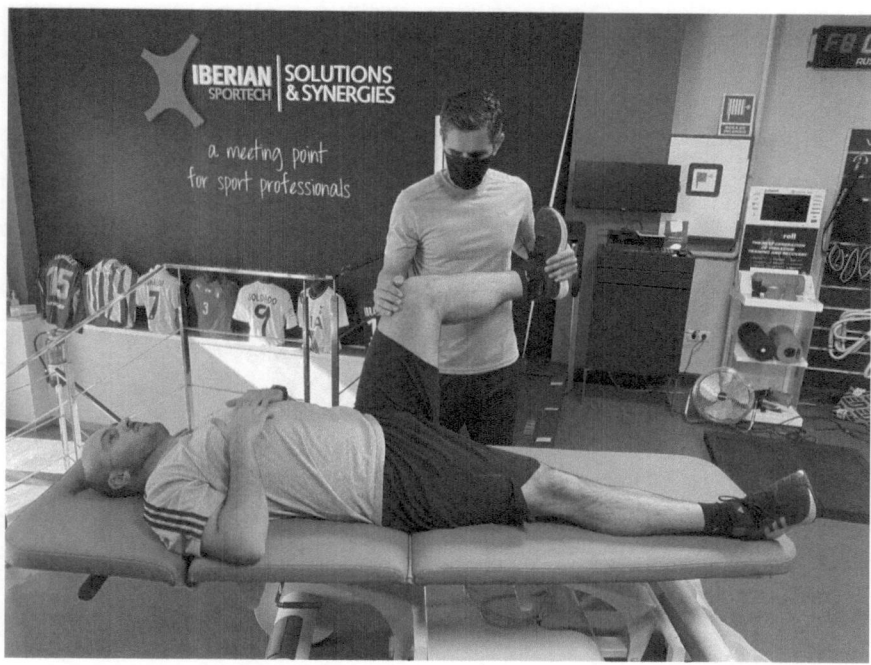

FIGURE 13.5   MTT of the hip internal rotator muscle chain [5].

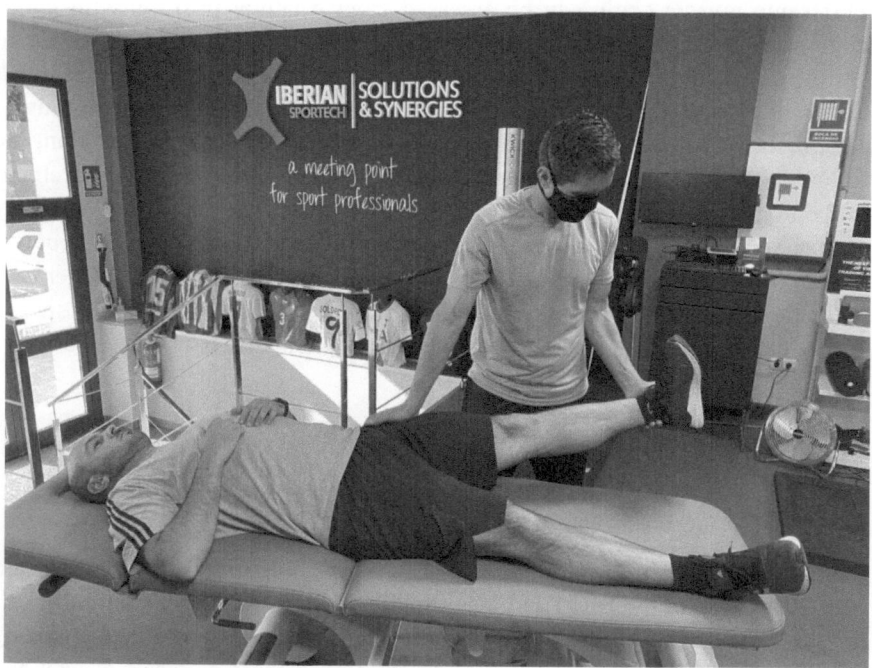

FIGURE 13.6   MTT of the supine hip abductor muscle chain [5].

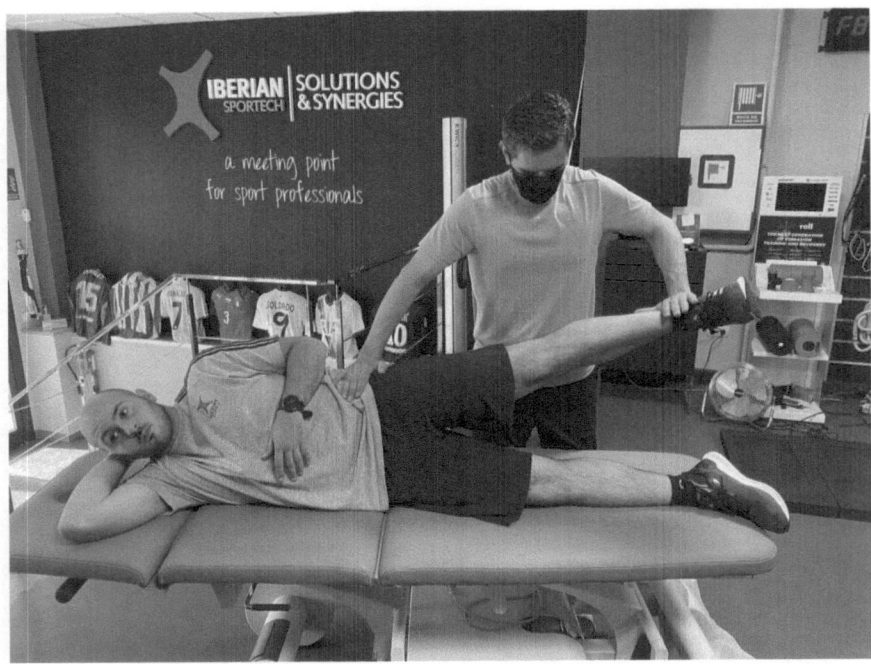

FIGURE 13.7 MTT of the hip abductor muscle chain in a lateral position [5].

This same muscle chain can be assessed from a lateral position with maximum knee and hip extension (Figure 13.7). The football player is asked to perform a hip abduction movement, separating one leg from the other as much as possible, focusing muscle tension and movement in the hip abductor muscle area, mainly the tensor fascia lata. This variant implies taking into account the following compensatory movements due to weakness of this muscular chain: (a) ruling out that a lateral flexion of the trunk is taking place, evidenced by causing an ascent of the hip and iliac pala that is in motion; (b) that the pelvis remains in a neutral position and does not tilt anteriorly (flexion) or posteriorly (extension).

The compensatory movements that we must avoid in this assessment are

- Hip flexion
- External hip rotation
- Lateral tilt of the trunk
- Increased lumbar lordosis

Similarly, by shortening the muscle chain, the lateral decubitus can be evaluated with 90° flexion of the knees and hips (Figure 13.8). In this case, from this position, the football player is asked to perform a hip abduction movement, separating the knees from each other as much as possible, focusing the muscle tension and

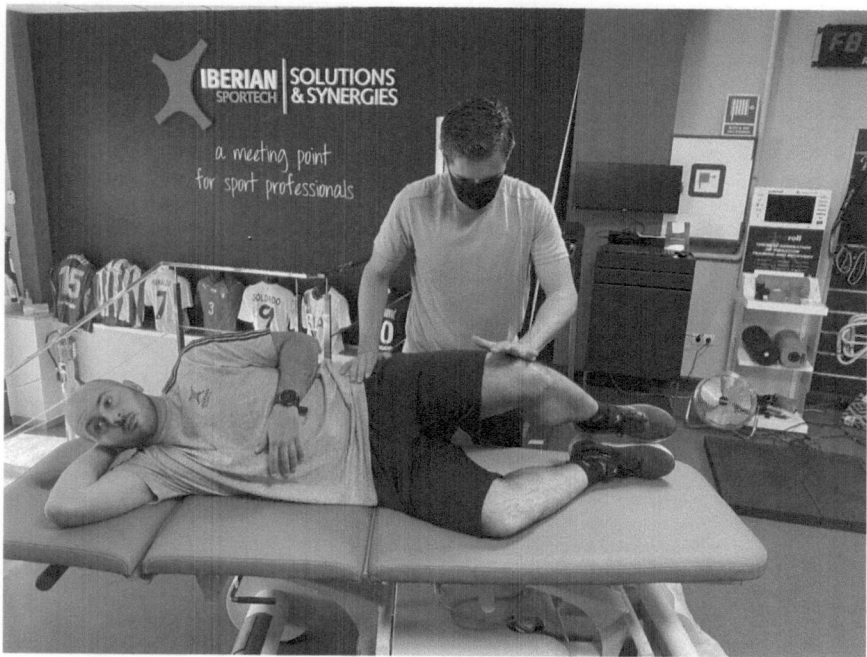

FIGURE 13.8   MTT of the hip abductor muscle chain in a lateral position with hips and knees flexed [5].

movement in the hip abductor muscle area, mainly the gluteus medius. It must be taken into account that the feet are not separated during the movement and that the lumbar spine is in slight pelvic anteversion.

The compensatory movements that we must avoid in this assessment are

- Pelvic retroversion
- The movement is directed by the knee and not by the hip

13.2.7   Hip adductor muscle chain

In a supine position on a stretcher, carry out a passive adduction movement, with the contralateral leg in knee flexion and slight abduction, reaching the maximum possible ROM, which allows us to articulate the hip without compensating with other structures (Figure 13.9).

The compensatory movements that we must avoid in this assessment are

- Hip flexion
- External hip rotation
- Knee flexion
- Hip abduction not assessed

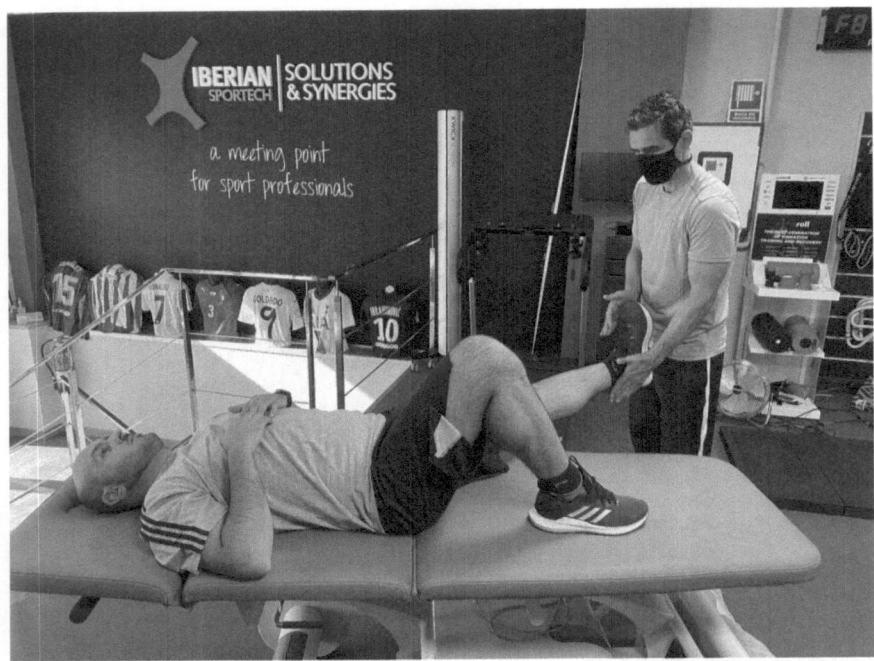

FIGURE 13.9 MTT of the supine adductor muscle chain [5].

13.2.8 *Hip flexor muscle chain*

In a supine position on a stretcher, perform a flexion movement with the leg in full extension, passive, with the contralateral leg in full extension, reaching the maximum ROM possible, which allows us to articulate the hip without compensating with other structures (Figure 13.10).

The compensatory movements that we must avoid in this assessment are

– External hip rotation
– Knee flexion

13.2.9 *Hip extensor muscle chain*

In the prone position on a stretcher, perform an extension movement with the leg in full extension, passive, with the contralateral leg in full extension, reaching the maximum ROM possible, which allows us to articulate the hip without compensating with other structures (Figure 13.11).

The compensatory movements that we must avoid in this assessment are

– External hip rotation
– Hip flexion not valued

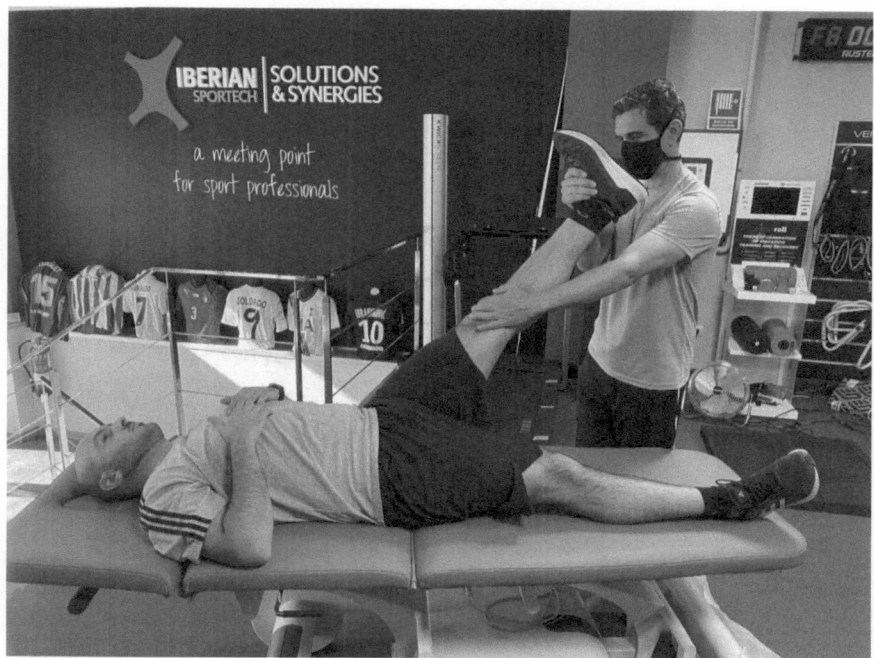

FIGURE 13.10   MTT of the supine ulnar hip flexor muscle chain [5].

The prone ulnar hip extensor muscle chain could also be assessed (Figure 13.12). In a prone position on a stretcher, perform a hip extension movement, with the contralateral leg in full extension, reaching the maximum ROM possible, which allows us to articulate the hip without compensating with other structures. From our point of view, this positioning offers us more information since through it, we must observe a greater tension in the gluteus maximus, followed by the hamstring and as a stabilizer to help the erectors. There should be no greater tension in the hamstrings and / or erectors than in the glutes.

The compensatory movements that we must avoid in this assessment are

- External hip rotation
- Knee flexion
- Increased lumbar lordosis

13.2.10   Knee extensor muscle chain

In a supine position on a stretcher and with both legs in full knee extension, we place our knee, and a towel or cushion not very elevated in the posterior knee area (popliteal). We ask the player to perform a knee extension movement with dorsal flexion of the foot, focusing muscle tension and movement in the knee extensor

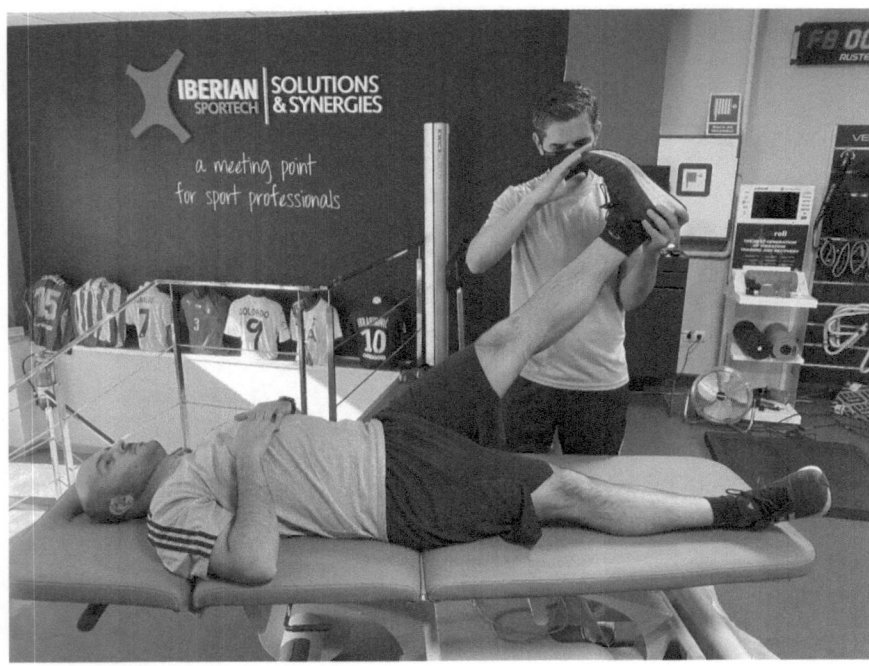

FIGURE 13.11 MTT of the supine hip extensor muscle chain [5].

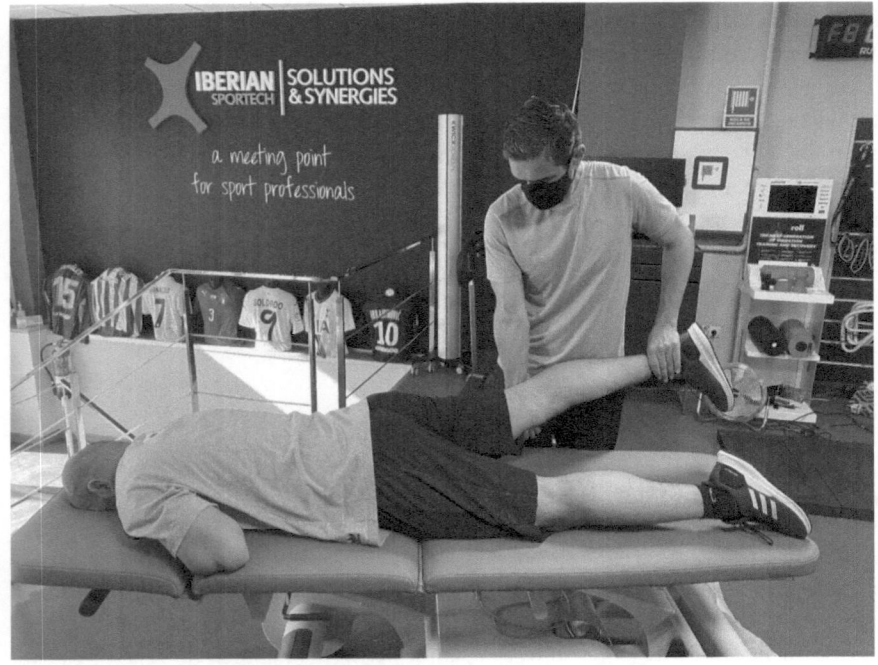

FIGURE 13.12 MTT of the hip extensor muscle chain in the prone position [5].

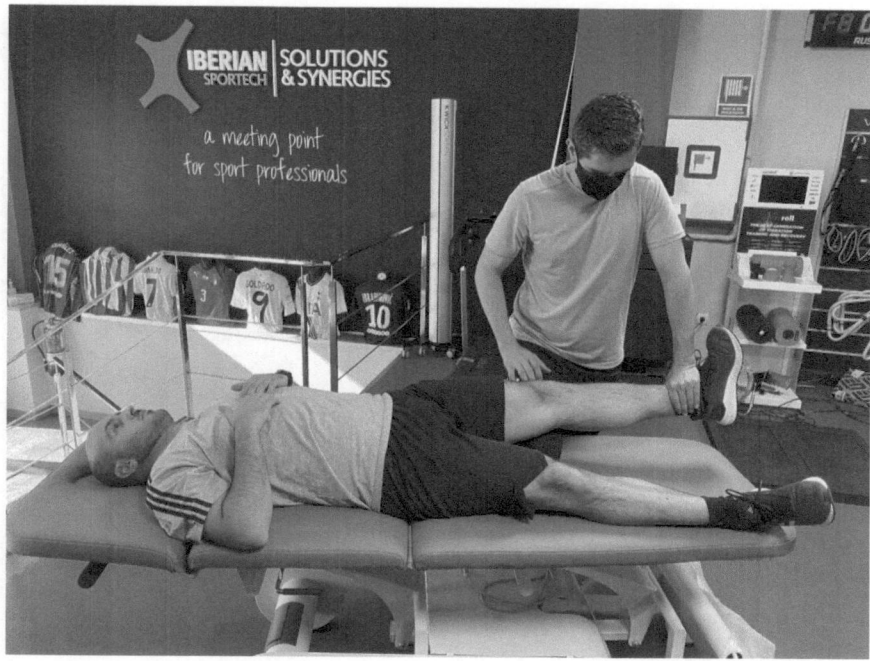

FIGURE 13.13 MTT of the supine knee extensor muscle chain [5].

musculature area, mainly the vastus medialis. This positioning based on the last degrees of knee extension will allow us to differentiate a predominant tension in the vastus medialis over the vastus lateralis and rectus femoris. We must bear in mind that if there is a lot of stretching tension in the hamstring area, it could indicate that the starting knee flexion is too high (Figure 13.13).

The compensatory movements that we must avoid in this assessment are

- Internal hip rotation
- Hip flexion

13.2.11   Knee flexor muscle chain in knee flexion

In the prone position on a stretcher, perform a flexion movement with the leg in knee flexion at 90°, passive, with the contralateral leg in full extension, reaching the maximum ROM possible, which allows us to articulate the hip without compensating with other structures (Figure 13.14).

The compensatory movements that we must avoid in this assessment are

- External hip rotation
- Hip adduction
- Increased lumbar lordosis

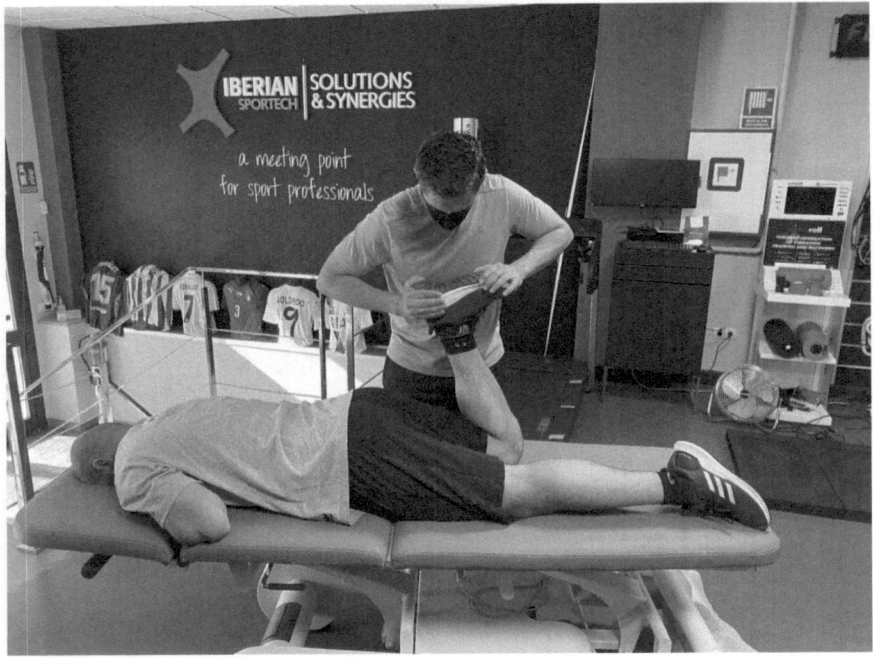

FIGURE 13.14 MTT of the flexor muscle chain of the prone knee [5].

Although it could also be assessed in the supine position, with the hip flexed at 90° and keeping the contralateral leg in extension (Figure 13.15), in this case, knee flexion would be more favored by the forces of gravity than in the previous case.

The compensatory movements that we must avoid in this assessment are

– External hip rotation
– Hip adduction
– Increased lumbar lordosis

Quantification and interpretation of MTT results.

During an MTT, if we do not have any means of objective evaluation, the evaluator will subjectively establish a score from 0 to 3 according to the degree of force perceived in the assessed muscle (Table 13.2).

In the case of having a manual pressure force gauge for the objective registration of the force exerted by the football player in each valued movement (Figure 13.16), the force exerted by the football player in maintaining the position and the force necessary to overcome their resistance to movement are measured.

We recommend that during the first two evaluations, the objective value of strength obtained is recorded, but that it be assessed based on the subjective criteria described previously since we do not know if what you have achieved is too much or

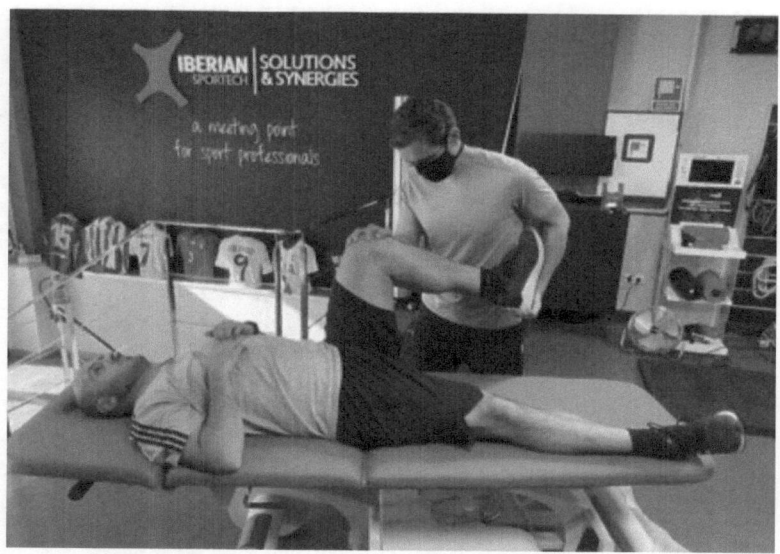

FIGURE 13.15 MTT of the supine knee flexor muscle chain [5].

TABLE 13.2 Subjective assessment equivalence criterion

0	Very weak muscle chain
1	Weak muscle chain
2	Strong muscle chain
3	Very strong muscle chain

too little for your ability. It is from the third assessment, when taking as a reference the average force data obtained in the two previous assessments, we will compare the objective data obtained to check if the state of said muscle chain is above or below its average. In the analysis of the muscular chain of the same leg, if the current measurement is + 6% of the average obtained in the two previous evaluations, we will consider that it is within its usual state; if this measurement is between 6% and 10% higher or lower than the average, we will consider it to be strong (+) or weak (−), respectively; if it is 10% higher or lower than the average, we will consider it to be very strong (++) or weak (−), respectively. In the analysis of a muscle chain in both legs, consider that if the differences between both legs are < 10%, they would be within normality; if the differences between both legs are between 10% and 15%, we would consider them to be unbalanced; if the differences between both legs are > 15%, we would consider it to be very unbalanced.

When should an MTT be done?

As one of our objectives is to know the state of the injured player with respect to the one he had when he was healthy and that the proposed MTT itself can serve as a

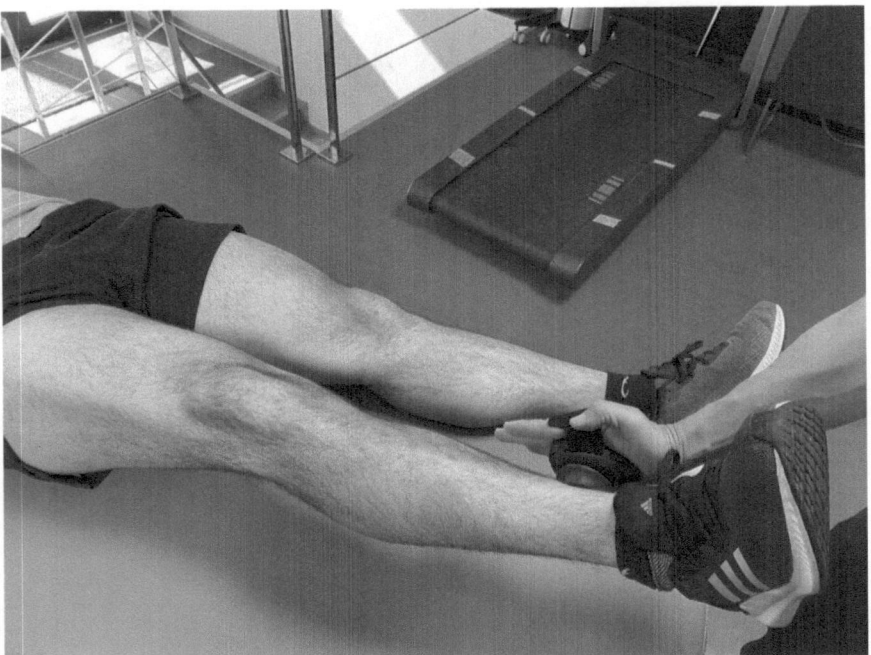

FIGURE 13.16 Using a dynamometer in MTT.

means to start the work of the deficit muscle chains in the football player, each 3–4 weeks in the healthy football player, and every 2–3 days in a football player with an imbalance in one of his muscular chains or injured, it is important to determine which muscle chains can be assessed according to the existing injury. Therefore, in this case, we must maintain close communication with the medical services to determine the said process.

13.3 Considerations to take into account in the evaluation of the football player based on the type of tissue damaged in the injury

13.3.1 Muscle, myofascial, and myotendinous tissue

In the physical rehabilitation of a muscle injury, one of the most useful assessments is the establishment of the unilateral strength deficit with respect to the uninjured leg [7]. As we know, muscle injury has a biological regeneration process that will last in proportion to the damage produced. From the readjustment of injuries, we test the unilateral deficit in order to determine if that player is predisposed to go from exercises in shortening (that is, based on the concentric phase of movement) to exercises in muscle elongation (that is, request in the eccentric phase of movement) [8]. The test protocol will be determined by the affected muscles and if we want to perform an assessment at its angle of maximum effectiveness or throughout its entire movement. In the first case, we determine a positioning at the most effective angle of the muscle, and we oppose it with a pressure force gauge with resistance well above the football player's maximum strength capacity (in this case we could use the MMT posture). We record the maximum isometric force value with his injured and uninjured leg. If the unilateral deficit between both legs is < 10%, we could start eccentric work on said muscles. In the second case, we monitor the exercise we use to strengthen the damaged muscles, either with a strain gauge or any other validated record that records the speed or power with which we mobilize the load, both with a damaged leg and with the nondamaged leg, and we also establish a unilateral deficit between both legs < 10%, giving way to eccentric exercises.

How do we calculate the unilateral DU deficit? We use a very simple formula where "IL" is the value obtained for the muscle chain measured in the injured leg and NL is the value obtained for the muscle chain measured in the uninjured leg [7]:

$$DU = 100 - ((IL \times 100)/UL)$$

13.3.2 Tendon or ligament tissue

In our case, when we address tendon or ligament injuries, we do not develop a specific test to determine the evolution of the degenerated tendon or ligament. Our performance is based on the control of the functionality of the tendon or the stabilization of the joint in natural movements of the football player during his game action. In this functionality, the force exerted by the muscles that mobilize said tendon or joint is compared with respect to the contralateral one or with respect to the values it had before the injury (MTT), the fluidity, ranges of movement, and speed of their movements, but above all, there is a strict control of the pain perceived during the proposed mobilizations. It is the perceived pain that guides the progression of the rehabilitation work in terms of strength, range of motion, or speed required in the exercise. For this, we use a verbal rating scale, which categorizes the existence of possible pain between 0 and 10 points, with 0 being the non-existence of pain and 10 being the most unbearable pain that could be suffered [9]. We understand that in a process of readapting a tendon or ligament injury, especially in the initial stages, the football player must live with a certain tolerance to pain during and after exercise and that in no case should exceed level 5 of the verbal rating scale. The evaluation of this pain is carried out throughout the entire process on an ongoing basis. As a reference value, until this pain is reduced to level 2, we do not increase the functional requirements of the exercise in terms of strength, range of motion, or speed. At the same time, in some cases, it is interesting to have a record of the evolution of the specific rehabilitation process. That is why, in the specific case of tendon injury, with a frequency of 2–3 weeks, we fill out VISA-P [10] or VISA-A

[11] if we are readapting from patellar or Achilles tendinopathy, respectively. Or we even select activities to be measured from the patient-specific functional scale in order to adapt to the movements in which the injury we are treating could have a higher incidence [9].

References

1. Loturco I, Pereira LA, Kobal R, Kitamura K, Ramírez-Campillo R, Zanetti V, Cal Abad CC, Nakamura FY. Muscle contraction velocity: A suitable approach to analyze the functional adaptations in elite soccer players. *J Sports Sci Med.* 2016; 15(3): 483–491.
2. Muñoz-López A, De Hoyo M, Nuñez FJ, Sañudo B. Using tensiomyography to assess changes in knee muscle contraction properties after concentric and eccentric fatiguing muscle actions. *J Strength Cond Res.* 2022; 36(4):935–940. doi:10.1519/jsc.0000000000003562
3. Glassbrook DJ, Fuller JT, Alderson JA, Doyle TLA. Measurement of lower-limb asymmetry in professional rugby league: A technical note describing the use of inertial measurement units. *PeerJ.* 2020; 8:e9366. doi:10.7717/peerj.9366
4. Hagglund M, Walden M, Ekstrand J. Risk factors for lower extremity muscle injury in professional soccer: The UEFA Injury Study. *Am J Sports Med.* 2013; 41(2):327–335. doi:10.1177/0363546512470634
5. Kendall FP, McCreary EK, Provance P, Rodgers M, Romani W. *Muscles: Testing and function,* with posture and pain (Kendall, Muscles). LWW, Netherlands, 2005.
6. Cuthbert SC, Goodheart GJ Jr. On the reliability and validity of manual muscle testing: A literature review. *Chiropr Osteopat.* 2007; 15:4. doi:10.1186/1746-1340-15-4
7. Núñez JF, Fernandez I, Torres A, García S, Manzanet P, Casani P, Suarez-Arrones L. Strength conditioning program to prevent adductor muscle strains in football: Does it really help professional football players? *Int J Environ Res Public Health.* 2020; 17:17. doi:10.3390/ijerph17176408
8. Taberner M, Cohen DD. Physical preparation of the football player with an intramuscular hamstring tendon tear: Clinical perspective with video demonstrations. *Br J Sports Med.* 2018; 52(19):1275–1278. doi:10.1136/bjsports-2017-098817
9. Moreno C, Mattiussi G, Núñez FJ. Therapeutic results after ultrasound-guided intratissue percutaneous electrolysis (EPI®) in the treatment of rectus abdominis-related groin pain in professional footballers: A pilot study. *J Sports Med Phys Fitness.* 2016; 56(10):1171–1178.
10. Hernandez-Sánchez S, Hidalgo MD, Gomez A. Cross-cultural adaptation of VISA-P score for patellar tendinopathy in Spanish population. *J Orthop Sports Phys Ther.* 2011; 41(8):581–591. doi:10.2519/jospt.2011.3613
11. Robinson JM, Cook JL, Purdam C, Visentini PJ, Ross J, Maffulli N, Taunton JE, Khan KM; Victorian Institute Of Sport Tendon Study Group. The VISA-A questionnaire: A valid and reliable index of the clinical severity of Achilles tendinopathy. *Br J Sports Med.* 2001; 35(5):335–41. doi: 10.1136/bjsm.35.5.335

14

GENOTYPIC ANALYSIS OF FOOTBALL PLAYERS

Luis Carrasco Páez and Inmaculada C. Martínez-Díaz

14.1   Introduction. Genes and sports: a scientific approach

Sports genomics is a relatively new scientific discipline focusing on the organization and functioning of the genome of elite athletes. The era of sports genomics began in the early 2000s after deciphering the human DNA structure and discovery of first genetic markers associated with athletic performance [1–6].

In all issues of the fitness gene map, endurance performance was a major focus. In the evolution, in the status of the endurance-related phenotypes, the number of articles began increasing from the year 2000. From 2018, more than 1,000 research papers per year have been published, and currently there are nearly 10,000 articles dealing with genes and sports.

Case–control studies remain the most common study design in sports genomics and generally involve determining whether one allele of a DNA sequence (gene or noncoding region of DNA) is more common in a group of elite athletes than it is in the general population, thus implying that the allele boosts performance [7].

Nevertheless, a fundamental resource for understanding the relationship between genes and sports is the series "The Human Gene Map for Performance and Health-Related Fitness Phenotypes." It began in 2001 [8], followed by six updates until the last installment in 2009 [9]. The final update contains tables of all publications with positive genetic associations to performance and fitness phenotypes. It included 214 autosomal gene entries and quantitative trait loci (QTLs) plus seven others on the X chromosome. In addition, 18 mitochondrial genes that influenced performance and fitness phenotypes were cited [9].

DOI: 10.4324/9781032637006-14

14.1.1 But what is a gene?

The gene is the basic physical–chemical unit of inheritance, consisting of the famous deoxyribonucleic acid (DNA), configured as a double helix of paired complementary strands, as deduced by Watson and Crick in 1953. The total DNA of a single cell is approximately 2.5 m in length (if stretched out straight) and 3 billion base pairs. Considering that an estimated 100 trillion cells make up the human body, the amount of DNA is massive. DNA encodes instructions for the development and function of the entire human being, producing the nickname, the "blueprint of life."

The definition of a gene was, until the Human Genome Project, a piece of DNA that encodes the amino acid sequence of a single protein, hence the cliche, "one gene—one protein," and the estimated total of 100,000 genes, the numbers of distinct human proteins. When the entire sequence of all nucleotides found in all nuclear DNA was analyzed, the definition of a human gene has become a physical–chemical one, based on the typical structure of a human gene (Figure 14.1). The estimated number of human genes has been revised downward to 25,000, with the realization that each stretch of DNA can code for an average of three proteins.

A chromosome contains a single, long DNA molecule, only portions of which correspond to single genes. This organization results in all human genes being arranged on 23 pairs of chromosomes in the cell nucleus, in addition to 37 genes which are located in the mitochondria in the cell cytoplasm.

Each DNA strand is made of four chemical units, called nucleotide bases, which comprise the DNA "alphabet." The bases are adenine (A), thymine (T), guanine (G), and cytosine (C). Binding is restrictive and complementary, resulting in a scenario where an adenine (A) on one strand always binds to a thymine (T) on the opposite strand. Similar binding occurs with guanine (G) and cytosine (C).

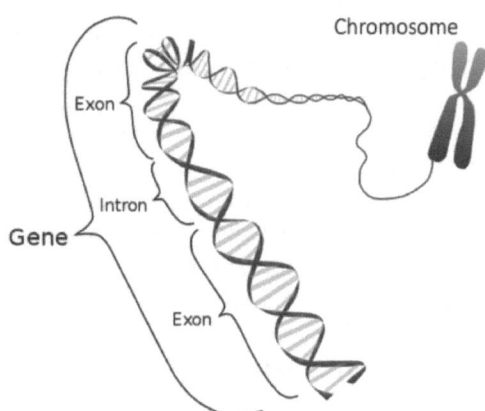

FIGURE 14.1 Human gene structure.

The order of these nucleotide bases (e.g., the As, Ts, Cs, and Gs) determines the meaning of the information encoded in that part of the DNA molecule.

Genes direct the production of proteins with the assistance of enzymes and messenger molecules. Specifically, an enzyme called an RNA polymerase copies the information in a gene's DNA into a molecule called messenger ribonucleic acid (mRNA). The mRNA travels out of the nucleus and into the cell's cytoplasm, where the mRNA is read by ribosomes. The information located on mRNA and read by ribosomes directs the specific linking of various amino acids in the right order to form a specific protein.

Mitochondrial DNA (mtDNA) is a 16,569-nucleotide, closed-circular molecule, located within the mitochondrial matrix and present in thousands of copies per cell. This mtDNA contains 37 genes: two ribosomal RNAs, 22 transfer RNAs (tRNAs) that can interpret the entire mtDNA genetic code (which differs slightly from the nuclear genetic code) and 13 genes that code for key polypeptides in oxidative phosphorylation. Other structural and functional proteins, estimated to be around 1,500, including many that take part in oxidative phosphorylation, are nuclear-encoded, and transported into the mitochondria. While nuclear genes encoding mitochondrial functions follow Mendelian inheritance patterns, genes encoded by mtDNA do not: mtDNA is strictly maternally inherited.

14.1.2   *Epigenetic regulation on gene expression: the role of exercise*

The term "epigenetic" implies changes that can regulate gene expression patterns "on top of genetics," but do not alter the DNA nucleotide sequence itself. Epigenetics is concerned with heritable changes in DNA not determined by the genetic code, but instead by such mechanisms as DNA methylation and chromatin modification. DNA in humans is packaged using histone proteins to form nucleosomes, with double-stranded DNA wrapped twice around an octameric core of four histones (H2A, H2B, H3, and H4) [10]. Chromatin modification involves conformational changes of the DNA–histone complexes, thus enhancing or diminishing transcription. The core histones are subject to posttranslational modification, including methylation and acetylation, and depending on the pattern of modification signals enhance or decrease gene expression.

DNA methylation (in humans restricted to cytosine–phosphate–guanine [CpG]-dinucleotides) is established and maintained by DNA methyltransferases, enzymes that transfer a methyl group from S-adenosyl methionine to the 5′ position of cytosine bases. Generally, methylated CpG islands are associated with gene silencing, as this occurs in imprinted regions of the human genome and in the inactivated X chromosome in females. Although much of the DNA methylation is cleared and reestablished in each generation [11], some DNA methylation marks escape this reprogramming and are transmitted epigenetically for at least three generations [12, 13].

A broad spectrum of environmental factors—such as nutrition, exposure to certain chemicals, emotional challenges, or physical activity—can influence a cell's epigenetic signature [14]. In fact, physical fitness seems to be influenced by epigenetic factors that include 214 gene single-nucleotide polymorphisms (SNPs) in nuclear DNA (nDNA) considered to be potential genetic markers associated with physical capacity [9]. As it has been reported by several authors, exercise training may induce changes in the methylation status of key genes involved in muscle function, thus possibly shaping a long-lasting favorable expression pattern for increased trainability [15, 16].

14.2 Key genes and polymorphisms associated with football performance

In general, observational studies have reported several positive associations between specific gene polymorphisms and football player's status [17–21]. Eynon et al. [17] and Santiago et al. [21] found that one of the most studied gene, the α-actinin 3 (ACTN3) gene RR genotype, and the −786 C allele of the nitric oxide synthase 3 (NOS3) gene were over-represented in Spanish elite football players in comparison with controls. On the other hand, Micheli et al. [20] observed that the ff genotype of the vitamin D receptor (VDR) gene was significantly more represented in young Italian football players than in a matched sedentary population. Furthermore, two independent studies have shown that Spanish and Lithuanian football players have a significantly higher percentage of the ACE (angiotensin I-converting enzyme) ID genotype when compared to non-athletic population [18, 19].

14.2.1 Muscle power: jump and sprint abilities

In their study, Micheli et al. [20] investigated the association between ACE and VDR gene polymorphisms, bioelectrical impedance analysis parameters, anthropometric features, and athletic performance in young male soccer players. One hundred twenty-five medium–high-level male soccer players were genotyped for ACE ID and vitamin D receptor (VDR) gene polymorphisms. Athletic performance was evaluated by squat jump, countermovement jump (CMJ), 2-kg medicine ball throw, and 10- and 20-m sprint time. No correlation was observed between ACE or VDR genotypes and 2-kg medicine ball throw, and 10- and 20-m sprint times. Nevertheless, the ID genotype of ACE was associated with the best performances in squat jump and CMJ.

Explosive strength is a vital predictor for intensive physical effort, and its heritability varies from 74 to 84% [22]. Since skeletal muscles, constituting approximately 33–40% of total body mass, are the greatest and the major site of the metabolism in the human body [23], genes encoding its building particles (e.g., proteins) responsible for maintaining a proper structure and functioning have been considered to be important agents that affect athletic performance [22]. Indeed, α-actinin-3 gene (ACTN3) polymorphism was one of the first that evidenced the association between the genotype and athletic performance [21, 24–26]. Although a number of genetic variants—over 69—have been associated with elite speed-power athlete status [27, 28], the most well-known of these occurs within ACTN3, which encodes for a protein found exclusively within type-II muscle fibers. A common polymorphism within this gene (R577X; rs1815739) results in a premature stop codon, denoted by the X allele. Individuals homozygous for the X allele (i.e., XX genotypes) cannot produce ACTN3. Such an outcome appears to be disadvantageous for speed-power performance [29], as demonstrated by the relative lack of XX genotypes reported in elite speed-power athletes [30]. However, the frequency of the XX-null genotype appears to be higher in endurance athletes than in controls but with contradictory results [31]. In any case, all seems to indicate that the null allele (XX) of the ACTN3 gene is related to a lower sprint/power performance, while RR and RX are associated to a higher sprint/power performance [32].

The study conducted by Koku et al. [33] aimed to determine the distribution of ACTN3 R577X gene polymorphism in soccer players and sedentary individuals and to investigate the relationship of this distribution with performance tests. A total of 100 soccer players and 101 sedentary individuals were enrolled in the study. Standing long jump and countermovement jump performance were recorded. ACTN3 R577X genotype distribution was found to have no effect on sprint and endurance characteristics in amateur soccer players.

Domańska-Senderowska et al. [34] analyzed the ACTN3 gene expression during a 2-month training cycle in soccer players and its correlation with the countermovement jump (CMJ) and squat jump (SJ). The study group consisted of 22 soccer players (aged 17–18). There was an increase in performance of both jumps: SJ ($p = 0.020$) and CMJ ($p = 0.012$) at the end of the training cycle. A simultaneous increase in the ACTN3 gene expression level and height in both jump tests was observed in 73% of athletes ($p > 0.05$). However, there were no significant relationships between the ACTN3 gene expression level and CMJ and SJ performance.

On the other hand, patellar tendon compliance seems to be a key physiological determinant of horizontal-forward jump performance in under 18-year-old (U-18) and U-21 elite male youth soccer players (ESP) [35] and has previously been associated with sprint performance [36]. The COL5A1 (rs12722) SNP has been associated with the extensibility of the tendon-aponeurosis structures of the knee extensors in some [37], but not all [38] studies. Other collagen SNPs, such as COL1A1 (rs2249492) and COL2A1 (rs2070739), which are variants of the genes encoding the alpha 1 chain of procollagen types I and II, respectively, may also influence tendon properties and, therefore, power performance, but this has yet to be investigated.

In contrast to horizontal forward jump performance, one of the main physiological determinants of vertical jump performance in soccer players is quadriceps femoris muscle volume [39]. The NOS3 (rs2070744) T [40] and AGT (rs699) G [41] alleles have both been associated with elite power athlete status and are thought to exert their favorable effect on power performance by promoting skeletal muscle hypertrophy [40, 41].

Maximal power during sprinting and jumping is not only governed by muscle-tendon properties but also neuromuscular activation [39, 42]. Brain-derived neurotrophic factor (BDNF) is a neurotrophin that regulates neuronal survival, growth, maintenance, neurogenesis, and synaptic plasticity, and the BDNF (rs6265) C > T SNP has been associated with BDNF serum concentration in response to exercise [43]. It is possible that this SNP might influence neural adaptation and, therefore, the ability to activate the relevant muscles and generate more power during jump and sprint performance [44]. Furthermore, the AMPD1 (rs17602729) GG genotype has been associated with elite power athlete status [24] and the VDR (rs2228570) GG genotype, on the other hand, has been associated with average- to high-level youth soccer playing status [20].

Recently, Murtagh et al. [44] investigated the association of multiple SNPs with athlete status and power/speed performance in ESP ($n = 535$; aged 8–23 years) and control participants (CON; $n = 151$; aged 9–26 years) at different stages of maturity. ESP and CON were genotyped for 10 SNPs and grouped according to years from predicted peak-height-velocity (PHV), i.e., pre- or post-PHV, to determine maturity status. Participants performed bilateral vertical countermovement jumps, bilateral horizontal-forward countermovement jumps, 20-m sprints, and modified 505-agility tests. The results demonstrated that power, acceleration, and sprint performance were associated with five SNPs, both individually and in combination, possibly by influencing muscle size and neuromuscular activation.

14.2.2   Endurance capacity: VO_{2max}

Some genes that show allelic differences that appear positively associated with endurance athlete status are those encoding the peroxisome proliferator-activated receptors (PPARs). PPARs are members of the nuclear hormone receptor superfamily involved in lipid metabolism and glucose homeostasis. In particular, PPARα regulates expression of genes involved in multiple steps of the lipid metabolism such as fatty acid uptake, transport, and oxidation. Consequently, PPARα shows increased expression in tissues involved in fatty acid utilization such as the liver, skeletal muscle, and cardiac muscle [45, 46]. Moreover, the regulation of expression of this gene may enhance skeletal muscle oxidative capacity in relation to endurance training [47].

With the aim to determine the prevalence of G allele of the PPARα intron 7 G/C polymorphism (rs4253778) in football players, 60 professional players and 30 sedentary volunteers were enrolled in the study conducted by Proia et al. [48]. These authors found variations in the genotype distribution of PPARα polymorphism between professional soccer players and sedentary volunteers. Particularly, G alleles and the GG genotype were significantly more frequent in soccer players compared with healthy controls (64% versus 48%). Although no significant correlations were found between lipid profile and genotype background, the authors, based on previous results, suggested an association of intron 7 G allele as well as the GG genotype in football players.

14.3 Muscle damage, soccer players' injuries, and genes: is there a real connection?

Noncontact muscle injuries are well-described disorders caused in the absence of a direct external trauma. A football professional-level team consists of 25 players can expect 15 muscle injuries each season, with 96% of them occurring in noncontact situations. About 92% of indirect muscle injuries affect the four major muscle groups of the lower limbs: namely, hamstrings (37%), adductors (23%), quadriceps (19%), and calf muscles (13%) [49].

Both physical performance and noncontact injuries are multifactorial domains including many intrinsic and extrinsic factors, which should also include the genetic profile [50, 51]. However, the effect of genetics on muscle injury predictors and neuromuscular performance is scarce in current research [52].

Some authors have shown an association between several genetic polymorphisms, which are located in the ACTN3, MCT1, VDR, and ESR1 genes, and the susceptibility to developing muscle damage and musculoskeletal injuries in professional football players [53, 54]. Among the genetic variants that have a potential influence on the pathogenesis of muscle injuries, one variant of interest is the insertion/deletion (I/D) polymorphism (rs1799752) in angiotensin I-converting enzyme (ACE), the first gene investigated in the context of human athletic performance [55]. Different concentrations of circulatory creatine kinase (CK) have also been observed among the different ACE I/D genotypes after eccentric exercise [56]. Moreover, there was an association of the D-allele with a lower CK response after triathlon [57] and marathon [58] competitions.

In a recent study, 710 male elite football players from Italy ($n = 341$) and Japan ($n = 369$) were recruited for DNA analysis. Genomic DNA was extracted from either the buccal epithelium or saliva using a standard protocol. Structural–mechanical injuries and functional muscle disorders were recorded from 2009 to 2018. In the Japanese cohort, the ACE I/D polymorphism was significantly associated with muscle injury using the D-dominant model (OR: 0.48, 95% CI: 0.24–0.97, P = 0.040). The meta-analysis showed that in the pooled model (Italian and Japanese populations), the frequencies of the DD + ID genotypes were significantly lower in the injured groups than in non-injured groups (OR: 0.61, 95% CI: 0.38 – 0.98, P = 0.04) with a low degree of heterogeneity (I2 = 0%). In conclusion, these findings suggest that the ACE I/D polymorphism could influence the susceptibility to developing muscle injuries among football players [59].

On the other hand, physical performance and the risk of injury have been associated with ligament and tendon properties, which are dependent on individual genotypes. The collagen alpha chain (COL5A1) gene has been associated with mechanical properties of tendon structure in the knee extensors in vivo [37] and tendon and ligament injuries [60]. Specifically, the COL5A1 rs12722 CT heterozygotes have been linked to poorer flexibility than CC and TT homozygotes [61] during a sit and reach test. Peroxisome proliferator–activated receptor alpha (PPARA) and growth differentiation factor (GDF5) genes have been associated with power performance [62], stress fractures [63], and muscle regeneration [64]. Specifically, it has been suggested that PPARA predicts anaerobic trainability [65] and aerobic trainability [66, 67], while GDF5 regulates the response of the proliferation satellite cell [64] (crucial after resistance training), meniscus injury incidents, and knee joint function recovery [68].

As it is well known, the musculotendinous structure plays a key role in the football-related injuries. The collagen tissue quality is genetically determined, among others, by genes encoding collagens, where the COL5A1 gene (rs12722, rs3196378, and rs11103544) seems to play a key role in the probability of knee and Achilles tendon injury and muscle flexibility [61].

The genetic predisposition for collagen production (COL5A1), carbohydrate and protein metabolism (PPARA), cell differentiation, and the transforming growth factor-b superfamily (GDF5) has a potential to determine overuse injuries or complex phenotypes related to tissue properties such as LS or RSI [69]. In this line, the study conducted by Stastny et al. [52] aimed to determine whether the COL5A1, PPARA, and GDF5 genes are associated with muscle functions and stretch-shortening cycle performance in athletes. The CT genotype in COL5A1 rs12722 is a possible predictor of functional movement disruption in the posterior hip muscle chain, causing shortening in the functional bend test and passive straight leg rise, which includes hamstrings' function. The CT genotype in COL5A1 rs12722 should be involved in programs targeting hamstring and posterior hip muscle chain.

14.4 Conclusions and perspectives

Considering the number of human genes (around 25,000) and the millions of DNA mutations, it is difficult to determine the exact genetic fundaments of sports performance. Nevertheless, there are many critical gene polymorphisms that have been reported to have a physiological impact on human performance.

The usability of genomics in football is mainly focused on two principal objectives: on the one hand, to analyze the genomic profile of football players related to muscle power/strength and endurance status, and on the other hand, to identify SNPs or mutations which could be involved in musculotendinous injuries. Regarding the first objective, and although there is not a full evidence base of research, ACE, ACTN3 (R577X), and AMPD1 seem to be genes that are able to modulate the muscle type and size and also the neuromuscular activation needed to high performance in football. In this same line, the PPARα (GG genotype) appears to be related with endurance capacity of elite football players. However, as the predictability of musculotendinous conditions by genetic factors is not sufficiently documented, it is difficult to identify genotypes that could play a specific role on players' muscle injuries. Further investigations should be focused on the influence of the COL5A1 gene on musculotendinous hamstring strain injuries.

Future studies based on genome-wide associations, whole-genome sequencing, and epigenic influence are needed to get a deeper understanding about the genetic effects on human physical ability in general and more particularly on football players' performance. Furthermore, as the number of studies increases, the use of Big Data or artificial intelligence procedures could allow sport scientists to establish optimal athlete gene profiles for different sports that could be used by football managers to select (or even reject) football players according to them.

References

1. De Moor MH, Spector TD, Cherkas LF, Falchi M, Hottenga JJ, Boomsma DI, De Geus EJ. Genome–wide linkage scan for athlete status in 700 British female DZ twin pairs. *Twin Res Hum Genet.* 2007; 10:812–820.
2. Lippi G, Longo UG, Maffulli N. Genetics and sports. *Br Med Bull.* 2009; 93:27–47.
3. Jung H, Lee N, Park S. Interaction of ACTN3 gene polymorphism and muscle imbalance effects on kinematic efficiency in combat sports athletes. *J Exerc Nutrition Biochem.* 2016; 20:1–7.
4. Ostrander EA, Huson HJ, Ostrander GK. Genetics of athletic performance. *Annu Rev Genomics Hum Genet.* 2009; 10:407–429.
5. Buxens A, Ruiz JR, Arteta D, et al. Can we predict top-level sports performance in power vs endurance events? A genetic approach. *Scand J Med Sci Sports.* 2011; 21(4):570–579.
6. Ahmetov II, Fedotovskaya ON. Sports genomics: Current state of knowledge and future directions. *Cellul Mol Exerc Physiol.* 2012; 1:e1. doi: 10.7457/cmep.v1i1.e1
7. Egorova ES, Borisova AV, Mustafina LJ, Arkhipova AA, Gabbasov RT, Druzhevskaya AM, Astratenkova IV, Ahmetov II. The polygenic profile of Russian football players. *J Sports Sci.* 2014; 32(13):1286–1293. doi: 10.1080/02640414.2014.898853
8. Rankinen T, Pérusse L, Rauramaa R, Rivera MA, Wolfarth B, Bouchard C. The human gene map for performance and health-related fitness phenotypes. *Med Sci Sports Exerc.* 2001; 33(6):855–867. doi: 10.1097/00005768-200106000-00001. PMID: 11404647.
9. Bray MS, Hagberg JM, Pérusse L, Rankinen T, Roth SM, Wolfarth B, Bouchard C. The human gene map for performance and health-related fitness phenotypes: the 2006-2007 update. *Med Sci Sports Exerc.* 2009 Jan; 41(1):35–73. doi: 10.1249/mss.0b013e3181844179. PMID: 19123262.
10. Rimoin D, Connor J, Pyeritz R, Krrf B. (Eds). *Emery and Rimoin's Principles and Practice of Medical Genetics, fourth edition.* Published by Churchill Livingston, 2002.
11. Reik W, Dean W, Walter J. Epigenetic reprogramming in mammalian development. *Science.* 2011; 293:1089–1093.
12. Delcuve GP, Rastegar M, Davie JR. Epigenetic control. *J Cell Physiol.* 2009; 219(2):243–250.
13. Gluckman PD, Hanson MA, Beedle AS. Non-genomic transgenerational inheritance of disease risk. *Bioessays.* 2007; 29:145–154.
14. Widmann M, Nieß AM, Munz B. Physical exercise and epigenetic modifications in skeletal muscle. *Sports Med.* 2019; 49:509–523.
15. Pareja-Galeano H, Sanchis-Gomar F, García-Giménez JL. Physical exercise and epigenetic modulation: elucidating intricate mechanisms. *Sports Med.* 2014; 44(4): 429–436.
16. Voisin S, Eynon N, Yan X, Bishop DJ. Exercise training and DNA methylation in humans. *Acta Physiol* (Oxf). 2015; 213(1):39–59.

17. Eynon N, Ruiz JR, Yvert T, Santiago C, Gómez-Gallego F, Lucia A, Birk R. The C allele in NOS3–786 T/C polymorphism is associated with elite soccer player's status. *Int J Sports Med.* 2012; 33:521–524.

18. Gineviciene V, Jakaitiene A, Tubelis L, Kucinskas V. Variation in the ACE, PPARGC1A and PPARA genes in Lithuanian football players. *Eur J Sport Sci.* 2014;14(supl 1):S289–295. doi:10.1080/17461391.2012.691117

19. Juffer P, Furrer R, González-Freire M, Santiago C, Verde Z, Serratosa L, Lucia A. Genotype distributions in top-level soccer players: A role for ACE? *Int J Sports Med.* 2009; 30:387–392.

20. Micheli ML, Gulisano M, Morucci G, Punzi T, Ruggiero M, Ceroti M, Pacini S. Angiotensin-converting enzyme/vitamin D receptor gene polymorphisms and bioelectrical impedance analysis in predicting athletic performances of Italian young soccer players. *J Strength Condition Res.* 2011; 25:2084–2091.

21. Santiago C, Gonzalez-Freire M, Serratosa L, Morate FJ, Meyer T, Gomez-Gallego F, Lucia A. ACTN3 genotype in professional soccer players. *Br J Sports Med.* 2008; 42(1), 71–73.

22. Eynon N, Hanson ED, Lucia A, Houweling PJ, Garton F, North KN, Bishop DJ. Genes for elite power and sprint performance: ACTN3 leads the way. *Sport Med.* 2013; 43:803–817.

23. Houweling PJ, Berman YD, Turner N, Quinlan KGR, Seto JT, Yang N, Lek M, Macarthur DG, Cooney G, North KN. Exploring the relationship between α-actinin-3 deficiency and obesity in mice and humans. *Int J Obes (Lond).* 2017; 41:1154–1157.

24. Cieszczyk P, Sawczuk M, Maciejewska-Karlowska A, Ficek K. ACTN3 R577X polymorphism in top-level Polish rowers. *J Exerc Sci Fit.* 2012; 10:12–15.

25. Pimenta EM, Coelho DB, Veneroso CE, Barros Coelho EJ, Cruz IR, Morandi RF, De A Pussieldi G, Carvalho MRS, Garcia ES, De Paz Fernández JA. Effect of ACTN3 gene on strength and endurance in soccer players. *J Strength Cond Res.* 2013; 27:3286–3292.

26. Kalinowski P, Bojkowski Ł, Śliwowski R. Motor and psychological predispositions for playing football. *TRENDS Sport Sci.* 2019; 2(26):51-54.

27. Ahmetov II, Egorova ES, Gabdrakhmanova LJ, Fedotovskaya ON. Genes and athletic performance: An update. *Med Sport Sci.* 2016; 61:41–54.

28. Maciejewska-Skrendo A, Cięszczyk P, Chycki J, Sawczuk M, Smo´ łka W. Genetic markers associated with power athlete status. *J Hum Kinet.* 2019; 68:17–36. https://doi.org/10.2478/hukin-2019-0053

29. Papadimitriou ID, Lucia A, Pitsiladis YP, et al. ACTN3 R577X and ACE I/D gene variants influence performance in elite sprinters: A multi-cohort study. *BMC Genomics.* 2016; 17:285.

30. Yang N, MacArthur DG, Gulbin JP, et al. ACTN3 genotype is associated with human elite athletic performance. *Am J Hum Genet.* 2003; 73:627–631.

31. Lucia A, Gómez-Gallego F, Santiago C, et al. ACTN3 genotype in professional endurance cyclists. *Int J Sports Med.* 2006; 27(11):880–884.

32. Berman Y, North KN. A gene for speed: the emerging role of alpha-actinin-3 in muscle metabolism. *Physiology (Bethesda).* 2010; 25(4):250–259.

33. Koku FE, Karamızrak SO, Arslan AS et al. The relationship between ACTN3 R577X gene polymorphism and physical performance in amateur soccer players and sedentary individuals. *Biol Sport.* 2019; 36(1):9–16.

34. Domańska-Senderowska D, Szmigielska P, Snochowska A, Jastrzębski Z, Jegier A, Kiszałkiewicz J, Jastrzębska J, Pastuszak-Lewandoska D, Cięszczyk P, Suchanecka A, Wilk M, Brzeziański M, Brzeziańska-Lasota E. Relationships between the expression

of the *ACTN*3 gene and explosive power of soccer players. *J Hum Kinet.* 2019 Oct 18; 69:79–87. doi: 10.2478/hukin-2019-0020.

35. Murtagh CF, Stubbs M, Vanrenterghem J, O'Boyle A, Morgans R, Drust B, et al. Patellar tendon properties distinguish elite from non-elite soccer players and are related to peak horizontal but not vertical power. *Eur J Appl Physiol.* 2018; 118:1737–1749. https://doi.org/10.1007/s00421-018-3905-0

36. Stafilidis S, Arampatzis A. Muscle–tendon unit mechanical and morphological properties and sprint performance. *J Sports Sci.* 2007; 25:1035–1046.

37. Kubo K, Yata H, Tsunoda N. Effect of gene polymorphisms on the mechanical properties of human tendon structures. *Springerplus.* 2013; 2:343. https://doi.org/10.1186/2193-1801-2-343

38. Foster BP, Morse CI, Onambele GL, Williams AG. Human COL5A1 rs12722 gene polymorphism and tendon properties in vivo in an asymptomatic population. *Eur J Appl Physiol.* 2014; 114:1393–1402. https://doi.org/10.1007/s00421-014-2868-z

39. Murtagh CF, Nulty C, Vanrenterghem J, O'Boyle A, Morgans R, Drust B, et al. The neuromuscular determinants of unilateral jump performance in soccer players are direction-specific. *Int J Sports Physiol Perform.* 2018; 13:604–611. https://doi.org/10.1123/ijspp.2017-0589

40. Gómez-Gallego F, Ruiz JR, Buxens A, Artieda M, Arteta D, Santiago C, et al. The −786 T/C polymorphism of the NOS3 gene is associated with elite performance in power sports. *Eur J Appl Physiol.* 2009; 107:565–569. https://doi.org/10.1007/s00421-009-1166-7

41. Zarębska A., Sawczyn S., Kaczmarczyk M., Ficek K., Maciejewska-Karłowska A., Sawczuk M., Leońska-Duniec A., Eider J., Grenda A., Cięszczyk P. Association of rs699 (M235T) polymorphism in the AGT gene with power but not endurance athlete status. *J Strength Condition Res.* 2013; 27:2898–2903.

42. Morin J-B, Gimenez P, Edouard P, Arnal P, Jiménez-Reyes P, Samozino P, et al. Sprint acceleration mechanics: the major role of hamstrings in horizontal force production. *Front Physiol.* 2015; 6:404. https://doi.org/10.3389/fphys.2015.00404

43. Egan MF, Kojima M, Callicott JH, Goldberg TE, Kolachana BS, Bertolino A, et al. The BDNF val66met polymorphism affects activity-dependent secretion of BDNF and human memory and hippocampal function. *Cell.* 2003; 112:257–269.

44. Murtagh CF, Brownlee TE, Rienzi E, Roquero S, Moreno S, Huertas G, et al. The genetic profile of elite youth soccer players and its association with power and speed depends on maturity status. *PLoS ONE.* 2020; 15(6): e0234458. https://doi.org/10.1371/journal.pone.0234458

45. Lemberger T, Braissant O, Juge-Aubry C, et al. PPAR tissue distribution and interactions with other hormone-signaling pathways. *Ann N Y Acad Sci.* 1996; 804: 231–251.

46. Braissant O, Foufelle F, Scotto C, Dauça M, Wahli W. Differential expression of peroxisome proliferator-activated receptors (PPARs): tissue distribution of PPAR-alpha, -beta, and -gamma in the adult rat. *Endocrinology.* 1996; 137(1):354–366.

47. Eynon N, Meckel Y, Sagiv M, et al. Do PPARGC1A and PPARalpha polymorphisms influence sprint or endurance phenotypes? *Scand J Med Sci Sports.* 2010; 20(1): e145–e150.

48. Proia P, Bianco A, Schiera G, Saladino P, Contrò V, Caramazza G, Traina M, Grimaldi KA, Palma A, Paoli A. PPARα gene variants as predicted performance-enhancing polymorphisms in professional Italian soccer players. *Open Access J Sports Med.* 2014; 5:273–8. doi: 10.2147/OAJSM.S68333. PMID: 25525399

49. Ekstrand J, Hagglund M, Walden M. Epidemiology of muscle injuries in professional football (soccer). *Am J Sports Med.* 2011; 39(6):1226–1232.

50. McCabe K., Collins C. Can genetics predict sports injury? The association of the genes GDF5, AMPD1, COL5A1 and IGF2 on soccer player injury occurrence. *Sports (Basel).* 2018; 6:E21.

51. Pearson DT, Naughton GA, Torode M. Predictability of physiological testing and the role of maturation in talent identification for adolescent team sports. *J Sci Med Sport.* 2006; 9:277–287.

52. Stastny P, Lehnert M, De Ste Croix M, Petr M, Svoboda Z, Maixnerova E, Varekova R, Botek M, Petrek M, Lenka K, Cieszczyk P. Effect of COL5A1, GDF5, and PPARA genes on a movement screen and neuromuscular performance in adolescent team sport athletes. *J Strength Cond Res.* 2019; 33(8):2057–2065.

53. Coelho DB, Pimenta EM, Rosse IC, Veneroso C, Pussieldi GA, Becker LK, Oliveira EC, Carvalho MRS, Silami-Garcia E. Alpha-actinin-3 R577X polymorphism influences muscle damage and hormonal responses after a soccer game. *J Strength Condition Res.* 2019; 33(10):2655–2664.

54. Massidda M, Voisin S, Culigioni C, Piras F, Cugia P, Yan X, Eynon N, Cal, CM. ACTN3 R577X polymorphism is associated with the incidence and severity of injuries in professional football players. *Clin J Sport Med.* 2019; 29(1):57–61.

55. Montgomery HE, Marshall R, Hemingway H, et al. Human gene for physical performance. *Nature.* 1998; 393(6682):221–222.

56. Yamin C, Amir O, Sagiv M, Attias E, Meckel Y, Eynon N, Sagiv M, Amir RE. ACE ID genotype affects blood creatine kinase response to eccentric exercise. *J Appl Physiol.* (1985) 2007; 103(6):2057–2061.

57. Del Coso J, Salinero JJ, Lara B, Gallo-Salazar C, Areces F, Herrero D, Puente C. Polygenic profile and exercise-induced muscle damage by a competitive half-ironman. *J Strength Condition Res.* 2020; 34(5):1400–1408. https://doi.org/10.1519/JSC.0000000000002303.

58. Del Coso J, Valero M, Salinero JJ, Lara B, Gallo-Salazar C, Areces F. Optimum polygenic profile to resist exertional rhabdomyolysis during a marathon. *PLoS One.* 2017; 12(3), e0172965.

59. Massidda M, Miyamoto-Mikami E, Kumagai H, Ikeda H, Shimasaki Y, Yoshimura M, Cugia P, Piras F, Scorcu M, Kikuchi N, Calò CM, Fuku N. Association between the ACE I/D polymorphism and muscle injuries in Italian and Japanese elite football players. *J Sports Sci.* 2020 Nov; 38(21):2423–2429.

60. September AV, Cook J, Handley CJ, et al. Variants within the COL5A1 gene are associated with achilles tendinopathy in two populations. *Br J Sports Med.* 2009; 43:357–365.

61. Collins M, Mokone GG, September AV, van der Merwe L, Schwellnus MP. The COL5A1 genotype is associated with range of motion measurements. *Scand J Med Sci Sports.* 2009; 19:803–810.

62. Petr M, Stastny P, Stastny P, et al. PPARA intron polymorphism associated with power performance in 30-s anaerobic Wingate Test. *PLoS One.* 2015; 10:e0134424.

63. Zhao L, Chang Q, Huang T, Huang C. Prospective cohort study of the risk factors for stress fractures in Chinese male infantry recruits. *J Int Med Res.* 2016; 44:787–795.

64. Hatazawa Y, Ono Y, Hirose Y, et al. Reduced Dnmt3a increases Gdf5 expression with suppressed satellite cell differentiation and impaired skeletal muscle regeneration. *FASEB J.* 2018; 32:1452–1467.

65. Aksenov MO, Ilyin AB. Training process design in weightlifting sports customized to genetic predispositions. *Teor Prakt Fiz Kult.* 2017; 6:75–77.

66. Nishida Y, Iyadomi M, Tominaga H, et al. Influence of single-nucleotide polymorphisms in PPAR-d, PPAR-g, and PRKAA2 on the changes in anthropometric indices and blood measurements through exercise centered lifestyle intervention in Japanese middle-aged men. *Int J Mol Sci.* 2018; 19:703.

67. Petr M, Stastny P, Zajac A, Tufano JJ, Maciejewska-Skrendo A. The role of peroxisome proliferator-activated receptors and their transcriptional coactivators gene variations in human trainability: A systematic review. *Int J Mol Sci.* 2018; 19:1472.

68. Ge W, Mu J, Huang C. The GDF5 SNP is associated with meniscus injury and function recovery in male Chinese soldiers. *Int J Sports Med.* 2014; 35:625–628.

69. Maffulli N, Margiotti K, Longo UG, Loppini M, Fazio VM, Denaro V. The genetics of sports injuries and athletic performance. *Muscles Ligaments Tendons J.* 2013; 3:173–189.

15

THE USE OF BIG DATA IN FOOTBALL PLAYERS' EVALUATION

Borja Sañudo Corrales and Moisés de Hoyo Lora

15.1 Introduction to Big Data

Smart Data, data science, machine learning, artificial intelligence, without a doubt, a clarification regarding the numerous terms associated with what has been agreed to call "Big Data" are necessary [1]. Roughly, Big Data refers to the data set whose size exceeds the capacity of conventional database software to capture, store, process, and analyze it [2]. In fact, and while the term "Big Data" seems to be generalized, in its beginnings, it was called "The Petabyte Age", alluding to massive data storage. There is no doubt that in today's society, everything we do will leave a digital trace and, therefore, there are plenty of data that could be used and analyzed. Big Data will offer greater precision and predictive power to numerous domains of the human behavior such as healthcare, business, urban planning, product design, or the sport industry [3]. Consequently, different authors consider that "The era of Big Data has only just begun" [4]. In fact, these authors consider that there is a need for further research on Big Data in general, and the effective use of data in sports is still under development [5].

In fact, it is so in development that we lack even a clear definition of the phenomenon of Big Data. Although the size of the data to be analyzed was alluded to in the previous paragraph, this term has traditionally been described by its characteristics [6, 7]. There are certain characteristics (the so-called three Vs) that must be considered: volume, velocity, and variety [7, 8].

a Volume (magnitude of the data): this term refers to the size of datasets, being able to overcome even zettabytes of data, typically encoded using Extensible Markup Language (XML). This volume will be increased with the addition of different sources (e.g., positioning or physiological data). Therefore, common

DOI: 10.4324/9781032637006-15

solutions for us, such as the use of an Excel sheet, do not usually have the capacity to manage these data.

b Velocity (data production rate): the speed at which novel data are being generated and processed to meet the user's demands. As will be summarized below, different technologies specifically are now available to process and store high velocity data.

c Variety (heterogeneity of data). This term refers to different data formats and data sources that are divided into (a) structured, (b) semi-structured, and (c) unstructured data. Structured data has a clearly predefined schema, and semi-structured data lacks a predefined structure but may have a variable schema which is often part of the data itself, while unstructured data lacks a definite schema (e.g., video data or text messages). Depending on the data type, different storage and analytical methods might be used.

From the Big Data perspective, the data originate from multitude of sources and require continuous processing. This massive volume of data generated by millions of users must be captured, stored, indexed, and processed [9]. In the following section, a brief review of the acquisition and storage is provided.

15.2 Data acquisition and management

As reported above, Big Data requires to effectively collect, organize, and analyze data generated from multiple sources. An important volume of information must be handled, and therefore, the demands for adequate storage capabilities are high [10]. These data are typically collected from multiple sport-relevant resources and can be either quantitative or qualitative. In the sport area, videos, performance data, biographical data, medical reports, or even scouting reports can be collected [11]. Once the data are collected, different metrics are used to standardize, centralize, integrate, and analyze them (Figure 15.1).

With the rise of new technologies and the evolution of wearable technologies, there is an increasing amount of data being generated and transmitted from numerous sensors. Our own mobile phone incorporates a GPS sensor, accelerometers, gyroscope, and proximity or ambient sensors, among others. Therefore, the storage needs of this data are high, and several open source software repositories are available for hosting data sets and facilitate further analysis. Platforms such as Machine Learning Open Source Software (MLOSS) or OpenML can be highlighted and include not just visualization tools or training and test sets but also facilitate reproducible research in *machine learning* [12] integrating applications such as Weka [13]. Machine learning is seen as a subset of *artificial intelligence* and could be defined as the algorithms and statistical models designed on the basis of sample data ("training data") to build a mathematical model able to make predictions or decisions without being explicitly programmed to perform the task [14]. However, prior to providing insightful information, we must be clear on how to

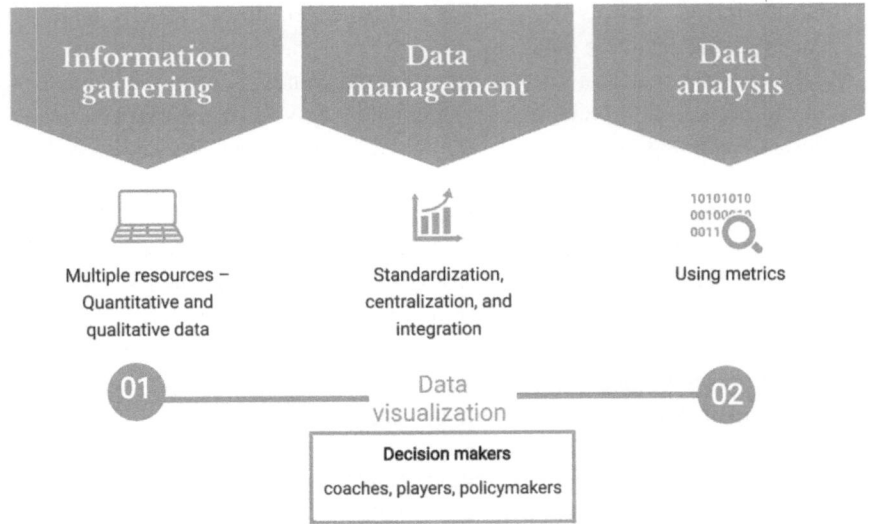

FIGURE 15.1   Data analytics framework in sports (adapted from Claudino et al. [5]).

obtain such information and, therefore, how to collect the data [15]. These artificial intelligence techniques must accumulate the large amount of data and transform them into practical solutions [16]. In this sense, different integrated platforms are being developed to bring together the information from the different technologies, measuring multiple signals at the same time, and often real-time processing. In the next section, different data management software platforms that meet all of these needs will be described.

Brad and Rob Millington entitled a manuscript published in 2015 *The Datafication of Everything* [17]. Authors explored the role of Big Data in sport and postulated that the presence of advanced analytics in this field is a progressive trend supported not just by the proliferation of tracking technologies but also for the desire to monitoring human activity. As stated above, data collected by athletes and teams come from numerous sensors (i.e., wearable devices) including global positioning and accelerometry data (e.g., distance, speed, accelerations, decelerations, changes in direction, and jumping), physiological data (e.g., heart rate, heart rate variability, and energy expenditure), and wellness (i.e., sleep data or feeling of recovery), to cite only some examples [18]. This proliferation of tracking systems in sports and the greater availability of data leads to some sports organizations to invest in the use of Big Data to make faster decisions compared with the past. Performance analysts and exercise scientists have now the difficult task of making sense of these data [19]. Consequently, data science has appeared as a strategical area in sports science aiming to fill some gaps left by traditional statistical methods.

15.3   Analysis of sports data

The classic notational analysis popularized in the 1960s, together with the technological developments in the 1980s, has allowed sports analytics to develop extensively, enabling professionals to objectively assess competitive performance gradually entering from the mid-1990s in the Big Data era [20]. The rise of player tracking technologies greatly increases data availability [21, 22], and examples of data analytics in sports are increasingly common, providing sports teams with insights to encourage data-based sport decision strategies. These advanced data analytics are frequently employed to provide sporting advantages in numerous fields, such as marketing, scouting, and performance [15, 23]. One of the main examples of these approaches is the relationship with the customers, and clubs such as the Manchester City Football Club develop numerous very successful marketing strategies with its clients (e.g., the stadium has a system that interacts with the customers' cards), developing strategies to engage their fans [24]. The Premier League is a benchmark in the use of these data, and they have a very deep analysis of their fans, even analyzing their behavior on social networks (i.e., Facebook) to shed some light about their human behavior patterns, allowing organizations to develop new strategies [25]. These technologies can also be used to facilitate social interactions such as real-time tracking or social sport challenges [8]. Further, the sports betting industry is another key sector where Big Data is used to predict outcomes of future events [11]. In cycling (e.g., Movistar Team) or basketball [26], wearable accelerometer technologies are able to quantify the load; these are examples on how advanced data analyses (Big Data, artificial intelligence, and machine learning) are used to create analytical tools to provide additional team performance knowledge for competitions.

Machine learning is based on artificial intelligence aimed at imitating learning abilities to predict outcomes. It was defined as building systems that learn from data [27]. In order to predict an outcome, both supervised algorithms, which require input and output data to develop a predictive model (e.g., classification and regression), and unsupervised algorithms, based on input data only (e.g., clustering), are used [28]. For example, with the supervised algorithms, we would be able to predict injury risk combining different inputs (e.g., injury and fatigue threshold). We can use conditional variables such as 10 m speed, countermovement jump height, and peak power together with arthro-muscular results to predict injuries (Figure 15.2).

Machine learning approaches are proliferating exponentially in different areas of football including injury risk prevention, tactics evaluation, and player activity assessment; providing knowledge to athletes and sport professionals, supporting their decisions. Platforms such as IBM Watson (https://www.ibm.com/watson), SAP Predictive Analytics (https://www.sap.com/products/analytics/predictive-analytics.html), Qlik (https://www.qlik.com/es-es), SAS (https://www.sas.com/es_es/home.html), or Pentaho BI Suite (https://community.hitachivantara.com/s/pentaho) use artificial intelligence to predict and shape future outcomes. For instance, in the Bundesliga,

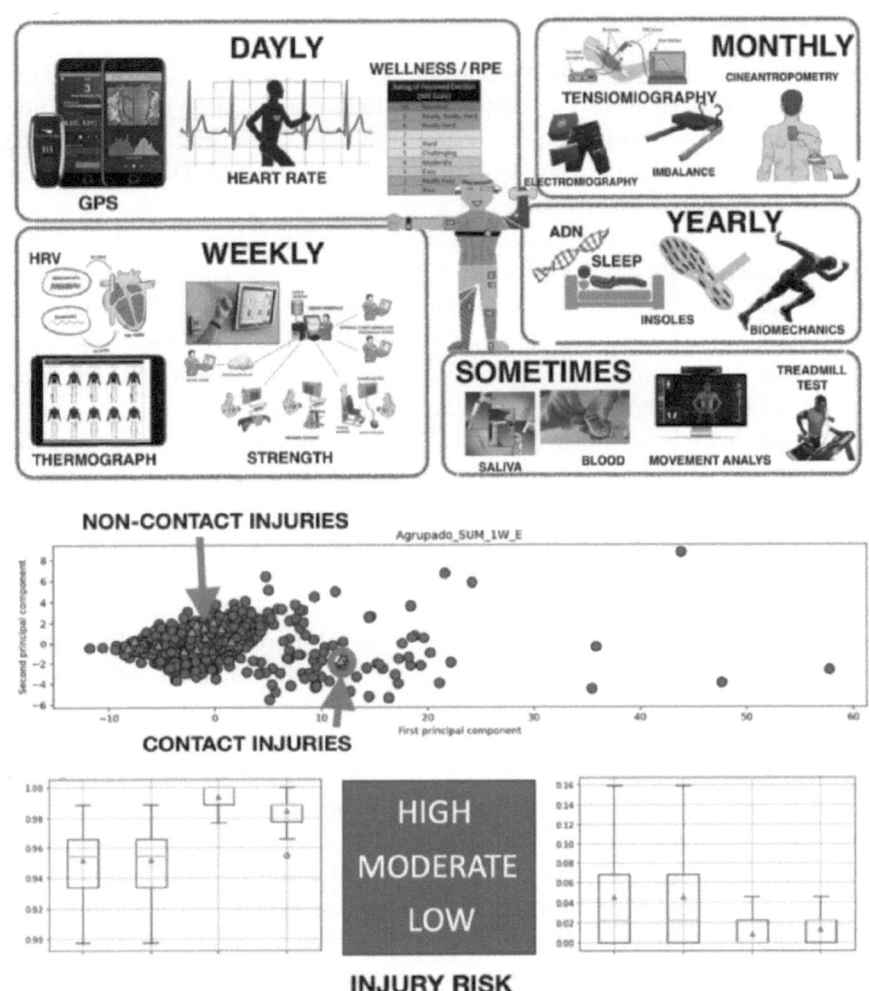

FIGURE 15.2 Example of inputs used to predict injuries using data mining.

TSG 1899 Hoffenheim utilizes SAP to enhance player performance and outcomes, whereas in the Premier League, SAS is employed to analyze team performance.

In football, the players are monitored almost 24 hours a day by wireless sensors technologies that can even be used to track player positions and physiological parameters during competitions [29]. As reported above, different tracking systems are available, allowing analysis of technical, tactical, and physical demands in elite football both during training and competition. Thus, one of the main challenges we face in this area is how to deal with the enormous amount of data. Given the needs of professional football today (time constraints), professionals, coaches, and technicians need highly visual and summary information (Figure 15.3). This is an

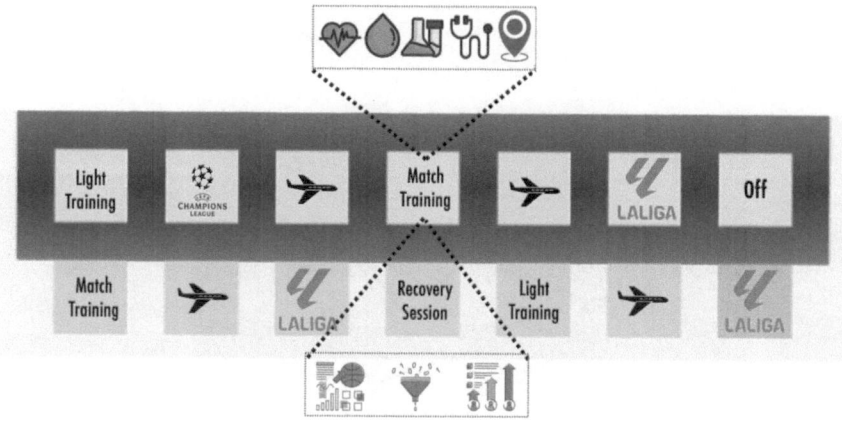

FIGURE 15.3   Quantification of variables and presentation of data during a typical week
in La Liga.

area that has experienced significant growth in recent years, especially in football
[30], and numerous visualization techniques (e.g., digital match tracking, computer
graphics, and image manipulation) are available to improve understanding (visually attractive or useful content).

This technological advance in the football industry would not be understood
without the role of numerous trading platforms such as Opta, Wyscout,[1] Instat,[2]
Kinduct,[3] Zephyr Technologies,[4] Edge10,[5] Kitman Labs[6], or Stats,[7] official data
providers are in charge of collecting, processing, and providing customized pack-
ages of information for clubs, broadcasters, and federations in numerous sports.
These advanced information systems provide the decision maker with numerous types of events, the start and end location of the event, the players who are
involved, or even heat maps and visualizations of ball movements on the pitch
(e.g., Opta Sports), making predictions based on those relationships. Optical tracking or wearable sensors can be highlighted: the first use optical tracking systems
to record the locations of the players and the ball during matches (e.g., Stats LLC
or ChyronHego)[8] and wearable technologies use sensors to monitor the players
(e.g., Catapult[9] or Wimu).[10] Most of these devices include GPS, accelerometer,
gyroscope, or magnetometer, able to provide data on locations, accelerations/
decelerations, and change of direction or jump performed. In some cases, sensors
to assess physiological data (i.e., heart rate) are also integrated. Further, these systems used to be complemented with additional data such as wellness scores (e.g.,
muscle soreness) or recovery (e.g., visual analogue scales or rating of perceived
exertion). Based on these data, sport analysts might develop models for improving
performance [11, 31], predicting the risk of injury [32, 33], or return to play protocols [34]. For example, these companies assist the team's scouting staff in football
or basketball [11], and others like Microsoft Power BI (free in its desktop version)

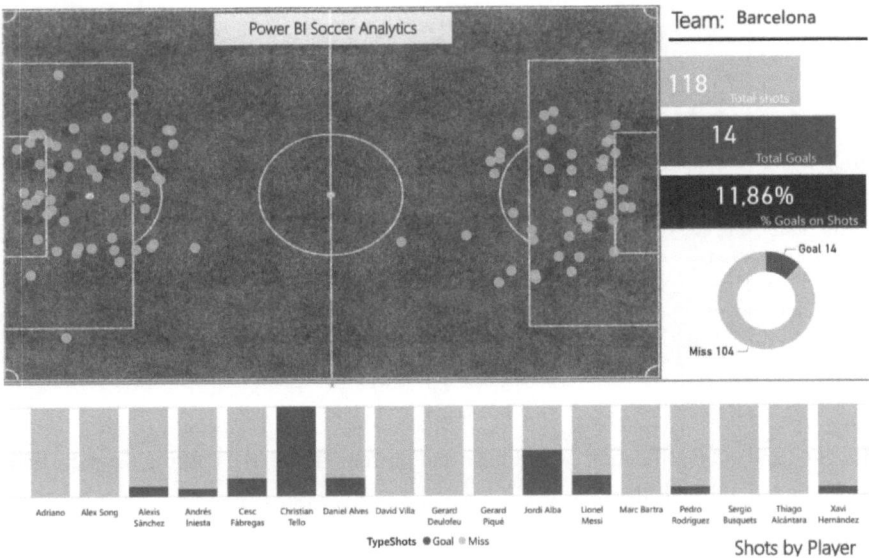

FIGURE 15.4 Example of data representation using Microsoft Power BI.

allow generating very intuitive reports, and it is used by different football clubs at an international level. On the basis of a tool called POP (https://powerbi.microsoft.com/es-es/partner-showcase/pop-pop-sports-science-and-analytics/), data from multiple data sources can be aggregated to understand the impact of training to muscle soreness or how players are performing relative to positional groups. These tools can be integrated with the open source environment R (cran.r-project.org), allowing for deeper data exploration and customization. The analytical tools of R offer statistical techniques and functions to analyze sport data (e.g., time-series accelerometer data). Other common open-source tools (e.g. XML and JSON formats) that incorporate different features to interpret game data and also allow others to analyze their own data are also used by these platforms [35]. With these tools, it would also be possible to analyze what has happened in a game or explore different scenarios of what could happen in a particular moment in the game (Figure 15.4).

15.4 Data analysis in football players: applications in physical performance and injury prevention

Predicting the outcomes of sporting events has been the subject of intensive research for many years; however, and despite the first examples of football outcome prediction in the 1960s [36], to date, few studies have investigated artificial intelligence approaches for football outcome prediction [37]. The availability of data in football is very wide. For example, the Open International Football Database (https://osf.io/kqcye/) contains the match reports of more than 2000,000 matches from 52 football leagues in 35 countries covering the years 2000–2018 designed to use machine learning to predict the outcome of future football matches. Different sport analytics techniques (i.e., machine learning techniques or modern statistical modeling) have been mainly used to predict injuries [18, 38] or to rate overall performance [15]. In a recent review, Claudino et al. [5] proposed to identify which artificial intelligence approaches have been applied to investigate sport performance and injury prevention in sport. Different artificial intelligence techniques were described in 12 different team sports. Among them, 43 artificial intelligence studies focused on sport performance, and the remaining 15 were related to injury risk. The methods used in preventing injuries or enhancing sporting performance mostly include artificial neural networks, support vector machine, decision tree classifier, or Fuzzy clustering [5]. In football, artificial intelligence was used to predict outcomes in different levels (i.e., from academy to professional players) and artificial neural network [39, 40], Bayesian network [41, 42], and decision tree classifier [32, 43–46], fuzzy clustering [47], or K-means clustering [48] can be highlighted (Figure 15.5).

There is increasing evidence suggesting that these approaches can help predict injury by identifying risk factors in sports [18]. Predictions in non-contact injury [46], hamstring injuries [32, 49], or knee injuries [50] have been reported. Injuries used to be multifactorial, and several factors have been identified, usually interacting among themselves, influencing his appearance [51]. Numerous risk factors associated with the occurrence of muscle injuries are being described in the literature [32], and therefore, recent machine learning approaches are able to understand the complexity of injury events by integrating numerous variables [52]. For example, Ayala et al. [49] combined information from numerous risk factors to develop a robust model able to predict hamstring injuries. Accumulated workloads are known to be associated with injury risk [53] allowing coaches and scientist to implement prevention programs. Determining both the internal and external loads of all players during training and match would allow monitoring players' health [23]. Using the systems reported in the previous section let professionals to assess the level of intensity performed by players obtaining information of the external load (e.g., using GPS and accelerometer) or the internal load (i.e., physiological response to the activity) by measuring the heart rate or computing the rating of perceived exertion (e.g., photoplethysmography). For example, we reported that GPSs are being used to measure player accelerations and decelerations, and these outcomes have been used as a measure of accumulated workloads (i.e., acceleration changes and distance covered) in relation with injury risk in elite youth football players in the UK and Australia [54]. Further, they have been used in relation with perceived wellness [46, 55] to improve recovery or optimize training routines.

When a large number of factors are involved, contemporary statistical approaches (e. g., supervised learning algorithms) are applied to predict these outcomes and identify athletes at high risk. In a recent study, López-Valenciano et al. [32] compared different machine learning techniques in order to find the best model for predicting muscle injuries in professional football and handball players.

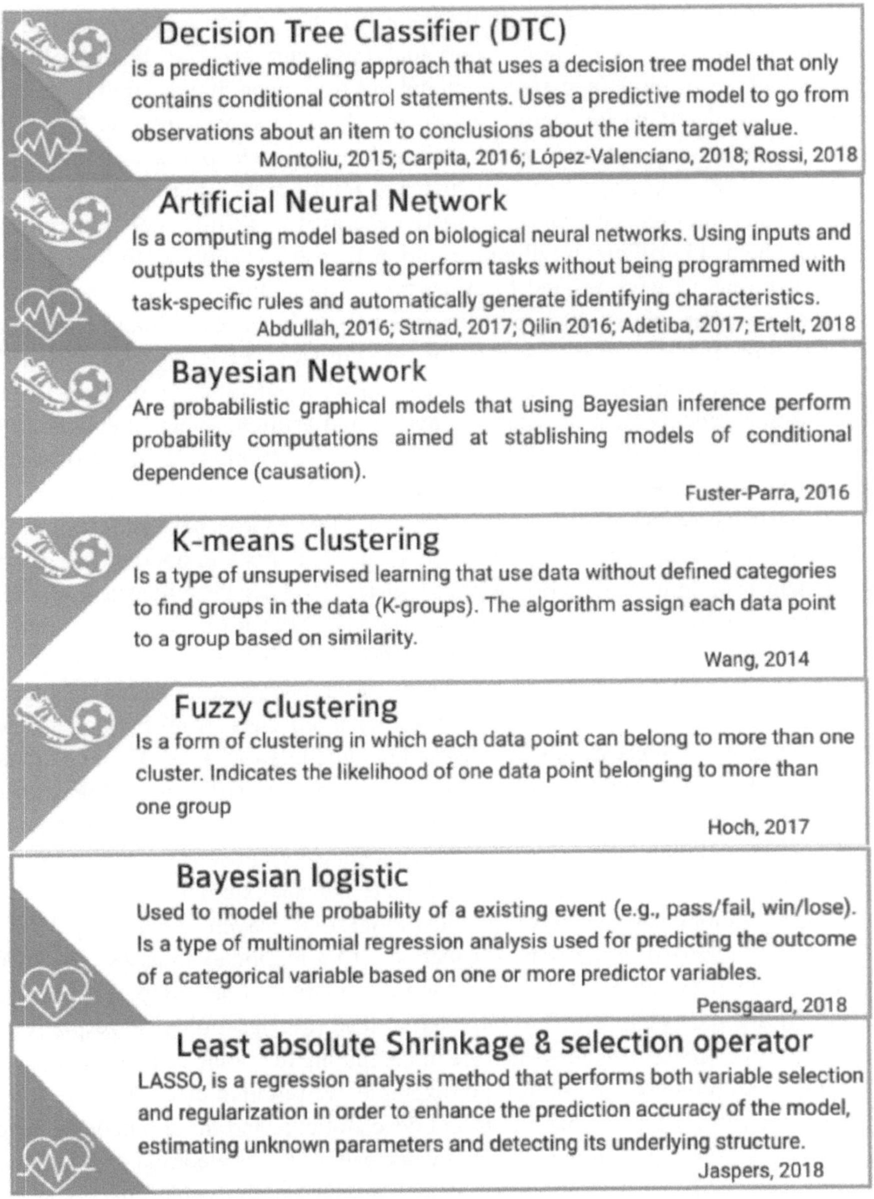

Decision Tree Classifier (DTC)

is a predictive modeling approach that uses a decision tree model that only contains conditional control statements. Uses a predictive model to go from observations about an item to conclusions about the item target value.

Montoliu, 2015; Carpita, 2016; López-Valenciano, 2018; Rossi, 2018

Artificial Neural Network

Is a computing model based on biological neural networks. Using inputs and outputs the system learns to perform tasks without being programmed with task-specific rules and automatically generate identifying characteristics.

Abdullah, 2016; Strnad, 2017; Qilin 2016; Adetiba, 2017; Ertelt, 2018

Bayesian Network

Are probabilistic graphical models that using Bayesian inference perform probability computations aimed at stablishing models of conditional dependence (causation).

Fuster-Parra, 2016

K-means clustering

Is a type of unsupervised learning that use data without defined categories to find groups in the data (K-groups). The algorithm assign each data point to a group based on similarity.

Wang, 2014

Fuzzy clustering

Is a form of clustering in which each data point can belong to more than one cluster. Indicates the likelihood of one data point belonging to more than one group

Hoch, 2017

Bayesian logistic

Used to model the probability of a existing event (e.g., pass/fail, win/lose). Is a type of multinomial regression analysis used for predicting the outcome of a categorical variable based on one or more predictor variables.

Pensgaard, 2018

Least absolute Shrinkage & selection operator

LASSO, is a regression analysis method that performs both variable selection and regularization in order to enhance the prediction accuracy of the model, estimating unknown parameters and detecting its underlying structure.

Jaspers, 2018

FIGURE 15.5 Main machine learning approaches to assess injury risk or performance in football (adapted from Claudino et al. [5]).

Authors aimed at assessing the behavior of the algorithms based on a supervised learning perspective and used a large number of risk factors (i.e., personal, psychological, and neuromuscular) assessed during the preseason training periods and the muscle injuries accounted within the following 9 months. Their ROC analysis demonstrated an AUC of 0.747, and the model developed (Figure 15.6) was able

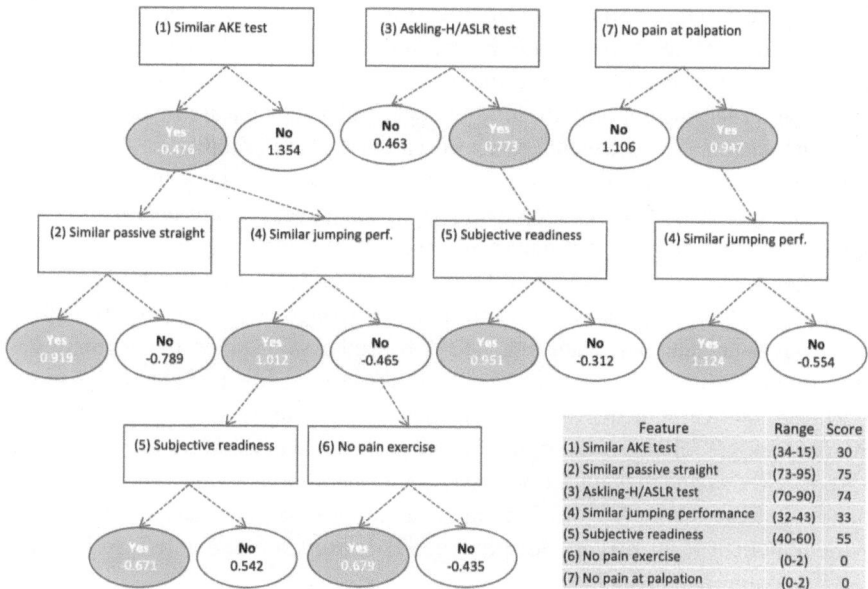

Feature	Range	Score
(1) Similar AKE test	(34-15)	30
(2) Similar passive straight	(73-95)	75
(3) Askling-H/ASLR test	(70-90)	74
(4) Similar jumping performance	(32-43)	33
(5) Subjective readiness	(40-60)	55
(6) No pain exercise	(0-2)	0
(7) No pain at palpation	(0-2)	0

FIGURE 15.6 Graphical representation of the first classifier of the predictive model for muscle injuries.

to show good true negative rates of 79.1% and true positive rates of 65.9%. In the same line, and reinforcing the idea of the multifactorial etiology of muscle injuries, Ayala et al. [49] assessed a model with 229 features that was finally reduced in the final model to 66 considered to be relevant. Authors classified the potential injury risk factors into three main categories (psychological, personal, and neuromuscular) and developed an algorithm with an AUC score of 0.837 and with true positive and negative rates of 77.8 % and 83.8 %, respectively. In the same line, a recent study by Rommers et al. [45] used a machine learning approach to assess injury risk in elite-level youth football players. Authors analyzed a total of 734 players (U-10 to U-15). The generated model was able to identify the injured players with 85% precision (sensitivity: 0.85 and accuracy: 0.85). The algorithm was even able to distinguish overuse from acute injuries with high accuracy.

Studies modeling sports performance mainly implemented the application of predictive analytic models to identify specific data patterns in large datasets, enabling decision makers in gaining a competitive advantage modifying certain aspects of the game [11]. The recent approach for tactical match analysis in elite football try to use machine learning to implement theoretical models by integrating information from different domains including tactics, physiological, or performance data [56]. One of the main machine learning approaches in the football literature are neural networks [31]. These models allow at incorporating a priori information to predict team tactical behaviors. And one of the main features is its capacity to integrate physiological, tactical, and performance-related information. Predictions of performance are mainly applied to monitoring of players actions (i.e., team or opponent tactics) such as scoring opportunities, predicting the probability of scoring based on the features of the shot (e.g., location, angle to the goal) [57] or determine the effectivity of a team creating scoring opportunities [58]. Supervised machine learning has been used to predict whether a shoot would result in scoring a goal in football [59]. Attacking sequences leading to a goal were also evaluated using algorithms able to combine event data type and event location data [60]. Similar results were obtained by Fernando et al. [58] using cluster analysis of game sequences.

Passing behavior has also been the subject of in-depth investigation [61, 62], classifying different types of passes [63] or predicting the success of a pass [64]. Using Bayesian analyses, Wang et al. [62] assessed passing position information in La Liga (Spanish First League, season 2013–2014) and generated a model that was able to automatically identify different tactical patterns across teams. In the English Premier League, changes in physiological performance variables across several seasons and evidenced a significant increase in the number of passes, resulting in changes in team tactics [65]. In fact, other examples look at defense strategies [66] or the opponent team players' locations [59] or team formations [67, 68] mainly based on ball movements [59].

15.5 Conclusions

From the aforementioned evidence, it has become clear that success in team sport (i.e., football) depends on a proper use of data based on evidence-based knowledge. This seems to be an effective manner to develop the decision-making process for injury risk reduction and athletes' performance optimization [69]. To date, these approaches are mainly based on conclusions from relatively small samples of athletes, mostly considering training load variables. Despite this, these analyses would optimize the range of variables required to identify injury risk [49] or scoring opportunities [57], what would considerably optimize training processes. From the sport science and medicine staff perspective, future collaborations with computer scientists are warranted in order to provide a more in-depth application of artificial intelligence models for injury risk assessment and performance prediction.

Notes

1 https://wyscout.com/
2 https://instatsport.com/football
3 https://www.kinduct.com/
4 https://www.zephyranywhere.com/
5 https://www.edge10group.com/
6 https://www.kitmanlabs.com/
7 https://www.statsperform.com/
8 https://chyronhego.com/
9 https://www.catapultsports.com/
10 http://www.realtracksystems.com/

References

1. Memmert D, Rein R. Match analysis, big data and tactics: Current trends in elite soccer. *Deutsche Zeitschrift Für Sportmedizin*. 2018(03): 65–72. https://doi.org/10.5960/dzsm.2018.322

2. Snijders C, Matzat U, Reips U. "Big Data": Big gaps of knowledge in the field of internet science. *Int J Internet Sci*. 2013; 7(1): 1–5.

3. Spaaij R, Thiel A. Big data: Critical questions for sport and society. *Eur J Sport Soc*. 2017; 14(1): 1–4. https://doi.org/10.1080/16138171.2017.1288374

4. Boyd Danah, Crawford K. Critical questions for big data. *Inf. Commun. Soc.* 2012; 15(5): 662–679. https://doi.org/10.1080/1369118X.2012.678878

5. Claudino JG, Capanema DO, de Souza TV, Serrão JC, Machado Pereira AC, Nassis GP. Current approaches to the use of artificial intelligence for injury risk assessment and performance prediction in team sports: A systematic review. *Sports Med – Open*. 2019; 5(1): 28. https://doi.org/10.1186/s40798-019-0202-3

6. Baro E, Degoul S, Beuscart R, Chazard E. Toward a literature-driven definition of big data in healthcare. *BioMed Res Int*. 2015; 2015: 639021. https://doi.org/10.1155/2015/639021

7. Noor AM, Holmberg L, Gillett C, Grigoriadis A. Big data: The challenge for small research groups in the era of cancer genomics. *Br J Cancer*. 2015; 113: 1405–1412. https://doi.org/10.1038/bjc.2015.341

8. Cortés R, Bonnaire X, Marin O, Sens P. *Sport trackers and big data: Studying user traces to identify opportunities and challenges* (November 2014). Retrieved from https://hal.inria.fr/hal-01092242

9. Chen M, Mao S, Liu Y. Big data: A survey. *Mob Netw Appl*. 2014; 19(2): 171–209. https://doi.org/10.1007/s11036-013-0489-0

10. Davalos S. Big data has a big role in biostatistics with big challenges and big expectations. *BBOAJ*. 2017; 1(3): 555563. https://doi.org/10.19080/bboaj.2017.01.555563

11. Morgulev E, Azar OH, Lidor R. Sports analytics and the big-data era. *Int J Data Sci Anal*. 2018; 5: 213–222. https://doi.org/10.1007/s41060-017-0093-7

12. Vanschoren J, van Rijn JN, Bischl B, Torgo L. OpenML: Networked science in machine learning. *ACM SIGKDD Explorations Newsletter*. 2014; 15(2): 49–60. https://doi.org/10.1145/2641190.2641198

13. Hall M, Frank E, Holmes G, Pfahringer B, Reutemann P, Witten IH. The WEKA data mining software: An update. *ACM SIGKDD Explorations Newsletter*. 2009; 11(1): 10–18.

14. Bishop CM. Information science and statistics. *Pattern Recognit Machine Learn*. 2006. Retrieved from https://www.springer.com/gp/book/9780387310732

15. Gabbett TJ, Nassis GP, Oetter E, Pretorius J, Johnston N, Medina D, Ryan A. The athlete monitoring cycle: A practical guide to interpreting and applying training monitoring data. *Br J Sports Med*. 2017; 51(20): 1451–1452. https://doi.org/10.1136/bjsports-2016-097298

16. Mehta N, Pandit A, Shukla S. Transforming healthcare with big data analytics and artificial intelligence: A systematic mapping study. *J Biomed Inf*. 2019; 100:103311. https://doi.org/10.1016/j.jbi.2019.103311

17. Millington B, Millington R. 'The Datafication of Everything': Toward a sociology of sport and big data. *Soc Sport J*. 2015; 32(2): 140–160. https://doi.org/10.1123/ssj.2014-0069

18. Sikka RS, Baer M, Raja A, Stuart M, Tompkins M. Analytics in sports medicine. *J Bone Jt Surg*. 2019; 101(3): 276–283. https://doi.org/10.2106/JBJS.17.01601

19. Rein R, Memmert D. Big data and tactical analysis in elite soccer: Future challenges and opportunities for sports science. *SpringerPlus*, 2016; 5(1): 1410. https://doi.org/10.1186/s40064-016-3108-2

20. Hughes M, Franks IM. *Notational analysis of sport: Systems for better coaching and performance in sport*. Routledge. 2004.

21. Castellano J, Alvarez-Pastor D, Bradley PS. Evaluation of research using computerised tracking systems (Amisco® and Prozone®) to analyse physical performance in elite soccer: A systematic review. *Sports Med.* 2014; 44(5): 701–712. https://doi.org/10.1007/s40279-014-0144-3

22. Lu WL, Ting JA, Little JJ, Murphy KP. Learning to track and identify players from broadcast sports videos. *IEEE Transactions on Pattern Analysis and Machine Intelligence*. 2013; 35(7): 1704–1716. https://doi.org/10.1109/TPAMI.2012.242

23. Berrar D, Lopes P, Davis J, Dubitzky W. Guest editorial: Special issue on machine learning for soccer. *Machine Learning*. 2019; 108: 1–7. https://doi.org/10.1007/s10994-018-5763-8

24. Shreffler MB. Sport analytics: A data-driven approach to sport business and management. *Int J Sport Commun.* 2017; 10(3): 421–422. https://doi.org/10.1123/ijsc.2017-0069

25. Bagić Babac M, Podobnik V. A sentiment analysis of who participates, how and why, at social media sport websites. *Online Inf Rev.* 2016; 40(6): 814–833. https://doi.org/10.1108/OIR-02-2016-0050

26. Schelling X, Torres L. Accelerometer load profiles for basketball-specific drills in elite players. *J Sports Sci Med.* 2016; 15(4): 585–591. Retrieved from https://www.ncbi.nlm.nih.gov/pubmed/27928203

27. Tiwari AK. Introduction to machine learning. In *Deep learning and neural networks: concepts, methodologies, tools, and applications* (pp. 41–51). 2020. IGI Global Eds. https://doi.org/10.4018/978-1-7998-0414-7.ch003

28. Bunker RP, Thabtah F. A machine learning framework for sport result prediction. *Appl Comp Inf.* 2019; 15(1): 27–33. https://doi.org/10.1016/j.aci.2017.09.005

29. Buchheit M, Allen A, Poon TK, Modonutti M, Gregson W, Di Salvo V. Integrating different tracking systems in football: Multiple camera semi-automatic system, local position measurement and GPS technologies. *J Sports Sci.* 2014; 32(20): 1844–1857. https://doi.org/10.1080/02640414.2014.942687

30. Fischer MT, Keim DA, Stein M. Video-based analysis of soccer matches. *MMSports 2019 – Proceedings of the 2nd International Workshop on Multimedia Content Analysis in Sports, Co-Located with MM* 2019: 1–9. https://doi.org/10.1145/3347318.3355515

31. Bishop CM. Model-based machine learning. *Philosophical Transactions of the Royal Society A: Mathematical, Physical and Engineering Sciences*, 2013; 371: 20120222. https://doi.org/10.1098/rsta.2012.0222

32. López-Valenciano A, Ayala F, Puerta JM, De Ste Croix MBA, Vera-Garcia FJ, Hernández-Sánchez S, Myer GD. A preventive model for muscle injuries: A novel approach based on learning algorithms. *Med Sci Sports Exerc.* 2018; 50(5): 915–927. https://doi.org/10.1249/MSS.0000000000001535

33. Shreffler MB. Sport analytics: A data-driven approach to sport business and management. *Int J Sport Commun.* 2017; 10(3): 421–422. https://doi.org/10.1123/ijsc.2017-0069

34. Ekstrand J, Krutsch W, Spreco A, van Zoest W, Roberts C, Meyer T, Bengtsson H. Time before return to play for the most common injuries in professional football: A 16-year follow-up of the UEFA elite club injury study. *Br J Sports Med.* 2020; 54(7): 421–426. https://doi.org/10.1136/bjsports-2019-100666

35. Delibas E, Uzun A, Inan MF, Guzey O, Cakmak A. Interactive exploratory soccer data analytics. *INFOR.* 2019; 57(2): 141–164. https://doi.org/10.1080/03155986.2018.1533204

36. Angelini G, De Angelis L. PARX model for football match predictions. *J Forecast.* 2017; 36(7): 795–807. https://doi.org/10.1002/for.2471

37. Dubitzky W, Lopes P, Davis J, Berrar D. The open international soccer database for machine learning. *Machine Learning*, 2019; 108(1): 9–28. https://doi.org/10.1007/s10994-018-5726-0

38. Carey DL, Ong K, Whiteley R, Crossley KM, Crow J, Morris ME. Predictive modelling of training loads and injury in Australian football. *Int J Comp Sci Sport.* 2018; 17(1): 49–66. https://doi.org/10.2478/ijcss-2018-0002

39. Abdullah MR, Maliki ABHM, Musa RM, Kosni NA, Juahir H. Intelligent prediction of soccer technical skill on youth soccer player's relative performance using multivariate analysis and artificial neural network techniques. *Int J Advan Sci Engin Inf Tech.* 2016; 6(5): 668. https://doi.org/10.18517/ijaseit.6.5.975

40. Strnad D, Nerat A, Kohek Š. Neural network models for group behavior prediction: A case of soccer match attendance. *Neural Comp Appl.* 2017; 28(2): 287–300. https://doi.org/10.1007/s00521-015-2056-z

41. Fuster-Parra P, García-Mas A, Cantallops J, Ponseti F, Luo Y. Ranking features on psychological dynamics of cooperative team work through Bayesian networks. *Symmetry*, 2016; 8(5): 34. https://doi.org/10.3390/sym8050034

42. Link D, Hoernig M. Individual ball possession in soccer. *PLOS ONE*, 2017; 12(7): e0179953. https://doi.org/10.1371/journal.pone.0179953

43. Carpita M, Sandri M, Simonetto A, Zuccolotto P. Discovering the drivers of football match outcomes with data mining. *Qual Tech Quan Manag.* 2015; 12(4): 561–577. https://doi.org/10.1080/16843703.2015.11673436

44. Montoliu R, Martín-Félez R, Torres-Sospedra J, Martínez-Usó A. Team activity recognition in association football using a bag-of-words-based method. *Human Mov Sci.* 2015; 41: 165–178. https://doi.org/10.1016/j.humov.2015.03.007

45. Rommers N, Rössler R, Verhagen E, Vandecasteele F, Verstockt S, Vaeyens R, Witvrouw E. A machine learning approach to assess injury risk in elite youth football players. *Med Sci Sports Exerc.* 2020; 52(8): 1745–1751. https://doi.org/10.1249/MSS.0000000000002305

46. Rossi A, Pappalardo L, Cintia P, Iaia FM, Fernàndez J, Medina D. Effective injury forecasting in soccer with GPS training data and machine learning. *PLOS ONE*, 2018; 13(7): e0201264. https://doi.org/10.1371/journal.pone.0201264

47. Hoch T, Tan X, Leser R, Baca A, Moser BA. A knowledge discovery framework for the assessment of tactical behaviour in soccer based on spatiotemporal data. *Math Comp Model Dynam Sys.* 2017; 23(4): 384–398. https://doi.org/10.1080/13873954.2017.1336634

48. Wang M. Evaluating technical and tactical abilities of football teams in euro 2012 based on improved information entropy model and SOM neural networks. *Int J Multimed Ubiquitous Engin.* 2014; 9(11): 293–302. https://doi.org/10.14257/ijmue.2014.9.11.29

49. Ayala F, López-Valenciano A, Gámez Martín JA, De Ste Croix M, Vera-Garcia F, García-Vaquero M, Myer G. A preventive model for hamstring injuries in professional soccer: Learning algorithms. *Int J Sports Med.* 2019; 40(05): 344–353. https://doi.org/10.1055/a-0826-1955

50. Ardestani MM, Chen Z, Wang L, Lian Q, Liu Y, He J, Jin Z. Feed forward artificial neural network to predict contact force at medial knee joint: Application to gait modification. *Neurocomputing*, 2014; 139: 114–129. https://doi.org/10.1016/j.neucom.2014.02.054

51. Mendiguchia J, Alentorn-Geli E, Brughelli M. Hamstring strain injuries: Are we heading in the right direction? *Br J Sports Med.* 46(2): 81–85. https://doi.org/10.1136/bjsm.2010.081695

52. Chen T, Guestrin C. XGBoost: A scalable tree boosting system. *Proceedings of the ACM SIGKDD International Conference on Knowledge Discovery and Data Mining.* 2016. https://doi.org/10.1145/2939672.2939785

53. Bowen L, Gross AS, Gimpel M, Li FX. Accumulated workloads and the acute: Chronic workload ratio relate to injury risk in elite youth football players. *Br J Sports Med.* 2017; 51(5): 452–459. https://doi.org/10.1136/bjsports-2015-095820

54. Gastin PB, McLean O, Spittle M, Breed RVP. Quantification of tackling demands in professional Australian football using integrated wearable athlete tracking technology. *J Sci Med Sport.* 2013; 16(6): 589–593. https://doi.org/10.1016/j.jsams.2013.01.007

55. Op De Beéck T, Jaspers A, Brink MS, Frencken WGP, Staes F, Davis JJ, Helsen WF. Predicting future perceived wellness in professional soccer: The role of preceding load and wellness. *Int J Sports Physiol Perform.* 2019; 14(8): 1074–1080. https://doi.org/10.1123/ijspp.2017-0864

56. Sarmento H, Marcelino R, Anguera MT, CampaniÇo J, Matos N, LeitÃo JC. Match analysis in football: A systematic review. *J Sports Sci.* 2014; 32(20): 1831–1843. https://doi.org/10.1080/02640414.2014.898852

57. Eggels HPH. *Expected Goals in Soccer: Explaining Match Results using Predictive Analytics.* Eindhoven University of Technology. 2016.

58. Fernando T, Wei X, Fookes C, Sridharan S, Lucey P. *Discovering Methods of Scoring in Soccer Using Tracking Data.* KDD Workshop on Large-Scale Sports Analytics. 2015.

59. Lucey P, Oliver D, Carr P, Roth J, Matthews I. *Assessing team strategy using spatiotemporal data.* Proceedings of the 19th ACM SIGKDD International Conference on Knowledge Discovery and Data Mining - KDD '13, 1366 pp. 2013. https://doi.org/10.1145/2487575.2488191

60. Hirano S, Tsumoto S. *Grouping of soccer game records by multiscale comparison technique and rough clustering.* Fifth International Conference on Hybrid Intelligent Systems (HIS'05), Rio de Janeiro, 6 pp. 2005. https://doi.org/10.1109/ICHIS.2005.53

61. Bekkers J, Dabadghao S. Flow motifs in soccer: What can passing behavior tell us? *J Sports Anal.* 2019; 5(4): 299–311. https://doi.org/10.3233/jsa-190290

62. Wang Q, Zhu H, Hu W, Shen Z, Yao Y. *Discerning tactical patterns for professional soccer teams: An enhanced topic model with applications.* Proceedings of the ACM SIGKDD International Conference on Knowledge Discovery and Data Mining, Sidney, 2015. https://doi.org/10.1145/2783258.2788577

63. Chawla S, Estephan J, Gudmundsson J, Horton M. Classification of passes in football matches using spatiotemporal data. *ACM Transactions on Spatial Algorithms and Systems.* 2017; 3(2): 1–30. https://doi.org/10.1145/3105576

64. Vercruyssen V, De Raedt L, Davis J. *Qualitative spatial reasoning for soccer pass prediction.* CEUR Workshop Proceedings. Riva del garda, Italy. 2016.

65. Bush M, Barnes C, Archer DT, Hogg B, Bradley PS. Evolution of match performance parameters for various playing positions in the English Premier League. *Human Mov Sci.* 2015; 39: 1–11. https://doi.org/10.1016/j.humov.2014.10.003

66. Knauf K, Memmert D, Brefeld U. Spatio-temporal convolution kernels. *Machine Learning,* 2016; 102(2): 247–273. https://doi.org/10.1007/s10994-015-5520-1

67. Bialkowski A, Lucey P, Carr P, Yue Y, Sridharan S, Matthews I. *Identifying Team Style in Soccer Using Formations Learned from Spatiotemporal Tracking Data.* 2014 IEEE International Conference on Data Mining Workshop, Shenzhen, China, 9–14. 2014. https://doi.org/10.1109/ICDMW.2014.167
68. Van Haaren J, Van den Broeck G. Relational learning for football-related predictions. In Muggleton S and Watanabe H (Eds). *Latest Advances in Inductive Logic Programming.* 2014. Imperial College Press. https://doi.org/10.1142/9781783265091_0025
69. Nassis GP. Leadership in science and medicine: Can you see the gap? *Sci Medicine Football*, 2017; 1: 195–196. https://doi.org/10.1080/24733938.2017.1377845

16

COMPREHENSIVE EVALUATION OF FOOTBALL PLAYERS

The biopsychosocial model

Tomás García-Calvo, Jesús Díaz-García,
Ana Rubio-Morales and Miguel Ángel López-Gajardo

16.1   Introduction to the biopsychosocial model in football

Traditionally, football-related analyses have been performed from a conditional viewpoint. It has been been widely explained in other chapters of this book. Meanwhile, the importance of psychological (e.g., motivation or mental fatigue) and social (e.g., group cohesion, team resilience) aspects in football performance has also been demonstrated. Thus, in the present chapter, we are going to highlight the importance of including psychological and social aspects in football players' assessments. Specifically, we are going to integrate these aspects in the contents shown in the rest of the chapters of this book from an ecological viewpoint through the biopsychosocial model.

The biopsychosocial model suggests the importance of synergizing the assessment of the conditional, mental, and social demands to obtain a global analysis of football players (see Figure 16.1). In this model, Blascovich and Mendes [1] indicated that sport situations produce motivational, emotional, cognitive, and physiological responses that players experience during sport situations. Therefore, to obtain an ecological analysis of football situations and an optimal training plan, experts and coaches should assess all these variables. Also, it seems important for this analysis to be individualized.

Concerning the importance of performing an analysis of these variables, previous studies have reported the importance of psychological and social aspects in sport performance. Bangsbo et al. [2] found that coaches may observe a decrease in their players' performance with no physiological explanation, and subsequently, Van Cutsem et al. [3] confirmed the role of the brain in this result. These authors defined the role of emotions and cognitive load in mental fatigue,

DOI: 10.4324/9781032637006-16

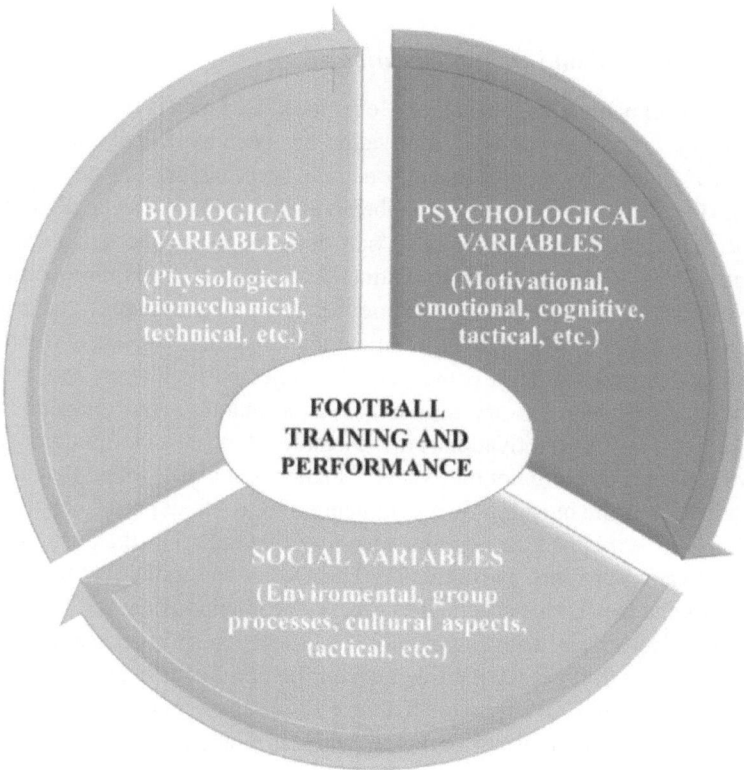

FIGURE 16.1 Biopsychosocial model applied to football.

and McCormick et al. [4] also confirmed the negative influence of mental fatigue in the ratio of perceived exertion. Meanwhile, McMorris [5] indicated that high levels of motivation might decrease the negative influence of mental fatigue in sports performance by increasing the perception of tolerance for effort. On the other hand, Leo et al. [6] observed the importance of cohesion or collective efficacy, highlighting the role of social aspects in football performance. Hence, the need to assess, plan, and train all these mental and social aspects in football players has been widely demonstrated.

Next, we shall present the main psychosocial variables that have been related to performance in football, as well as several instruments to assess them. The information is divided into three dimensions: motivational and emotional, cognitive, and social variables. We will offer information on the conceptualization and evaluation of mental load and fatigue, and we will conclude with some practical applications to start implementing them in a real competition context.

16.2 Main psychosocial variables in football

16.2.1 Motivational and emotional variables

Motivation can explain human behavior. Being motivated means to be moved to do something [7]. In the sport context, motivation has been explained from different perspectives. One of the most frequently used in sports is the self-determination theory (SDT) [7]. The SDT proposes that behavioral regulation can be divided into three blocks, ranging from higher to lower self-determination: autonomous motivation, controlled motivation, and amotivation. Autonomous motivation comprises intrinsic motivation and identified regulation (players who engage in the training sessions and matches for the feelings of enjoyment, pleasure, interest, and satisfaction). Controlled motivation is composed of introjected regulation and external regulation (e.g., players who try to avoid guilt or shame, avoid punishment, or obtain rewards). Lastly, amotivation is the lowest level of self-determination, associated with players who are not motivated. Chamorro et al. [8] found that autonomous motivation is the most highly recommended for football performance.

McMorris [5] explained the neural mechanism that underlies the positive influence of motivation in sports performance. This author suggested that the facilitation system enhances their participation (i.e., catecholamines) in the presence of high levels of motivation, with several positive effects on sports performance like an increase in the effort perception tolerance or the optimization of cognitive processes [9]. Barte et al. [10] suggested that motivation may counteract the negative effects of fatigue in football performance, whereas Slimani et al. [11] noted the importance of motivation in football performance.

Concerning the emotions in sports, they can be caused by specific sport situations (e.g., pre-competitive anxiety, rumination about consecutive or previous failures, or positive emotions associated with success). Anxiety and stress are two of the most researched negative emotions in sports [12]. Slimani et al. [11] suggested that although normal levels of these variables may be positive, over-anxiety and over-stress have a negative effect on football performance (i.e., physiological failures associated with an overload of cortisol). In this sense, the ideal emotional state has been defined as the *flow state*, with strong positive consequences for sport performance [13]. To prepare a competition adequately and get into a flow state, it may be necessary to improve psychological coping skills (PCSs). These were identified by Smith et al. [14] as the mechanisms that are used to help a player navigate mental lapses during practices and games. Previous research has shown that athletes who possessed PCSs exhibited greater athletic success, and the use of PCSs positively predicted athletic performance.

16.2.2 Cognitive variables

Cognitive issues are very important for football practice and performance [15], including variables like perceptual skills, decision-making, and executive functions.

In the field of research on perceptual skills in football, the psychological variables of attention and concentration stand out as they influence the coding of external and internal stimuli and the selection, organization, and execution of the motor response [16]. Various authors emphasize that attentional processes are determinants of competitive success or failure in football [17]. Also, several studies have shown that visual attention has a positive impact on the variety of rare and flexible decisions in team sports [18].

Decision-making is defined as the ability to select and execute an appropriate action in a given situation, taking into account the available time [19]. It is based on the players' ability to notice and integrate mobile information on the field, as well as their actions. It is also related to specific knowledge of sports and tactical mastery. Therefore, it is also influenced by perceptual-cognitive skills, like attention and concentration. Within decision-making, anticipation, defined as the performer's ability to predict what is likely to happen before it occurs [20], has been widely studied. Anticipation is closely related to visual behavior and is characterized as an essential ability in football because football is played in environments with a deficit of time and space. Several studies have confirmed that skilled football players have a higher ability to anticipate and make decisions than less skilled players [21]. These players execute visual strategies that imply few visual fixations, albeit of great duration, which are assumed to be more effective to initiate a prompt and precise response.

Lastly, executive functions (EFs) are a set of cognitive processes that are affected by social, emotional, and physical variables. EFs are necessary for the cognitive control of behavior, as well as to execute effective and creative behaviors. They can be divided into core and higher-order EFs. Core EFs comprise three sub-functions: working memory (monitoring, manipulating, and updating online information), cognitive flexibility (ability to flexibly switch between different mental operations or schemas), and inhibitory control (ability to deliberately control or inhibit the production of predominant automatic responses when the situation requires it). Higher-order EFs, which are based on the core EFs, comprise reasoning, problem-solving, and planning. It has been shown that elite youth football players have better inhibitory control, cognitive flexibility, and higher-order EFs than sub-elite players [22]. In addition, Vestberg et al. [23] found a significant correlation between the results of the EF test and the number of goals and assists the top-football players scored two seasons later.

16.2.3 Social variables

Considering that football is a collective sport, where players are nested in sports teams, it is very important to know how the players interact with each other. In this regard, psychological group processes may be one of the triggers of the achievement of sports objectives [24]. Numerous variables have shown a relationship with team performance and can help optimize collective functioning.

First, we shall examine variables that have a closer relationship with social aspects (union, friendship, interpersonal relationships, etc.), such as group cohesion [25], intra-group conflict [26], social identity, or team identification and social belonging [27]. The construct of group cohesion is made up of two main dimensions: (a) task cohesion, which reflects the degree to which team members work together to achieve common purposes, and (b) social cohesion, which reflects the degree to which team members have empathy toward each other and enjoy comradeship within the group [24]. These dimensions have different effects on performance, depending on the context in which the performers play. In performance contexts, it seems that task cohesion has a closer relationship with team performance, whereas social aspects are more relevant when players interact in more recreational or educational contexts [24]. If players feel integrated and identify with their team, they will be more united and will achieve better performance.

Second, some variables are related to teamwork and the functions of each player, such as the team's mental model [28], roles [29], transactive memory system [30], team work [31], and team resilience [32]. All these variables have been associated with better performance in different contexts. For example, it has been shown that teams that trust the group's skills the most during competitions [33] were better organized and coordinated, work better as a team [6], are better prepared to resolve adverse situations [32], and more likely to achieve higher performance.

Finally, the leadership behaviors, both the coach's (coach leadership; 34) and the players' (athlete leadership; 27), are related to the team's behavior, and they affect other players. Specifically, good coach and athlete leadership have been associated with higher satisfaction with team performance [35]. Thus, when team leaders perform their functions well, remembering which tasks must be performed, supporting their players on the field, promoting positive group relationships, and managing external aspects, the team will be more likely to perform well. Also, coaches should promote athlete leadership as it improves individual and team performance in team sports [35].

16.3 Instruments and procedures for psychosocial evaluation

In football, to measure the psychosocial aspect, different instruments and procedures have been used, such as questionnaires, observation, or technologies, from a quantitative [33] and qualitative [32] perspective. Next, we will review some of these tools generated for each of the relevant variables from the biopsychosocial model.

16.3.1 Motivational and emotional variables

Several instruments have been designed to quantify the motivational and emotional variables. To measure the motivational aspect, the Behavioral Regulation in Sport

Questionnaire (BRSQ: 36), the adaptation of the Motivational Questionnaire in Sport Context [37], or the Coach Interpersonal Style Observational System [38] analyze motivation types and the coaches' motivational support.

On the other hand, there are several options to quantify emotions. For example, the Competitive Anxiety Inventory 2 (CSAI-2: 39) or the State-Trait Anxiety Inventory (STAI: 40) were developed to measure anxiety. Meanwhile, the CSAI-2 was mainly oriented for concentration, and the STAI allows to obtain the effects of anxiety on self-confidence.

To study the flow state, the most frequently used measure is the Flow State Scale-2 [41]. Regarding coping skills, Smith et al. [14] developed the Athletic Coping Skills Inventory-28 (ACSI-28) to explore athletes' use of seven skills (i.e., coping with adversity, peaking under pressure, goal-setting preparation, concentration, freedom from worry, confidence, and coachability).

16.3.2 Cognitive variables

Referring to the evaluation of cognitive variables in football, some of the instruments mentioned in the evaluation of motivational variables include perceptual variables that can be measured through them, such as concentration. In addition, other instruments have been developed for the study of attention, like the eye-tracker device, which detects and records the player's visual fixations at all times and in all game actions [42] and with which the pupillometry technique is used to investigate attention effort, or the allocation of attention resources during the quiet eye phenomenon (QE), which is the time that elapses between the last fixation on a specific goal and the subsequent initiation of a motor response relevant to athletes [43]. It should be noted that visual fixations are also studied to analyze their subsequent relationship with the ability to anticipate.

Continuing with the evaluation of decision-making, it has long been characterized by limitations related to its methodology. In this sense, we emphasize that more coherent and representative protocols concerning players' real performance in match contexts should be applied. For example, the System of Tactical Assessment in Football (FUT-SAT; 44), which assesses the main defensive and offensive tactical principles of football. Machado and da Costa [45] have also recently developed and validated the TacticUP video test, which contains video sequences in which the subject is shown situations of 11 versus 11 of each tactical principle, both in offensive and defensive phases. For each scene, participants had to choose the most appropriate solution from four possible options.

Ending with the evaluation of executive functions, we highlight the following instrument: (a) the Stroop Test, which measures inhibitory control and information processing speed/accuracy [46]; (b) the Design Fluency Test (DFT), which evaluates planning, cognitive flexibility, creativity, and working memory [47]; and (c) the Trail Making Test (TMT) to measure the cognitive domains of processing speed, sequencing, mental flexibility, and visual-motor skills [48].

16.3.3 Social variables

To measure the interactions between players, questionnaires have been the most used by researchers in the scientific literature, through the quantitative methodology. For example, to measure group cohesion, different measurement instruments have been developed, among which is highlighted the Group Environment Questionnaire (GEQ), originally developed and validated by Carron et al. [49]. This original questionnaire has been adapted to various languages, for instance, to Portuguese [50], Spanish [51], or French [52].

On the other hand, as team sports are characterized by a multifactorial structure, access to the information can be difficult. In this vein, qualitative research can be particularly helpful to increase our knowledge about team performance [53]. To extract information about the players' opinions of the relevant interactions to achieve sporting success, semi-structured interviews have been conducted to analyze their personal experiences [26].

In addition, other techniques are the sociogram and the ludogram. They are useful to determine the preferences of the members of a group concerning different stimuli-people that are part of their environment [54]. Also, they are used to determine the relationships among members of a group, their intensity, the position of each member with the others, or the informal structure they present as a collective [55]. Ludograms are very useful tools to analyze the relationships among players, and they are used through games and recreational activities within training sessions. In the scientific literature, these tools are also known as network analysis [35].

16.4 Mental load and mental fatigue in football: conceptualization and evaluation from a biopsychosocial perspective

Taking into account the global assessment and applications proposed by the biopsychosocial model, we shall now present the effects of these variables on football training and competition load. Conditional load in football is caused by movements, skills, or shots, among others. Although motivation, cognitive, or social aspects also influence physical load, the specific load caused by these variables is the mental load, which produces mental fatigue. Mental and physical fatigue synergize in the football context. Therefore, as other chapters of this book have defined the physical aspects, we shall explain mental load and fatigue in football.

Mental fatigue could be defined as a psychobiological state caused by emotional or cognitive demands with subjective (i.e., higher feelings of fatigue), behavioral (i.e., reaction time impairments), and physiological (i.e., alterations in EEG) outcomes [56]. It has been shown that mental fatigue impairs technical accuracy [57] and tactical decisions [58], through the impairment of cognitive processes. Also, mental fatigue impairs physical performance in football players by an increase in the reported perception of effort [58]. Coutinho et al. [59] performed a global analysis of the influence of mental fatigue on football performance. These authors reported that mental fatigue increased the feelings of fatigue in football players, and, consequently, these players decreased the distance between team-mates, producing poor tactical performances. Therefore, we conclude that mental fatigue impairs football performance.

Various instruments have been designed to assess mental fatigue. For example, to quantify players' reported subjective mental fatigue, the most employed instrument is the Visual Analog Scale. Since, there may be a large variation instruments for the analysis of the behavioral consequences of mental fatigue. For example, the Psychomotor Vigilance Task may be used to quantify the influence of mental fatigue on reaction time. The effect of mental fatigue on sleep can be included as a behavioral response either through subjective (i.e., Pittsburgh Sleep Quality Index) or objective (i.e., tracking bands) measures. Indeed, the technical or tactical performance may be included as behavioral consequences of mental fatigue. Both subjective and behavioral aspects have been mainly used in football because physiological variables are difficult to implement in this context (i.e., expensive, long time to obtain results, and they could not be implemented in real conditions). From a physiological viewpoint, blood samples of cortisol, testosterone, and adenosine, and the implementation of electroencephalography have been the variables most used in this topic. Specifically, the accumulation of adenosine seems a good candidate to explain the effects of mental fatigue on the ratio of perceived exertion.

Less information has been provided about the causes of mental fatigue. Similar to physical fatigue, where physical efforts have been defined as the causes of physical fatigue, there is an increasing interest in the term "mental load" in the football context. García-Calvo et al. [60] defined mental load in football as the mental effort necessary to solve the objective of the tasks in a certain period of time, influenced by physical, cognitive, and emotional aspects. However, this variable is more difficult to assess than mental fatigue. The main instrument used to quantify mental load in football has been the NASA-Task Index Load, an instrument adapted from the psychology of organizations. However, this instrument is not specific to the sport context. To quantify the specific mental load, Díaz-García et al. [61] validated the Questionnaire to Quantify the Mental Load in Team Sports. These authors designed a four-item questionnaire to measure the physical, cognitive, emotional, and interdependence efforts.

16.5 Practical applications

Starting from an ecological training perspective, it seems logical to think that the inclusion of psychobiological and social factors is essential to achieve an adequate adaptation to competition. Thus, it is not possible to develop a certain workload from the physiological perspective, without taking into account the players' cognitive, emotional, affective, or motivational situation, and including these variables holistically in training sessions. It is also necessary to control and evaluate these variables comprehensively, to know their levels and impact on athletes' behavior and performance as much as possible.

Returning to the ideas of the psychobiological model, football players analyze (i) the perceived complexity of the situation and (ii) their self-confidence to resolve it. As such, higher levels of motivation and positive emotions can enhance players' participation in a perceived challenge. For this purpose, coaches may also need to present negative emotions or performance failures during football training. Díaz-García et al. [62] indicate that coaches should imagine the perceptions or analysis that players are going to perform about the next match to planning the psychological and social aspects. If they are going to identify the next match as a challenge, coaches should reinforce this with the tasks of the week. On the contrary, if they are going to identify it as a threat (or like a very easy match), coaches should re-educate them, for example, by the implementation of negative emotions.

In this sense, the main problem associated with mental load and fatigue (and other psychological and social variables) in the football studies performed is that most of these studies did not use an ecological manipulation of these variables. Based on Martin et al. [59], the treatment of mental load and fatigue should imply ecological contexts and football-specific strategies. Thus, coaches should manipulate the mental load and fatigue by designing a sport-specific context. Constraints are a widely used strategy for this purpose.

Coaches may vary the mental load of football tasks by constraints to cause more or fewer difficulties in the tasks. Specifically, more difficulties in the tasks (i.e., high number of players) lead to higher cognitive efforts. However, less is known about the influence of constraints on mental responses. García-Calvo et al. [60] found higher levels of mental fatigue in non-oriented football tasks than in oriented tasks in female football players. The explanation of this result was that higher levels of entropy and uncertainty increase mental load and fatigue. García-Calvo et al. [60] also studied the impact of modifying the punctuation system as a constraint. These authors reported higher levels of mental load and fatigue when score a goal in the first (×2) or final (×3) minutes of the tasks had a higher impact in the score than in normal condition (×1 during the full task). This could also be caused by the uncertainty or higher values of attention during the first of final minutes. Díaz-García et al. [62] also reported higher values of mental load and fatigue when coaches used general positive advice than when coaches did not participate. The main explanation is that coaches' advice was perceived as judgments, although it was positive.

In conclusion, the information provided by these previous studies allows coaches to manipulate the psychological and social load according to their objectives. For example, when one team is going to play versus another very important team, certain players could perceive this match as a threat. In this case, the use of the normal football score or positive feedback may reduce the mental load of these players. On the contrary, if this team is going to play versus a team with poor results, certain players may perceive this match like an easy challenge; meanwhile this idea could cause performance decreases associated to an increase in self-confidence and relaxation. In this case, the use of constraints that enhance the mental load could enhance the participation of the facilitation system, improving the performance.

With respect to the planning of evaluation, it is necessary to differentiate those evaluations that are necessary for the daily control of the training load from those that allow us to determine generic aspects from the biopsychosocial perspective. The assessment of more specific variables (e.g., cognitive state) is recommended at specific times of the season to gain knowledge of the players' psychosocial processes, which complements observation and other measures (e.g., start, mid-, and end of the season). For this purpose, besides the instruments used to assess these issues, it is necessary to determine when these variables are going to be evaluated and to plan appropriately throughout the season.

With respect to the daily measure of these aspects, the assessment of mental load and fatigue, complemented with the quantification of the physical load, can help us control the level of global demand of training and competition, as well as to modulate the training load and adapt it to the athletes' needs. This reveals the importance of complementing the data of the most complex assessment systems (i.e., GPS and VTS) with the athletes' perceptions [63]. Evaluating these variables is quite simple, affording an acceptable control of the players' workload perception (e.g., mental fatigue). The first thing to note is that players should not be overloaded with a multitude of measures, so it is usually more advisable to use observational instruments or those that do not involve excessive additional effort for the athletes. Meanwhile, mental fatigue is normally measured both at the start and at the end of the training session, and mental load is normally quantified at the end.

References

1. Blascovich J, Mendes WB. Challenge and threat appraisals: The role of affective cues. In J. Forgas (Ed.), *Feeling and thinking: The role of affect in social cognition* (pp. 59–82). Cambridge University Press, 2000.
2. Bangsbo J, Iaia FM, Krustrup P. Metabolic response and fatigue in soccer. *International Journal of Sports Physiology and Performance* 2007; 2(2): 111–127.
3. Van Cutsem J, Roelands B, Pluym B, Tassignon B, Verschueren JO, DE Pauw K, Meeusen R. Can creatine combat the mental fatigue-associated decrease in visuomotor skills? *Medicine and Science in Sports and Exercise* 2020; 52(1): 120–130.
4. McCormick A, Meijen C, Marcora S. Psychological determinants of whole-body endurance performance. *Sports Medicine* 2015; 45(7): 997–1015.
5. McMorris T. Cognitive fatigue effects on physical performance: The role of interoception. *Sports Medicine* 2020; 50(10): 1703–1708.
6. Leo FM, González-Ponce I, García-Calvo T, Sánchez-Oliva D. The relationship among cohesion, transactive memory systems, and collective efficacy in professional soccer teams: A multilevel structural equation analysis. *Group Dynamics: Theory, Research, and Practice* 2019; 23: 44–56.
7. Deci EL, Ryan RM. The "what" and "why" of goal pursuits: Human needs and the self-determination of behavior. *Psychological Inquiry* 2000; 11: 227–268.

8. Chamorro JL, Moreno R, García-Calvo T, Torregrosa M. The influence of basic psychological needs and passion in promoting elite young football players'development. *Frontiers in Psychology* 2020; 11: 570–584.

9. Herlambang MB, Taatgen NA, Cnossen F. The role of motivation as a factor in mental fatigue. *Human Factors* 2019; 61(7): 1171–1185.

10. Barte J, Nieuwenhuys A, Geurts S, Kompier M. Motivation counteracts fatigue-induced performance decrements in soccer passing performance. *Journal of Sports Sciences* 2019; 37(10): 1189–1196.

11. Slimani M, Bragazzi NL, Tod D, Dellal A, Hue O, Cheour F, Taylor L, Chamari K. Do cognitive training strategies improve motor and positive psychological skills development in soccer players? Insights from a systematic review. *Journal of Sports Sciences* 2016; 34(24): 2338–2349.

12. Thompson CJ, Noon M, Towlson C, Perry J, Coutts AJ, Harper LD, Skorski S, Smith MR, Barrett S, Meyer T. Understanding the presence of mental fatigue in English academy soccer players. *Journal of Sports Sciences* 2020; 38(13): 1524–1530.

13. García-Calvo T, Cervelló-Gimeno E, Jiménez-Castuera R, Iglesias-Gallego D, Santos-Rosa FJ. La implicación motivacional de jugadores jóvenes de fútbol y su relación con el estado de flow y la satisfacción en competición. *Revista de Psicología del Deporte* 2005; 14(1): 21–42.

14. Smith RE, Schutz RW, Smoll FL, Ptacek JT (1995). Development and validation of a multidimensional measure of sport-specific psychology skills: The Athletic Coping Skills Inventory-28. *Journal of Sport and Exercise Psychology* 1995; 17: 379–398.

15. Cappuccio ML. *Handbook of embodied cognition and sport psychology*. The MIT Press, 2019.

16. González-Campos G, Valdivia-Moral P, Cachón Zagalaz J, Romero Ramos O. La motivación y la atención-concentración en futbolistas. Revisión de Estudios. *SPORT TK-Revista EuroAmericana de Ciencias Del Deporte* 2016; 5(2): 77.

17. De la Vega R. Principales consideraciones acerca del entrenamiento de la concentración en el fútbol. *Lecturas de Educación Física y Deportes* 2003. Recovered from https://www.efdeportes.com/efd60/atencion.htm

18. Memmert D. Sports and creativity. In M. A. Runco & S. R. Pritzker (Eds.), *Encyclopedia of creativity* (2nd ed., pp. 373–378). Academic Press. 2017.

19. Williams AM, Ford PR, Eccles DW, Ward P. Perceptual-cognitive expertise in sport and its acquisition: Implications for applied cognitive psychology. *Applied Cognitive Psychology* 2011; 25: 432–442. https://doi.org/10.1002/acp.1710

20. Roca A, Williams AM, Ford PR. Developmental activities and the acquisition of superior anticipation and decision making in soccer players. *Journal of Sports Sciences* 2012; 30(15): 1643–1652.

21. Vaeyens R, Lenoir M, Williams AM, Mazyn L, Philippaerts RM. Mechanisms underpinning successful decision making in skilled youth soccer players: An analysis of visual search behaviours. *Journal of Motor Behavior* 2007; 39: 395–408.

22. Huijgen BCH, Leemhuis S, Kok NM, Verburgh L, Oosterlaan J, Elferink-Gemser MT, Visscher C. Cognitive functions in elite and sub-elite youth soccer players aged 13 to 17 years. *PLOS ONE* 2015; 10(12): e0144580.

23. Vestberg T, Gustafson R, Maurex L, Ingvar M, Petrovic P. Executive functions predict the success of top-soccer players. *PLoS ONE* 2012; 7(4): e34731.

24. Carron AV, Colman MM, Wheeler J, Stevens D (2002). Cohesion and performance in sport: A meta analysis. *Journal of Sport and Exercise Psychology* 2002; 24: 68–188.

25. Leo FM, Sánchez-Miguel PA, Sánchez-Oliva D, Amado D, García-Calvo T. Analysis of cohesion and collective efficacy profiles for the performance of soccer players. *Journal of Human Kinetics* 2013; 39: 221–229.
26. Paradis KF, Carron AV, Martin LJ. Athlete perceptions of intra-group conflict in sport teams. *Sport & Exercise Psychology Review* 2014: 10: 4–18.
27. Fransen K, Haslam AS, Steffens NK, Vanbeselaere N, De Cuyper B, Boen F. Believing in "Us": Exploring leaders' capacity to enhance team confidence and performance by building a sense of shared social identity. *Journal of Experimental Psychology: Applied* 2015; 21: 89–100.
28. Filho E, Tenenbaum G, Yang Y. Cohesion, team mental models, and collective efficacy: Towards an integrated framework of team dynamics in sport. *Journal of Sports Sciences* 2014; 33: 641–653.
29. Leo FM, González-Ponce I, Sánchez-Miguel PA, Ivarsson A, García-Calvo T. Role ambiguity, role conflict, team conflict, cohesion and collective efficacy in sport teams: A multilevel analysis. *Psychology of Sport and Exercise* 2015; 20: 60–66.
30. Leo FM, González-Ponce I, Alonso DA, González JJP, García-Calvo T. An approachment to group processes in female professional sport. *European Journal of Human Movement* 2016; 36: 57–74.
31. McEwan D. The effects of perceived teamwork on emergent states and satisfaction with performance among team sport athletes. *Sport, Exercise, and Performance Psychology* 2020; 9: 1–15.
32. Morgan PBC, Fletcher D, Sarkar M. Developing team resilience: A season-long study of psychosocial enablers and strategies in a high-level sports team. *Psychology of Sport & Exercise* 2019; 45: 101543.
33. Fransen K, Decroos S, Vanbeselaere N, Vande Broek G, De Cuyper B, Vanroy J, et al. Is team confidence the key to success? The reciprocal relation between collective efficacy, team outcome confidence, and perceptions of team performance during soccer games. *Journal of Sports Science* 2015; 33: 219–231.
34. De Backer M, Boen F, De Cuyper B, Høigaard R, Vande Broek G. A team fares well with a fair coach: Predictors of social loafing in interactive female sport teams. *Scandinavian Journal of Medicine and Science in Sports* 2015; 25: 897–908.
35. Fransen K, Haslam SA, Mallett CJ, Steffens NK, Peters K, Boen F (2017). Is perceived athlete leadership quality related to team effectiveness? A comparison of three professional sports teams. *Journal of Science and Medicine in Sport* 2017; 20: 800–806.
36. Lonsdale C, Hodge K, Rose EA. The behavioral regulation in sport questionnaire (BRSQ): Instrument development and initial validity evidence. *Journal of Sport & Exercise Psychology* 2008; 30(3): 323–355.
37. Pulido JJ, Sánchez-Oliva D, González-Ponce I, Amado-Alonso D, Montero Carretero C, García-Calvo T. Adaptation and validation of a questionnaire to assess motivation in the sport context. *Cuadernos de Psicología del Deporte* 2015; 15(3): 17–26.
38. Pulido JJ, Sánchez-Oliva D, Silva MN, Palmeira AL, García-Calvo T. Development and preliminary validation of the coach interpersonal style observational system. *International Journal of Sports Science & Coaching* 2019; 14(4): 471–479.
39. Ramis Y, Torregrosa M, Viladrich C, Cruz J. Adaptación y validación de la versión española de la Escala de Ansiedad Competitiva SAS-2 para deportistas de iniciación. *Psicothema* 2010; 22(4): 10004–1009.
40. Martens R, Vealey RS, Burton D, Bump L, Smith DE. Development and validation of the competitive state anxiety inventory-2. In R. Martens, R. S. Vealey, & D. Burton (Eds.), *Competitive anxiety in sport* (pp. 117–178). Human Kinetics, 1990.

41. García-Calvo T, Jiménez CR, Santos-Rosa F, Reina R, Cervelló E. Psichometric properties of the spanish version of the Flow State Scale. *The Spanish Journal of Psychology* 2008; 11(2): 660–669.
42. Aksum KM, Magnaguagno L, Bjørndal CT, Jordet G. What do football players look at? An eye-tracking analysis of the visual fixations of players in 11 v 11 elite football match play. *Frontiers in Psychology* 2020; 11:562995.
43. Moran A, Quinn A, Campbell M, Rooney B, Brady N, Burke C. Using pupillometry to evaluate attentional effort in quiet eye: A preliminary investigation. *Sport, Exercise, and Performance Psychology* 2016; 5(4), 365–376.
44. Teoldo I, Garganta J, Greco P, Mesquita I, Maia J. System of tactical assessment in soccer (FUT-SAT): Development and preliminary validation. *Motricidade* 2011;7: 69–83.
45. Machado G, da Costa IT. TacticUP video test for soccer: Development and validation. *Frontiers in Psychology* 2020; 11.
46. Sakamoto S, Takeuchi H, Ihara N, Ligao B, Suzukawa K. Possible requirement of executive functions for high performance in soccer. *PLOS ONE,* 2018; 13(8): e0201871.
47. Homack S, Lee D, Riccio CA. Test review: Delis-Kaplan executive function system. *Journal of Clinical and Experimental Neuropsychology* 2005; 27(5): 599–609.
48. Bowie CR, Harvey PD. Administration and interpretation of the Trail Making Test. *Nature Protocols* 2006; 1(5): 2277–2281.
49. Carron A, Widmeyer W, Brawley L. The development of an instrument to assess cohesion in sport teams: The group environment questionnaire. *Journal of Sport and Exercise Psychology* 1985; 7: 244–266.
50. Borrego CC, Leitão JC, Silva C, Alves J, Palmi J. Análise factorial confirmatória do Group Environment Questionnaire com atletas portugueses. *Avaliação Psicológica* 2010; 9: 359–369.
51. Leo FM, González-Ponce I, Sánchez-Oliva D, Pulido JJ, García-Calvo T. Adaptation and validation in Spanish of the group environment questionnaire (GEQ) with professional football players. *Psicothema* 2015; 27: 261–268.
52. Heuzé JP, Fontayne P. Questionnaire sur l'Ambiance du Groupe: A French–language instrument for measuring group cohesion. *Journal of Sport and Exercise Psychology* 2002; 24: 42–67.
53. Booroff M, Nelson L, Potrac P. A coach's political use of video-based feedback: A case study in elite-level academy soccer. *Journal of Sports Sciences* 2016; 34: 16–124.
54. Rodríguez A. El Sociograma, una técnica útil para representar las relaciones informales. In: En Rodríguez y Morera (Eds.), *El sociograma. Estudio de las relaciones informales en las organizaciones* (pp. 43–51). Pirámide, 2001.
55. Sabin SI, Mihai S, Marcel P. The importance and utility of the sociometric survey method in physical education research. *Procedia: Social and Behavioral Sciences* 2014; 117: 185–192.
56. Van Cutsem J, Marcora S, De Pauw K, Bailey S, Meeusen R, Roelands B. The effects of mental fatigue on physical performance: A systematic review. *Sports Medicine (Auckland, N.Z.)* 2017; 47(8): 1569–1588.
57. Badin OO, Smith MR, Conte D, Coutts AJ. Mental fatigue: Impairment of technical performance in small-sided soccer games. *International Journal of Sports Physiology and Performance* 2016; 11(8): 1100–1105.
58. Coutinho D, Gonçalves B, Wong DP, Travassos B, Coutts AJ, Sampaio J. (2018). Exploring the effects of mental and muscular fatigue in soccer players' performance. *Human Movement Science* 2018; 58: 287–296.

59. Martin K, Meeusen R, Thompson KG, Keegan R, Rattray B. Mental fatigue impairs endurance performance: A physiological explanation. *Sports Medicine* 2018; 48(9): 2041–2051.
60. García-Calvo T, González-Ponce I, Ponce-Bordón JC, Tomé-Lourido D, Vales-Vázquez A. Incidence of the tasks scoring system on the mental load in football training. *Revista de Psicología del Deporte* 2019; 28(4): 79–86.
61. Diaz-García J, González-Ponce I, Ponce-Bordón JC, López-Gajardo MA, Garcia-Calvo T. Design and validation of a questionnaire to quantify the mental load in teams sports (QMLST). *Cuadernos de Psicología del Deporte* 2021; 21(2): 138–145.
62. Díaz-García J, Pulido JJ, Ponce-Bordón JC, Cano-Prado C, López-Gajardo MA, García-Calvo T. Coach encouragement during soccer practices can influence players′ mental and physical demands. *Journal of Human Kinetics*, 2021; 79: 277–288.
63. Jeffries AC, Wallace L, Coutts AJ, McLaren SJ, McCall A, Impellizzeri FM. Athlete-reported outcome measures for monitoring training responses: A systematic review of risk of bias and measurement property quality according to the COSMIN guidelines. *International Journal of Sports Physiology and Performance* 2020; 15(9): 1203–1215.

INDEX

Note: **Bold** page numbers refer to tables and *italic* page numbers refer to figures.

5 jump test (5JT) 91–92
5-0-5 agility test 94–96, 96
30–15 intermittent fitness test (30–15 IFT) 112–113

Abalakov test 87, *88,* 137, 141, *142*
achilles injury 203
acromioclavicular joint (ACJ) sprain 199
active knee extension (AKE) test 61–62, *62, 63*
acute:chronic workload ratio (ACWR) 165–166
adductor injuries 208
aerobic metabolism 43
agility development 134–137, *136*
aging process 1–2
ankle dorsiflexion 55–60; gait biomechanics 55; goniometer 58, *59;* inclinometer *57,* 57–58, *58;* soccer-related injuries 55; tape measure 58, 60, *60;* weight-bearing lunge test 55–57, *56*
ankle injury 203
apophysitis/apophyseal avulsion fractures 201
articular muscle assessment 225
artificial intelligence 253–254, 259, *260*
athlete-tracking technologies 157
Australian Football League (AFL) 178
autonomic nervous system (ANS) 182–183

balance-based tests 128, *129*
Balance Error Scoring System 119
Banister's model 175, *176*
bent knee fall out test 65, *65*
bilateral symmetry 24
biochemical stresses 176
biopsychosocial model *269;* cognitive variables 270–271; emotions and cognitive load 268–269; mental load and fatigue 274–275, 277; motivational and emotional variables 270; SDT 270; social variables 271–272; *see also* psychosocial evaluation
blood biomarkers: CK evolution 179, *179;* intramuscular enzymes 178; ROS 180; stress-response hormesis theory 179
body composition analysis: aging process 1–2; anthropometric data collection 2–4; anthropometric traits and sport performance 1–2; cultural and social factors 4; equations 5–6; measurement process 3–4; muscle mass/fat mass ratio 1; skinfolds 4, *5;* somatotype 6–8; UEFA Consensus document 2
bone mass (BM) 6
brain derived neurotrophic factor (BDNF) 244

calf injury 213–215
carbohydrates (CHO): competition day 10, *11;* glycogen stores 9; hydration 10,

11; post-match goals 11; requirements
11–12, *12*; sweat rates 10
cardiorespiratory fitness testing: aerobic
metabolism 43; fatty acid oxidation
47; heart rate assessment 48–49, *49*;
isocapnic buffering phase 46; maximal
aerobic speed 44–45; maximal oxygen
uptake 44–45; measurements 49, **50**;
mechanical efficiency 47–48, *48*;
respiratory compensation phase 47;
ventilatory threshold 46–47
catabolic/anabolic-related hormonal
homeostasis 180
change-of-direction (COD): deficit 135,
149; evaluations of 134–135; 505 test
135; T-test (modified) 135; Y-shaped
COD 135, *136*, 137; zigzag COD 135
clavicle fracture 198
comprehensive evaluation: biopsychosocial
model 268–269, *269*; cognitive
variables 270–271; ecological training
perspective 275; mental load and fatigue
274–275; psychobiological model
276; psychosocial evaluation 272–274;
psychosocial variables 270–272
concussion 197–198
Copenhagen adduction exercise 209, *210*
countermovement jump (CMJ) 140, *141*
cumulative head trauma 198

data analytics framework 253–254, *254*
data mining 255, *256*
design fluency test (DFT) 273
double leg lowering test 127–128, *128*
drop jump test 87, *89*, 141, *142*
dynamic neuromuscular control *120*, 120–121
dynamometer 234, *236*

ectomorphy 7
elbow dislocation/sprain 199
electromyography (EMG) 19–20; *see also*
surface electromyography (sEMG)
endomorphy 7
English Premier League (EPL) 178
equivalent distance index (EDI) 160
evidence-based decisions 157
executive functions (EFs) 271
exponentially weighted moving average
(EWMA) model 165
eye injuries 198

fat mass (FM) 5, 6
fatty acid oxidation 47

field-based core stability tests 126;
balance-based tests 128, *129*; double
leg lowering test 127–128, *128*; lumbar
pelvic stability 128; muscular-based
tests 127, *127*
field testing: 5-0-5 agility test 94–96, *96*;
hexagonal agility test 96–97, *97*; illinois
test 93–94, *95*; 5 jump test 91–92; L-run
test 96, *96*; power test 91–92, *92*; pro
agility shuttle/5-10-5 shuttle test 93; 10 ×
5 m shuttle test 93, *93*; sprint test 92–93;
standing kick test 92; throwing-in test
92, *92*; T-test 94, *95*; zigzag test 93, *94*
fitness testing in professional football
players: cardiorespiratory 43–50; during
injury periods 219–238
football injuries: achilles injury 203; ankle
injury 203; apophysitis/apophyseal
avulsion fractures 201; extrinsic
factors 196–197; fractures 197;
goalkeeper injuries 204; groin sprains
200; hamstring sprains 201; head and
face injuries 197–198; incidence and
epidemiology 195; intrinsic factors 196;
knee injuries 201–202; medial ankle
injuries 203–204; meniscal injuries 202;
metatharsal stress fractures 204; muscle
strains 200; overuse injuries 202;
patellofemoral injuries 202; pubalgia
201; strained calf muscle 202–203; thigh
201; upper member injuries 198–200
football-specific endurance: aerobic fitness
assessment tests 109–110, 113–114;
30–15 IFT 112–113; laboratory tests 110;
physical training 109; YYIR 110–112
force-velocity-power (FVP) profiling:
jumping profile 142–143; loaded squat
jump 142, *143*; 2-load method 143, *144*;
sprinting profile 143–144, *145*
functional and physiological evaluation *see*
individual entries
functional symmetry 24–25

genotypic analysis: Big Data/artificial
intelligence 247; case-control studies
239; epigenetic regulation 241–242;
gene, definition 240; genetic markers
239; human gene structure 240, *240*;
mtDNA 241; muscle damage 245–246;
polymorphisms 242–244; RNA
polymerase 241
glenohumeral internal rotation deficit
(GIRD) 68

global positioning system (GPS) 157–158, 166–168, 220–221
goalkeeper injuries 204
goniometer 58, *59*
groin injuries 64–65, *65–68*, 200, 208; bent knee fall out test 65, *65*; hip abduction ROM test 66–67, *67*; hip flexion ROM test 66; hip rotation ROM test 65–66, *66*; multiple pathologies 64; sagittal plane tilt 67–68, *68*
growth differentiation factor (GDF5) 245–246

hamstring injuries 54–55, 61–64, 201, 210–212; AKE test 61–62, *62, 63*; incidence 61; PSLR 62–64, *63, 64*; tightness 61
head and face injuries 197–198
heart rate: ANS 182–183; assessment 48–49, *49*; intensity zones 181; TRIMP methods 181–182
heart rate variability (HRV) 182–184
Heath-Carter somatotype 6–7
hexagonal agility test 96–97, *97*
hip abduction ROM test 66–67, *67*
hip abductor muscle chain 226, *227–229*, 228–229
hip adductor muscle chain 229, *230*
hip extensor muscle chain 230–231, *232*
hip flexion ROM test 66
hip flexor muscle chain 230, *231*
hip rotation ROM test 65–66, *66*
Hoff test 115
hop tests 121–122

Illinois test 93–94, *95*
immunoglobulin A (IgA) salivary concentration 180–181
inclinometer *57*, 57–58, *58*
inertial measurement units (IMUs) 157, 158
injuries: achilles 203; adductor 208; ankle 203; calf 213–215; eye 198; goalkeeper 204; hamstring 54–55, 61–64, 201, 210–212; head and face 197–198; knee 201–202; medial ankle 203–204; meniscal 202; muscle *see* muscle injuries; muscular strain 70; nasal 198; overuse 202; patellofemoral 202; quadriceps 212–213; recto femoris 212; shoulder 67–69, *69*; tension 200; thigh 201
injury incidence, external load 164–166

injury periods: rehabilitation process 219–220; return to play 219–236; tissue damage 236–238
injury prevention 30, 33–34, 121, 166, 197, 209–213, 258–262, *260, 261*
injury risk identification 123, 262; *see also* muscle injuries
internal and external training load in football 114, 259; Banister's model 175, *176*; blood biomarkers 178–180; endocrine response 180–181; GPS technology 166–168; heart rate 181–184; injury incidence 164–166; microcycle planning 166–168; neuromuscular response 184–185; peak match demands 161–162; ROM 186–187; subjective measurements 176–178; time-motion analysis 158–164; TMG 185–186
International Society for the Advancement of Kinanthropometry (ISAK) 2–3
isokinetic dynamometers 20; fatigue 27; injury risk reduction 27–28; load range concept 26, *26*; muscular endurance 25–26; performance measurements 27; tests 26; time-torque curve 25
isometric knee flexion/extension 147–148, *148*
isometric midthigh clean pull (IMTP) *148*, 148–149

joint fracture 199
jumping assessment **139**; Abalakov test 137, 141, *142*; CMJ 140, *141*; drop jump 141, *142*; landing and eccentric phases 140; outcomes, soccer players **140**; RSI 138; SJ 141, *141*; take-off velocity 138; time in the air jump 138; vertical jumps 137, *137*; warm-up 140

kinematic and kinetic assessment in professional football players 86; agility 134–137; COD 134–137; FVP profiling 142–144; jumping assessment 137–141; linear sprinting assessment 133, **134**; RFD 144–149
knee control assessment 122–125; external rotator muscle chain 225, *226*; internal rotator muscle chain 226, *227*; knee flexor muscle chain 233–234, *234*, **235,** *235*
knee extensor muscle chain 231, 233, *233*
knee injuries 201–202

landing error scoring system (LESS) test 123, *124*

leg asymmetry assessment 121–122, *122*; biomechanical evidence 122; high knee abduction loads 122–123; LESS test 123, *124*; single leg jumps and hops test 121–122, *122*; tuck jump test 123–125, *125*

leg motion device 60, *60*

linear sprinting assessment: outcomes, soccer players 133, **134**; set-up and execution 133; warm-up 133

lower-back syndrome 126

lower limb assessment/injuries 55–60; change of direction 125–126; dynamic neuromuscular control *120*, 120–121; knee control assessment 122–125; leg asymmetry assessment 121–122, *122*; static neuromuscular control 119

L-run test 96, *96*

Ludograms 274

lumbar pelvic stability 128

machine learning 253, 255, 259–261

manual muscle testing (MMT): articular muscle assessment 225; dynamometer 234, *236*; external rotator muscle chain, 90° knee flexion 225, *226*; hip abductor muscle chain 226, *227–229,* 228–229; hip adductor muscle chain 229, *230*; hip extensor muscle chain 230–231, *232*; hip flexor muscle chain 230, *231*; internal rotator muscle chain, 90° knee flexion 226, *227*; knee extensor muscle chain 231, 233, *233*; knee flexor muscle chain, knee flexion 233–234, *234,* **235,** *235*; objectives 235–236; quantification and interpretation 234; ROM 224, 225

maximum isometric voluntary contraction (MIVC) 28, 33

mechanomyographic (MMG) methods 185

medial ankle injuries 203–204

meniscal injuries 202

mental load and fatigue 274–275, 277

mesomorphy 7

messenger ribonucleic acid (mRNA) 241

metacarpal and phalanx fracture 199

metacarpophalangeal (MCP) joint 199–200

metatharsal stress fractures 204

microcycle planning 166–168

Microsoft Power BI 258, *258*

mitochondrial DNA (mtDNA) 241

muscle injuries 200; adductor injuries 208; calf injury 213–215; Copenhagen adduction exercise 209, *210*; with elastic band 209, *209*; groin/hip injuries 208; hamstring injury 210–212; incidence 208; prevention programs 207, 209; quadriceps injury 212–213; risk factors 207

muscular-based tests 127, *127*

muscular functioning 21, 32, 70, 80, 122, 125–127, *127,* 224–225, 228, 235–236; *see also* soccer player musculature

muscular strain injuries 70

nasal injuries 198

NASA-Task Index Load 275

neuromuscular balance field-based assessments: lower limb assessment 119–126; trunk dominance assessment 126–128

neuromuscular response 184–185

new technologies and Big Data 247; characteristics 252; data acquisition and management 253–254, *254*; physical performance and injury prevention 258–262; ROC analysis 260–261, *261*; sports data analysis 255–258; variety 253; velocity 253; volume 252–253

nutrition: after competition 11; benefits 8; carbohydrate requirements 11–12, *12*; during competition 10, *11*; energy requirements 8–9; fat requirements 12–13; physical demand 8; pre-competition 9–10; protein requirements 12; technological devices 9

olecranon bursitis 199

overuse injuries 202

passive straight leg raise test (PSLR) 62–64, *63, 64*

patellofemoral injuries 202

peak match demands, external load 161–162

peroxisome proliferator–activated receptor alpha (PPARA) 245–246

peroxisome proliferator-activated receptors (PPARs) 244

player load monitoring 176, *177*

player preparation: alcohol 80; creatine monohydrate 80; familiarization 83; frequency and scheduling 81;

physiological capacities 79; planning 82; safety 82; specificity 83; stimulants 80; supplements 80; task familiarization 80; testing time 81; test order 81; training 80; warm-up 81–82
Poincaré plot analysis 183–184, *184*
polymorphisms: ACTN3 242–243; BDNF 244; endurance capacity 244; muscle power 242–244; patellar tendon compliance 243; VDR gene 242
predictive analytic models 261
pro agility shuttle/5-10-5 shuttle test 93
professional football players performance 201, 246–247, 268
psychological coping skills (PCSs) 270
Psychomotor Vigilance Task 275
psychosocial evaluation: cognitive variables 273; motivational and emotional variables 272–273; social variables 274
pubalgia 201

quadriceps injury 212–213

range of motion (ROM) 186–187; ankle dorsiflexion 55–60; flexibility *vs.* injury 54–69; groin injuries 64–68, *65–68*; hamstring injuries 54–55, 61–64; lower limb injuries 55–60; muscular strain injuries 70; shoulder injuries 68–69, *69*; soccer actions 69
rate of force development (RFD): ballistic isometric knee flexion/extension 147–148, *148*; execution 147; field-based context 144; IMTP *148*, 148–149; injury rehabilitation management 147; isometric ballistic test 146, *146*; metrics for 144, **145**; warm-up 147
rating of perceived exertion (RPE) 177
reactive oxygen species (ROS) 180
reactive strength index (RSI) 138
recto femoris injuries 212
reinjuries 195, 196
residual mass (RM) 6
return to play (RTP) process 21, 219; GPS 220–221; MMT 224–236; TMG 221–224; training monitoring 220; video analysis 220–221
rolling average (RA) model 165

Sahrmann core stability test 127–128, *128*
scaphoid fracture 200
scapholunate dissociation 200

self-determination theory (SDT) 270
sEMG *see* surface electromyography (sEMG)
session rating of perceived exertion (sRPE) 176–177
shoulder dislocation 198–199
shoulder injuries 68–69, *69*
shuttle test: 10×5 m shuttle test 93, *93*
skeletal muscle mass (SMM) 6
small-sided games (SSGs) 113–114
soccer player musculature: EMG 19–20, 28–34, *30–32, 35*; isokinetic dynamometers 20, 25–28, *26*; muscle contraction 19; neuromuscular assessment 19; technologies 19, *20*; TMG 20–25, *21, 24*; US imaging 34, *36, 36–37*
sonography 20
Spanish Kinanthropometry Group 5
sprint test 92–93
squat jump (SJ) test 85–86, *86*, 141, *141*
standing kick test 92
standing long jump test 87–88, *89*
star excursion balance test (SEBT) 120, 121
static neuromuscular control 119
stiffness measured with elastography (SWE) 37
strained calf muscle 202–203
strength and muscle power testing: Abalakov jump test 87, *88*; assessment 78; balance performance 98–99; bench press 90, *91*; countermovement jump test 86, *87*; drop jump test 87, *89*; exercise intensity 88–89; explosive training programs 97, 98; fatigue prevention 77; field testing 91–97; full squat 89–91; high-intensity actions 79; laboratory measurements 83; linear velocity transducer 90–91; loaded countermovement jump 86; maximal strength 99–101; multiple RM test benefits 89; player preparation 79–83; quality control 77; 1 repetition maximum 89–90; sprinting 78; squat jump test 85–86, *86*; standing long jump test 87–88, *89*; vertical jump measurements 85–88; vertical jump test 84–85, *85*
stress-response hormesis theory 179
Stroop Test 273
subjective measurements: blood biomarkers 178–180; endocrine response 180–181; heart rate 181–184; neuromuscular

response 184–185; ROM 186–187; RPE 177; sRPE 176–177; TMG 185–186
surface electromyography (sEMG): biceps femoris 34, *35*; detection materials 29; electrode montages 29, *30*; fatigue 29–30, *31*; hamstring muscle injuries 33; injury risk reduction 32–34; MIVC 28; motor unit 28; performance 30–32; quadriceps EMG *32*; SENIAM project 29
sympathetic-parasympathetic balance 183

Tensiomyography™ (TMG) 20, 185–186; fatigue 22–23; Henneman's size principal 22; injury risk reduction 23–25, *24*; lateral symmetry 223; maximum displacement 221, *222*; measurements 22; muscle contractile properties 21, *21*; muscle reference values 223, **224**; performance 23; player positioning 222, *223*; stimulated muscle fibers 221, *221*
tension injuries 200
thermal responses, posterior chain 185, *186*
thigh injuries 201
throwing-in test 92, *92*
time-motion analysis: acceleration thresholds 159; EDI 160; exercise-intensity continuum 163; individual thresholds 163, *164*; locomotor activities 158; metabolic power 159–160, *160*; physical performance 163; regression model 164
tissue damage: muscle, myofascial and myotendinous tissue 236–237; tendon/ligament tissue 237–238
tracking systems 256, *257*
trail making test (TMT) 273
training impulse (TRIMP) 181–182

training-induced fatigue 175
training load (TL) quantification: external 157–168; internal 175–187
training stress balance 165
trunk dominance assessment: balance-based tests 128, *129*; double leg lowering test 127–128, *128*; field-based core stability tests 126; lumbar pelvic stability 128; muscular-based tests 127, *127*; unstable sitting paradigms 126
trunk stability deficit 126
T-test 94, *95*

UEFA Consensus document 2
ultrasonography: analysis 34, *35*; muscle architecture 34, 36; muscle dimensions 36; muscle quality 36; SWE 37; tendon dimensions 37; tendon mechanical properties 37
University of Montreal Track Test 115

velocity intermittent fitness test (VIFT) 112–113
vertical jump test 84–85, *85*
vitamin D receptor (VDR) gene 242

weight-bearing lunge test 55–57, *56*; goniometer 58, *59*; inclinometer *57*, 57–58, *58*; maximal dorsiflexion 55–56, *56*
wellness questionnaire, internal load 176, *178*
wrist fracture 199

Y-balance test *120*, 120–121
Yo-Yo intermittent recovery test (YYIR) 110–112

zigzag test 93, *94*